Clinical Calculations

A Unified Approach

5th Edition

Approximate Equivalents

1 gr	=	60 mg
15 gr	=	1 g = 1000 mg
1000 mcg	=	1 mg
1 kg	=	2.2 lb
1 mL	=	15 minims
4 mL	=	1 dr
5 mL	=	1 tsp (t)
30 mL	=	1 oz = 2 tbs (T) = 6 tsp (t) = 8 dr
500 mL	=	1 pt (0) = 16 oz
1000 mL	=	1 L = 1 qt = 32 oz

Clinical Calculations

A Unified Approach

5th Edition

Joanne M. Daniels, RN, BSN, MSN
Professor Emeritus
SUNY College of Technology at Alfred

Loretta M. Smith, RN, BSN, M.Ed.
Professor Emeritus
SUNY College of Technology at Alfred

DELMAR
CENGAGE Learning™

Australia Canada Mexico Singapore Spain United Kingdom United States

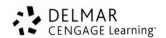

**Clinical Calculations:
A Unified Approach,
Fifth Edition**
by Joanne M. Daniels
and Loretta M. Smith

Vice President,
Health Care Business Unit:
William Brottmiller

Editorial Director:
Cathy L. Esperti

Executive Editor:
Matthew Kane

Developmental Editor:
Maria D'Angelico

Editorial Assistant:
Michelle Leavitt

Marketing Director:
Jennifer McAvey

Marketing Channel Manager:
Tamara Caruso

Marketing Coordinator:
Michele Gleason

Technology Director:
Laurie Davis

Technology Project Manager:
Mary Colleen Liburdi

Production Director:
Carolyn Miller

Art and Design Coordinator:
Alexandros Vasilakos

Production Coordinator:
Jessica McNavich

Project Editor:
David Buddle

Production Editor:
Jack Pendleton

> For product information and technology assistance, contact us at
> **Cengage Learning Customer & Sales Support, 1-800-354-9706**
>
> For permission to use material from this text or product,
> submit all requests online at **cengage.com/permissions**
> Further permissions questions can be emailed to
> **permissionrequest@cengage.com**

Library of Congress Control Number: 2005001046
ISBN-13: 978-1-4018-5849-0
ISBN-10: 1-4018-5849-X

Delmar Cengage Learning
5 Maxwell Drive
Clifton Park, NY 12065-2919
USA

Cengage Learning products are represented in Canada by Nelson Education, Ltd.

For your lifelong learning solutions, visit **delmar.cengage.com**

Visit our corporate website at **www.cengage.com**

Notice to the Reader
Publisher does not warrant or guarantee any of the products described herein or perform any independent analysis in connection with any of the product information contained herein. Publisher does not assume, and expressly disclaims, any obligation to obtain and include information other than that provided to it by the manufacturer. The reader is expressly warned to consider and adopt all safety precautions that might be indicated by the activities described herein and to avoid all potential hazards. By following the instructions contained herein, the reader willingly assumes all risks in connection with such instructions. The publisher makes no representations or warranties of any kind, including but not limited to, the warranties of fitness for particular purpose or merchantability, nor are any such representations implied with respect to the material set forth herein, and the publisher takes no responsibility with respect to such material. The publisher shall not be liable for any special, consequential, or exemplary damages resulting, in whole or part, from the readers' use of, or reliance upon, this material.

Printed in China
3 4 5 6 7 8 9 12 11 10 09 08

CONTENTS

Clinical Calculations offers learners and practitioners alike the opportunity to develop skill in solving dosage problems using the computation method of *dimensional analysis*. This method is a logical and systematic approach to solving any type of medication administration problem. The method can be used with any system of measurement and facilitates conversion from one system to another. It easily replaces all other procedures for calculating medication dosages.

The advantages of a unified approach to clinical calculations include protection and precision, as well as ease and efficiency. The variety of approaches to dosage computations can be confusing and perplexing. A logical system is needed to significantly reduce errors made when medications are administered or dispensed. Dimensional analysis is such a system.

The text applies this versatile method to a cross section of computational applications typical of the clinical setting. These applications include calculating adult and pediatric oral and parenteral dosages, as well as intravenous flow rates and infusion times. Numerous solved examples guide the learner in using the method for these applications. Self-quizzes provide the opportunity for learners to practice dimensional analysis.

In the fifth edition, all drug labels and references have been updated to ensure that only those drugs currently in use are included. A number of drug labels have been added as well as numerous diagrams of syringes and medicine cups to provide practice in calculating and measuring drug dosages. The IV chapter has been reorganized into smaller units, making a large amount of technical material more user-friendly and better adapted to self-study. The Performance Criteria checklists have been relocated, as tear-out sheets, to Appendix H.

A number of heretofore commonly used symbols, abbreviations, and dose designations have been deleted or replaced in accordance with advisory recommendations by the Joint Commission on Accreditation of Healthcare Organizations, the purpose of which is to minimize the danger of serious medication errors resulting from misuse or misinterpretation of these abbreviations and expressions.

Throughout the text, emphasis is placed on accuracy and accountability. In the presentation of dimensional analysis methodology, the writers frequently pose the question "Does my answer make sense?" Thus, learners are encouraged to examine and analyze computational problems and answers in terms of common sense as well as memorized rules, to anticipate logical answers, and to reduce the potential for medication errors.

The text includes a detailed review of the routes by which medications are administered, particularly as they relate to the different types of dosage calculations.

Performance criteria checklists for each route of administration provide a means of documenting learner progress in mastering the techniques.

This textbook is suitable for use in either traditional lecture classes, small group tutorial classes, or self-instruction. The text contributes to the self-instructional mode of learning, providing detailed explanations of dimensional analysis as it is used in different applications to help learners understand the method. To enhance practice in the reading of labels for identification of information essential to computations, a total of 160 labels appear in the text. These labels familiarize learners with commonly prescribed drugs and provide opportunities for hands-on computation practice. All drugs have been updated and identified by generic names.

Diagrams of syringes and medicine cups have been added throughout the text, providing practice for learners to measure out dosages.

Ample space for working problems has been provided throughout the text, making it usable as a workbook and helping to avoid errors in transcribing problems to a work sheet.

Content includes use of dimensional analysis for nutritional calculations and titration of infusions. Calculations applicable to critical care situations have been so identified. The writers have also included content on Celsius/Fahrenheit temperature conversions, fluid balance recording, computerized MAR, and use of the twenty-four hour clock.

Content

Chapter 1 introduces dimensional analysis, teaches the basic steps, and provides practice problems for each step as well as for the entire procedure.

Chapters 2–5 review the three systems of measurement (metric, apothecaries, and household) commonly used in prescribing medications and apply dimensional analysis to conversions within and between the systems.

Chapters 6 and 7 focus on medications administered by the oral route. Dimensional analysis is used in Chapter 6 to determine dosages of medications, both liquid and solid. In Chapter 7, general considerations related to safe and effective administration of oral medications are included, as are terms and abbreviations.

Chapters 8 and 9 apply dimensional analysis to dosage computations for medications administered parenterally (exclusive of intravenous administration), specifically via intradermal, subcutaneous, and intramuscular routes. General considerations, methodology, equipment, and location of sites are included in Chapter 9.

Chapters 10 and 11 focus on intravenous computations and administration. In Chapter 10 dimensional analysis is applied to the various computational problems associated with intravenous (IV) flow rate, infusion times, titrated medication additives, infusions, and parenteral nutrition. Chapter 11 describes the various routes of IV administration and includes sample problems.

Chapter 12 applies dimensional analysis to the calculation of pediatric dosages based on body weight or body surface area. Also included are general considerations related to administering medications to infants and children.

Chapter 13 summarizes the application of dimensional analysis. Two hundred twenty clinical problems offer a variety of examples of all of the preceding types of calculations. This unit can serve as a performance evaluation tool and a useful reference or review.

The appendix section of the text contains eight parts. Although it is assumed that learners using this text are familiar with elementary mathematics. Appendix A includes a variety of drill problems for review or practice in basic arithmetic processes. Learners who require additional review or remediation are encouraged to seek the assistance of faculty or other sources.

Appendices B to E contain miscellaneous information which, although unrelated to dimensional analysis, is typically encountered in the clinical situation, including conversion between Celsius and Fahrenheit temperatures, measuring and recording fluid balance, dimensional analysis variation, and twenty-four hour clock.

Appendix F applies dimensional analysis to the calculation of components for the preparation of percentage solutions.

Appendix G contains the answers to all of the self-quizzes and problems in the text.

Finally, Appendix H contains Performance Criteria checklists for 10 medication administration procedures. These are printed on tear-out sheets that can be used for practice or performance evaluation.

The text also includes an interactive CD-ROM multimedia presentation that shows sample problems, review questions, and a testing component. The program provides scoring, helpful hints, animations, and color photos and illustrations. It is designed for individual, self-paced learning at home or in the computer lab.

A valuable adjunct to the text for teachers looking for additional problems is an Instructor's Manual containing the answers to all quizzes and solutions to all practice problems, and a test bank covering Chapters 6–13 of the text with problem solutions. The Instructor's Manual also contains many useful and time-tested hints for effectively teaching the methodology. New features and teacher aids should make this edition particularly attractive to instructors.

Acknowledgments

We wish to express our sincere appreciation to the many individuals whose interest and assistance sustained and supported our efforts throughout the revision of this text.

We are especially grateful to our reviewers for their constructive and instructive critiques as well as their excellent ideas and suggestions, which have added new depth and dimension to the present edition.

Lisa Bauer, RN, MN, CRNP
Instructor
Pennsylvania State University
St. Mary's, Pennsylvania

Kathryn Carney, APRN, BC, MSN
Instructor
Pennsylvania State University, Worthington Scranton
Dunmore, Pennsylvania

Dr. Angelica Smith Collins, DSN, RN, CCNS, APRN, BC
Clinical Associate Professor
Capstone College of Nursing, University of Alabama
Tuscaloosa, Alabama

Trellis G. Moore, RN, MS
Clinical Instructor
Beth-El College of Nursing and Health Sciences, University of Colorado
Colorado Springs, Colorado

Duveen Woolbright
Director, Health Services
University of South Carolina, Spartanburg
Spartanburg, South Carolina

Last, but surely not least, our loving thanks to Stu and Ang for fealty, fortitude, and forbearance above and beyond the call of husbandry.

Chapter Opener and Objectives

Each chapter begins with a list of objectives to orient the learner to the topics covered in the chapter. These points can be used to guide self-study and assess comprehension of important topics.

CHAPTER 12

Pediatric Dosage

OBJECTIVES

Upon completion of this chapter, you should be able to:
- Identify special considerations related to safety and comfort when administering medications to infants and children.
- Identify adaptations and special considerations related to administration of oral and parenteral medications to infants and children and when giving intramuscular injections and intravenous infusions.
- Apply dimensional analysis to clinical calculations of pediatric dosage based on weight and body surface area.

Examples

Each new topic is explained and followed by step-by-step examples. An icon highlights examples so that the learner can easily locate them. Steps are broken down so that the learner can follow.

ROUNDING OFF

When Administering Tablets

- Tablets scored in halves or quarters may be broken in half or quarters in order to obtain as exact a dose as possible, Figure 6-1.

EXAMPLE If calculated dose is 1.5 tablets, give $1\frac{1}{2}$ tablets.
1.25 tablets, give $1\frac{1}{4}$ tablets
1.75 tablets, give $1\frac{3}{4}$ tablets

- If tablets are not scored, a pill splitter may be used if hospital policy permits. Because this can be a very inaccurate method, it should be used only when an alternative form (e.g., liquid) of the medication is not available. Check with the pharmacist regarding alternative dosage forms.
- Capsules, spansules, and enteric coated tablets cannot be divided. If the calculated dose is not a whole number, consult with the pharmacist or provider in regard to rounding.

Remember Boxes

Remember boxes summarize important safety issues pertaining to calculation lessons. The principles covered reinforce prevention of medication errors. They have a conspicuous, visually appealing design for easy identification.

REMEMBER

It is critically important to perform this final step, dividing by number of doses, in computations based on body weight. Consistency in this regard helps avoid errors when medication is to be given in divided doses. If this step is omitted, it is easy to forget to divide the total daily dose into the prescribed number of doses, thus greatly increasing the risk of administering an overdosage.

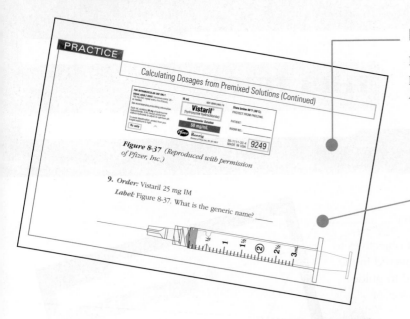

Figure 8-37 *(Reproduced with permission of Pfizer, Inc.)*

9. *Order:* Vistaril 25 mg IM
   Label: Figure 8-37. What is the generic name? _____

Practice Sets

Practice sets allow the learner to practice the concepts taught. Answers are included in Appendix G.

Labels and Syringes

Current drug labels and drawings of syringes appear throughout the practice sets and examples.

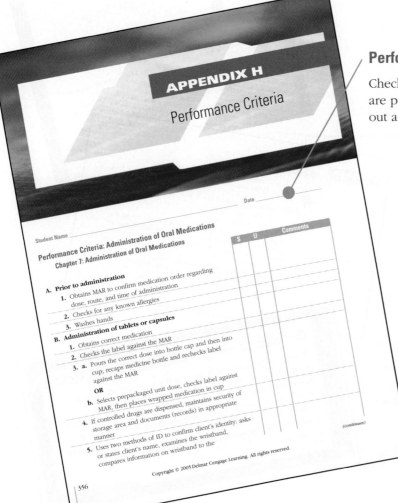

Performance Criteria Checklists

Checklists appear in Appendix H. Pages are perforated so that they can be torn out and used in a clinical setting.

HOW TO USE PRACTICE SOFTWARE

Using the Clinical Calculations Practice Software

We hope you enjoy the interactive CD-ROM that accompanies this book. Every attempt has been made to make it a fun, attractive, and effective learning environment for the user. Careful attention was paid to providing step-by-step solutions in a consistent format. By using this software, users will continuously expand their skills and confidence in performing dosage calcuations.

Organization and Features

The *Clinical Calculations Practice Software* is organized into seven parts:
(1) Dimensional Analysis,
(2) Metric, Apothecaries, and Household Systems of Measurement, (3) Oral Medications, (4) Parenteral Medications, (5) Intravenous Medications and Solutions, (6) Pediatric Dosage, and (7) Clinical Calculations Review Sets. The first six parts include Remember boxes and Practice Sets. Part 7 contains comprehensive sets of review questions that test all of the content in the book.

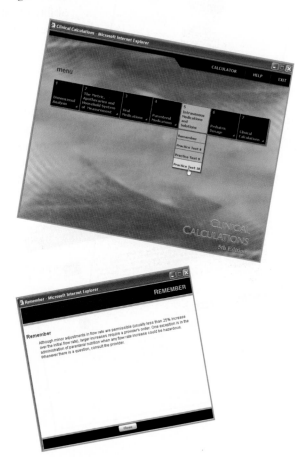

Practice Tests

Each part includes practice tests that incorporate labels and syringes for the most realistic and challenging practice experience. Practice problems allow the user two tries to enter the correct answer. If the correct answer is not entered on the second try, the answer and solution appear on the screen.

Scoring

Most of the problems are scored so that the user can assess strengths and weaknesses and determine which topics need further study.

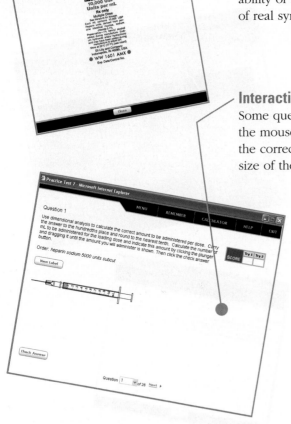

Labels and Syringes

Real, full-color labels are provided to aid recognition and read-ability of information needed to perform a calculation. Photos of real syringes are also provided.

Interactive Syringes

Some questions include the use of interactive syringes. With the mouse, users click and drag the syringe plunger to select the correct syringe measurement. All syringes duplicate the size of the actual syringes.

Dimensional Analysis

Upon completion of this chapter, you should be able to:

- Analyze computation problems in order to identify the starting factor and the answer unit.

- Analyze computation problems to identify equivalents given and equivalents needed.

- Set up an appropriate sequence of unit factors, called a conversion equation, whereby successive units can be cancelled.

- Correctly solve the conversion equation using cancellation and arithmetic to arrive at the answer in desired units.

This text presents a comprehensive approach to clinical calculations that is unique, uniform, and understandable. The term *clinical calculations* refers to the solving of computational problems associated with the administration of medications, specifically, determining the correct dosage to be given. Because these computations often involve converting from one system of measurement to another, it is essential that an accurate, reliable, and consistent method of solving conversion problems be utilized.

INTRODUCTION

Many drug and dose calculation textbooks dealing with mathematics relative to clinical practice use the methods of *ratio and proportion* and *desire over have times quantity* for the conversion of units of measure. Where two or more conversions are involved, these methods often become cumbersome and confusing to the learner. Frequently, the learner must remember a certain procedure or a different approach for each type of problem. This attempt to memorize several procedures involving similar units may be perplexing and discouraging. Furthermore, the additional steps in multiple calculation processes can predispose to error.

We attempt to bring order out of confusion by using a consistent method, dimensional analysis, for all conversion problems.

DIMENSIONAL ANALYSIS METHODOLOGY

Dimensional analysis is a computation method whereby one particular unit of measurement is converted to another unit of measurement by use of a conversion factor or factors. This method focuses on the particular quantity of units in a problem that needs to be converted to equivalent units in the same or in another system of measurement. This known quantity and unit is called the starting factor. With consistent practice, the learner soon develops the ability to find this key item (starting factor). From this point on, equivalent values, called conversion factors, are utilized to convert from one system of units to another, leading, finally, to the desired unit (answer). These conversion factors fall into two categories that have either been (1) learned or (2) obtained from tables. With practice, conversion factors become very familiar and recognizable to the learner and, soon, this familiarity facilitates almost automatic application of the method to all conversion problems. Once the technique has been mastered, all other formulas or methodologies can be discarded.

Other advantages of dimensional analysis include:

- Eliminating memorization of different procedures and formulas for various types of problems.
- Enhancing the ability to analyze all problems in a systematic manner.
- Requiring only one equation and simple arithmetic, resulting in a very powerful mathematical tool that is almost foolproof.
- Applying the method to clinical calculation is both rapid and facile. Many students are already familiar with dimensional analysis because it is a computational technique taught in basic chemistry courses.

DIMENSIONAL ANALYSIS

Definitions

1. Dimensional analysis is a computation method whereby one particular unit of measurement is converted to another unit of measurement by use of a conversion factor or factors.
2. A conversion factor is an equivalent value that can be used as a bridge between units of measurement without changing their value.

Steps in Dimensional Analysis

Dimensional analysis is composed of three steps:

1. Determining the starting factor and answer unit.
2. Formulating a conversion equation consisting of a sequence of labeled factors, in which successive units can be cancelled until the desired answer unit is reached.
3. Solving the conversion equation by use of cancellation and simple arithmetic.

STEP I DETERMINING THE STARTING FACTOR AND ANSWER UNIT

Initially, it is essential to determine exactly what information is sought. This information goal involves converting from one type of unit to another.

EXAMPLE   How many seconds are there in 5 minutes?

To answer this question, it is necessary to convert from minute units to seconds units. Therefore, the known quantity and its unit (5 min) that is to be converted is called the **starting factor.** The desired unit to which the starting factor will be converted is called the **answer unit.** These two items, the starting factor and the answer unit become, respectively, the first and the final items in the conversion equation. When the computation of the conversion equation has been completed, the two units of measurement (minutes and seconds) will have an equivalent relationship.

The starting factors and answer units are identified in the following:

EXAMPLE   How many feet are there in 12 yards?
This example requires converting from yards to feet.

Starting Factor	Answer Unit
12 yds	ft

EXAMPLE   How many inches are there in 29 feet?
This example requires converting from feet to inches.

Starting Factor	Answer Unit
29 ft	in

EXAMPLE   How many ounces are there in 6 cups?
This example requires converting from cups to ounces.

Starting Factor	Answer Unit
6 cups	oz

Quantities can be expressed in a variety of units. For example, milk can be purchased by the pint, quart, or gallon. Thus, the same starting factor can have a variety of answer labels depending on the units asked for.

EXAMPLE   Find the number of milliliters in 4 quarts.
How many ounces are contained in 4 quarts?
Determine the number of cups in 4 quarts.
Calculate how many pints equals 4 quarts.

In each of these instances, an equivalent amount is sought for the quantity and unit, 4 quarts. Thus, 4 quarts is a known quantity and unit that must be converted to an equivalent unit to solve a problem or answer a question. In the above examples, the starting factor is always 4 quarts but the answer labels are milliliters, ounces, cups, and pints. Each of the four computations results in equivalent relationships.

The following questions and answers further identify starting factors and answer units:

1. If you went to the bank and obtained 325 dollars worth of quarters, how many quarters would you receive?

Answer: 325 dollars is the known quantity and unit that must be converted to a desired unit (quarters). The starting factor, therefore, is 325 dollars and the answer unit is quarters and these two units will have an equivalent relationship.

2. You have 6 quarters but need dimes to use at the laundromat. How many dimes would you receive from 6 quarters?

Answer: 6 quarters is the known quantity and unit that must be converted to a desired unit (dimes). The starting factor, therefore, is 6 quarters and the answer unit is dimes and these two units will have an equivalent relationship.

3. How many milliliters are contained in 1 teaspoon?

Answer: 1 teaspoon is the known quantity and unit that must be converted to a desired unit (milliliters). The starting factor, therefore, is 1 teaspoon and the answer unit is milliliters and these two units will have an equivalent relationship.

4. What is the weight in kilograms of a child weighing 40 pounds?

Answer: 40 pounds is a known quantity and unit that must be converted to a desired unit (kilograms). The starting factor, therefore, is 40 pounds and the answer unit is kilograms and these two units will have an equivalent relationship.

5. How many 10 grain tablets are needed to administer 1 gram of medication?

Answer: 1 gram is the known quantity and unit that must be converted to a desired unit (tablets). The starting factor, therefore, is 1 gram and the answer unit is tablets and these two units will have an equivalent relationship.

REMEMBER

The starting factor is always the first item in the conversion equation. The answer unit is always the final item in the equation. When the conversion equation is solved, it will be seen that the starting factor and the labeled answer have formed an equivalent relationship. See also Appendix D, Dimensional Analysis Variation.

PRACTICE

Identifying the Starting Factor and Answer Unit

1. How many milligrams are there in 3 grains?

Starting Factor   Answer Unit

_____   _____

2. How many pounds are there in 5 kilograms?

Starting Factor   Answer Unit

_____   _____

PRACTICE

Identifying the Starting Factor and Answer Unit (Continued)

3. How many tablets should the client receive if the provider ordered 250 milligrams?

Starting Factor   Answer Unit

_____   _____

4. How many capsules should the client receive if the ordered dose was 0.5 gram?

Starting Factor   Answer Unit

_____   _____

5. How many milliliters should be administered if the dose is 250 milligrams?

Starting Factor   Answer Unit

_____   _____

6. How many quarters are equal to 650 pennies?

Starting Factor   Answer Unit

_____   _____

7. How many nickels are equal to 9 dimes?

Starting Factor   Answer Unit

_____   _____

8. What is the length in inches of a toothpick that measures 5.08 cm in length?

Starting Factor   Answer Unit

_____   _____

9. A marathon race is 26.2 miles. This would be equal to _____ kilometers.

Starting Factor   Answer Unit

_____   _____

10. An automobile gets 30 miles per gal and gasoline costs $1.50 per gal. What is the total cost of gasoline for a trip of 350 miles?

Starting Factor   Answer Unit

_____   _____

(*Note:* See Appendix G for answer key.)

STEP II FORMULATING THE CONVERSION EQUATION

The second step in dimensional analysis is to set up a sequential series of equivalent values called *conversion factors,* which function as bridges leading from the starting factor to the answer unit. This is the conversion equation. The conversion equation is written in a manner whereby successive units can be cancelled until the only unit remaining is the answer unit. It is essential that conversion factors contain only true (1:1) relationships; that is, the numerator and denominator of each factor must be of equivalent value. Multiplying a number by 1 does not change its value, and multiplying by a fraction equal to 1 also leaves the value unchanged. A fraction is equal to 1 when the numerator is equivalent to the denominator.

For example: 60 sec = 1 min

Therefore, $\dfrac{60 \text{ sec}}{1 \text{ min}} = 1$

Similarly, $\dfrac{1 \text{ min}}{60 \text{ sec}} = 1$

It is important to note that conversion factors may be constant or variable relationships. Constant relationships are absolutes; they do not vary regardless of the context in which they are used. On the other hand, variable relationships do not necessarily remain constant, as illustrated in the following examples. Note that all the following equivalent values are 1:1 relationships and when written as conversion factors, the denominators and numerators can be interchanged.

Constant Relationships

EXAMPLE Equivalent Value: 15 gr = 1 g

Conversion Factor: $\dfrac{15\text{ gr}}{1\text{ g}}$ or $\dfrac{1\text{ g}}{15\text{ gr}}$

EXAMPLE Equivalent Value: 1 kg = 2.2 lb

Conversion Factor: $\dfrac{1\text{ kg}}{2.2\text{ lb}}$ or $\dfrac{2.2\text{ lb}}{1\text{ kg}}$

EXAMPLE Equivalent Value: 1 tsp = 5 mL

Conversion Factor: $\dfrac{1\text{ tsp}}{5\text{ mL}}$ or $\dfrac{5\text{ mL}}{1\text{ tsp}}$

Variable Relationships

EXAMPLE Equivalent Value: 350 mg = 1 tab

Conversion Factor: $\dfrac{350\text{ mg}}{1\text{ tab}}$ or $\dfrac{1\text{ tab}}{350\text{ mg}}$

EXAMPLE Equivalent Value: 350 mg = 2.5 mL

Conversion Factor: $\dfrac{350\text{ mg}}{2.5\text{ mL}}$ or $\dfrac{2.5\text{ mL}}{350\text{ mg}}$

EXAMPLE Equivalent Value: 350 mg = 1 tsp

Conversion Factor: $\dfrac{350\text{ mg}}{1\text{ tsp}}$ or $\dfrac{1\text{ tsp}}{350\text{ mg}}$

Approximate Equivalents

In setting up conversion factors, the learner either must know the equivalent relationships in various systems of measurement or have this information available for reference. Because it is frequently necessary to convert from one system of measurement to another in the same problem, the use of exact equivalents for corresponding units often results in large and cumbersome fractions or decimals that are very inconvenient in calculations and that may contribute to error. Therefore, certain approximations have been accepted widely and are in general use as equivalents for converting between systems. Table 1-1 lists approximate equivalents that are most frequently used in the calculation of medication dosages or solutions.

Approximate equivalents sometimes fall within a range, for example, 60–65 mg = 1 gr, 4–5 mL = dr 1, 15–16 minim = 1 mL. In addition, the pint and quart equivalents are rounded from 480 mL to 500 mL and 960 mL to 1000 mL, respectively. For purposes of clinical calculations in this text, the numbers in Table 5-1 (chapter 5) will be used.

Table 1-1 *Approximate Equivalents*

1 gr	=	60 mg
15 gr	=	1 g = 1000 mg
1000 mcg	=	1 mg
1 kg	=	2.2 lb
1 mL	=	15 minims
4 mL	=	1 dr
5 mL	=	1 tsp (t)
30 mL	=	1 oz = 2 tbs (T) = 6 tsp (t) = 8 dr
500 mL	=	1 pt = 16 oz
1000 mL	=	1 L = 1 qt = 32 oz

Key to Abbreviations

gr = grain	lb = pound	oz = ounce
mg = milligram	gtt = drop	tbs (T) = tablespoon
g = gram	mL = milliliter	pt = pint
kg = kilogram	dr = dram	L = liter
	tsp (t) = teaspoon	qt = quart

Prior to formulating the conversion equation, the learner may find it helpful to list the equivalent values that will be used as conversion factors. These are the items that function as bridges leading from the starting factor to the answer unit.

EXAMPLE Find the number of yards in 1.5 miles.
Equivalents: 1 yd = 36 in
1 yd = 3 ft
5280 ft = 1 mi
These are *constant* relationships familiar to most students.

EXAMPLE How many 10 gr tablets are needed to administer 1 gram of medication?
Equivalents: 10 gr = 1 tab
15 gr = 1 g
(*Note:* 10 gr = 1 tab is a *variable* relationship. Information regarding variable relationships is obtainable from drug labels, handbooks, inserts, pharmacists, etc. Note also that the problem contains both constant and variable equivalents.)

Identifying Equivalents

Using Table 1-1, list all the equivalents needed to solve the following problems.

EXAMPLE How many 0.5 pint bottles can be filled by 4 quarts of solution?
Analysis of the question identifies 4 quarts as the starting factor and bottles as the answer label. Therefore, the equation involves going from 4 quarts to an equivalent number of bottles. The steps would include quarts to pints to bottles.
Equivalents: 1 qt = 2 pt, 1 bottle = 0.5 pt

EXAMPLE   Find the number of feet in 60 inches.
Equivalents: 12 in = 1 ft

EXAMPLE   How many miles would a runner complete in 1 hour if he runs the mile in 4 minutes?
Equivalents: 1 mi = 4 min, 60 min = 1 hr

EXAMPLE   Change 250 mg to g.
Equivalents: 1 g = 1000 mg

EXAMPLE   0.5 lb is equivalent to how many kg?
Equivalents: 2.2 lb = 1 kg

PRACTICE

Identifying Equivalents

1. How many feet are there in 12 yards?

   Equivalents:

2. How many inches are there in 29 feet?

   Equivalents:

3. How many quarters are there in $25.00?

   Equivalents:

4. How many nickels are equal to 9 dimes?

   Equivalents:

5. What is the length in inches of a toothpick that measures 5.08 cm in length? (See Table 5-1.)

   Equivalents:

6. How many milligrams are there in 3 grains?

   Equivalents:

7. How many pounds are there in 5 kilograms?

   Equivalents:

8. How many 0.5 gram tablets should the client receive if the provider ordered 250 milligrams?

   Equivalents:

9. How many 250 milligram capsules should the client receive if the ordered dose was 0.5 gram?

   Equivalents:

10. How many milliliters would be administered if the order was for 2 teaspoons?

    Equivalents:

Setting Up the Sequence of Conversion Factors

The conversion equation is formulated so that all unwanted units can be cancelled except the designated answer unit. Start with the known quantity and unit and apply the conversion factors as needed to get an answer in the desired unit. When the desired unit appears in the numerator, no more conversion factors are needed.

EXAMPLE   Find the number of minutes in 90 seconds.

Equivalents: 1 min = 60 sec

Starting	Conversion	Answer
Factor	Factor	Unit

Conversion Equation:

$$90 \text{ sec} \quad \times \frac{1 \text{ min}}{60 \text{ sec}} \quad = \_\_\_\_ \text{ min}$$

As long as conversion factors are true 1:1 relationships that equal 1, adding conversion factors to the equation does not change the value of the answer.

EXAMPLE   Convert 60 seconds to hours.

Equivalents: 1 min = 60 sec, 60 min = 1 hr

Starting	Conversion	Answer
Factor	Factor	Unit

Conversion Equation:

$$60 \text{ sec} \times \frac{1 \text{ min}}{60 \text{ sec}} \times \frac{1 \text{ hr}}{60 \text{ min}} = \_\_\_\_ \text{ hr}$$

Thus, it can be seen that units can be logically and sequentially cancelled, greatly reducing the chance of error or omission. In solving the problem, each numerator unit cancels the immediately following denominator unit, so that all unwanted units are removed until the desired unit for the answer is reached. For instance, in the first example, all units are cancelled until the desired unit (min) is reached, ending the equation. This is the answer unit that was identified in Step I. Similarly, in the second example, all units are cancelled until the desired unit (hr) is reached, which was previously identified as the answer unit. The conversion equation is shown in Figure 1-1.

Conversion Factors

$$\text{Known Quantity and Unit} \quad \times \frac{1}{1} \times \frac{1}{1} \times \frac{1}{1} \times \frac{1}{1} = \text{Answer (in desired unit)}$$
(Starting Factor)

Equivalent Relationship

Figure 1-1 Conversion Equation

Summary of Step II

EXAMPLE   Find the number of yards in 1.5 miles.

Equivalents: 1 mi = 5280 ft; 3 ft = 1 yd

Starting Factor	Conversion Factors	Answer Unit

$$1.5 \text{ mi} \times \qquad \frac{5280 \text{ ft}}{1 \text{ mi}} \times \frac{1 \text{ yd}}{3 \text{ ft}} \qquad = \underline{\quad} \text{ yd}$$

The following observations regarding this problem summarize Step II of dimensional analysis.

- The starting factor is 1.5 mi, because this is the known quantity and unit that must be converted to an equivalent unit.

- In the two conversion factors, the units mile and feet are placed in the denominators to cancel the corresponding units of the immediately preceding factors. (*Note:* Make it a cardinal rule that each factor cancels a unit in the preceding factor.)

- The two conversion factors, 5280 ft per mi and 1 yd per 3 ft are each equivalent relationships. That is, these factors have 1:1 value and do not change the actual value of the starting factor. Their purpose is to lead to an equivalent answer expressed in some other unit. The relationships in each factor must be true for the answer to be correct.

- The answer unit always appears in the numerator farthest to the right in the conversion equation (in the example above: yd).

REMEMBER

It is desirable that conversion factors be arranged in a sequence so that identical units are placed diagonally; that is, whatever unit appears in the numerator of one factor appears in the denominator of the factor immediately following.

Setting Up Conversion Equations

EXAMPLE   How many milligrams are there in 3 grains?

Equivalents: 60 mg = gr 1

$$\text{Conversion Equation: } \text{gr } 3 \times \frac{60 \text{ mg}}{\text{gr } 1} = \underline{\quad} \text{ mg}$$

EXAMPLE How many pounds are there in 5 kilograms?
Equivalents: 1 kg = 2.2 lb

Conversion Equation: $5 \text{ kg} \times \dfrac{2.2 \text{ lb}}{1 \text{ kg}} =$ _____ lb

EXAMPLE How many tablets should the client receive if the provider ordered 250 mg and each tablet contains 100 mg?
Equivalents: 1 tab = 100 mg

Conversion Equation: $250 \text{ mg} \times \dfrac{1 \text{ tab}}{100 \text{ mg}} =$ _____ tab

EXAMPLE How many capsules should be administered if the order states gr 2 and the medication label states 60 mg per capsule?
Equivalents: gr 1 = 60 mg, 60 mg = 1 cap

Conversion Equation: $\text{gr } 2 \times \dfrac{60 \text{ mg}}{\text{gr } 1} \times \dfrac{1 \text{ cap}}{60 \text{ mg}} =$ _____ cap

EXAMPLE Change 5 grains to grams.
Equivalents: 15 gr = 1 g

Conversion Equation: $5 \text{ gr} \times \dfrac{1 \text{ g}}{15 \text{ gr}} =$ _____ g

Note that the last equation shows the most direct route from grains to grams. However, it can be seen from Table 1-1 that other equivalent relationships exist between grains and grams.

EXAMPLE Equivalents: 15 gr = 1000 mg, 1000 mg = 1 g

Conversion Equation: $5 \text{ gr} \times \dfrac{1000 \text{ mg}}{15 \text{ gr}} \times \dfrac{1 \text{ g}}{1000 \text{ mg}} =$ _____ g

EXAMPLE Equivalents: 1 gr = 60 mg, 1000 mg = 1 g

Conversion Equation: $5 \text{ gr} \times \dfrac{60 \text{ mg}}{1 \text{ gr}} \times \dfrac{1 \text{ g}}{1000 \text{ mg}} =$ _____ g

Thus, there may be several routes leading from one starting factor to an equivalent end value. Insofar as possible, it is best to choose the most direct route (i.e., that which requires the fewest conversion factors). Because many of the equivalent relationships, as pointed out before, are *approximations,* the use of additional conversion factors may result in small differences in the end result values. *Therefore, in some instances, the learner may obtain a slightly different answer from the answer key in Appendix G.* Some multiple answers have been included in the key but, obviously, others are possible. When a discrepancy is found, the learner should recheck for accuracy of arithmetic and equivalents. If these are correct, the alternative answer is acceptable. When there is a question as to a safe margin for accuracy, a pharmacist or a drug reference manual should be consulted. *In any case, no more than a 10% difference should occur between the ordered dose of a medication and the amount administered.*

PRACTICE

Setting Up Conversion Equations

1. How many mL should be administered if the dose is 250 mg and the label states 500 mg per tsp?

Equivalents:

Conversion Equation:

2. How many milliliters should the client receive if the order states 125 mg and the medication strength is 250 mg per 5 mL?

Equivalents:

Conversion Equation:

3. How many milliliters are necessary to follow the order of 0.75 g if the medication label states 0.5 g per dr?

Equivalents:

Conversion Equation:

4. How many tablets (scored) will be administered if the ordered dose is gr ⅛ and the tablet strength is 15 mg per tab?

Equivalents:

Conversion Equation:

5. How many milligrams would the client receive if the order is for 15 mL and the medication strength is 300 mg per tsp?

Equivalents:

Conversion Equation:

6. What is the length in feet of a sofa that measures 84 inches?

Equivalents:

Conversion Equation:

PRACTICE

Setting Up Conversion Equations (Continued)

7. A newborn weighs 6.5 lb at birth. What is his weight in kilograms?

Equivalents:

Conversion Equation:

8. A recipe calls for 675 mL of milk. How many ounces of milk will you need?

Equivalents:

Conversion Equation:

9. How many milliliters are there in a 2.5 L bottle of soda pop?

Equivalents:

Conversion Equation:

10. If a provider ordered 10 mL of a cough medicine, how many tsp should be administered?

Equivalents:

Conversion Equation:

(**Note:** See Appendix G for answer key.)

STEP III SOLVING THE CONVERSION EQUATION

The third step in dimensional analysis involves the use of cancellation and simple arithmetic to solve the equation formulated in Step II. Cancellation of labels, reduction of numerical values, and simple multiplication are used to solve the conversion equation.

$$5 \, \cancel{\text{min}} \times \frac{60 \text{ sec}}{1 \, \cancel{\text{min}}} = 300 \text{ sec}$$

Note that the known quantity and unit (starting factor), 5 min, and answer in desired units (answer label), 300 sec, have now formed an equivalent relationship; that is, 5 minutes has been converted to 300 seconds. Thus, dimensional analysis has been applied to convert one particular unit of measurement to another unit of measurement without changing the values.

If the series of conversion factors has been set up so that corresponding units are in sequential numerator/denominator positions, the numerical values can likewise be cancelled or reduced to lowest terms and appropriately multiplied to solve the equation. The resulting answer should be reduced to lowest terms, converted to a decimal, or rounded off, as appropriate.

Solving the Conversion Equation

EXAMPLE How many tablets should be administered?
Order: Codeine 60 mg
Label: Codeine gr ½ per tab

Equivalents: 60 mg = gr 1, gr ½ = 1 tab

Conversion Equation: $60 \text{ mg} \times \dfrac{\text{gr } 1}{60 \text{ mg}} \times \dfrac{1 \text{ tab}}{\text{gr } \dfrac{1}{2}} = 2 \text{ tab}$

Does this answer make sense? Note the equivalent 60 mg = gr 1 and 1 tab = gr ½. If the order is for 60 mg, it is obvious that more than 1 tablet is required. Therefore, an answer of less than 1 tablet should be recognized as incorrect.

EXAMPLE How many milliliters should be administered?

Order: Vistaril 25 mg

Label: Vistaril (hydroxyzine hydrochloride) 100 mg per 2 mL

Equivalents: 100 mg = 2 mL

Conversion Equation: $25 \text{ mg} \times \dfrac{2 \text{ mL}}{100 \text{ mg}} = 0.5 \text{ mL}$

Does this answer make sense? Note the equivalent 100 mg = 2 mL. If the order is for 25 mg, it is obvious that less than 2 mL is required. Therefore, an answer of 2 mL or more would not make sense.

EXAMPLE How many 0.5 pint bottles can be filled by 4 quarts of solution?

Equivalents: 1 qt = 2 pt, 1 bottle = 0.5 pt

Conversion Equation: $4 \text{ qt} \times \dfrac{2 \text{ pt}}{1 \text{ qt}} \times \dfrac{1 \text{ bottle}}{0.5 \text{ pt}} = 16 \text{ bottles}$

Does this answer make sense? It can be seen that a bottle is a much smaller container than a quart. Therefore, the number of bottles in the answer must be larger than the number of quarts.

EXAMPLE Change 250 mg to g.

Equivalents: 1 g = 1000 mg

Conversion Equation: $250 \text{ mg} \times \dfrac{1 \text{ g}}{1000 \text{ mg}} = 0.25 \text{ g}$

Does this answer make sense? If it takes 1000 mg to make 1 g, it makes sense to expect that 250 mg would be less than 1 g.

EXAMPLE What is the equivalent in kilograms of 0.5 lb?

Equivalents: 2.2 lb = 1 kg

Conversion Equation: $0.5 \text{ lb} \times \dfrac{1 \text{ kg}}{2.2 \text{ lb}} = 0.23 \text{ kg}$

Does this answer make sense? If 1 kg is equivalent to 2.2 lb, it is obvious that 0.5 lb would be far less than 1 kg.

(**Note:** Refer to Appendix A for basic arithmetic review.)

The learner who is having difficulty solving equations should seek remedial assistance before proceeding further.

REMEMBER

1. *Be sure the starting factor is the first item and the answer unit is the last item in the conversion equation.*
2. *Use only conversion factors that have a 1:1 relationship.*
3. *Set up the conversion equation so that cancellable labels (units) appear in consecutive numerator/denominator positions.*
4. *When solving the conversion equation:*
   * *cancel units first.*
   * *reduce numbers to lowest terms.*
   * *multiply/divide to solve the equation.*
   * *reduce the answer to lowest terms, convert to decimal, or round off.*
5. *Always ask yourself if your answer makes sense.*

PRACTICE

Solving Conversion Equations

1. Order: Lanoxin 0.250 mg

Label: Lanoxin (digoxin) 0.125 mg per tab

Question: How many tablets should the client receive? _____

Equivalents:

Conversion Equation:

Does your answer make sense?

2. Order: Nembutal gr ½

Label: Nembutal (pentobarbital) 30 mg per cap

Question: How many capsules should the nurse give? _____

Equivalents:

Conversion Equation:

Does your answer make sense?

PRACTICE

Solving Conversion Equations (Continued)

3. Order: Tolinase 250 mg

Label: Tolinase (tolazamide) 0.5 g per tab (scored)

Question: How many tablets should be administered? _____

Equivalents:

Conversion Equation:

Does your answer make sense?

4. Order: Morphine sulfate gr ⅙

Label: Morphine sulfate gr ¼ per 1.4 mL

Question: How many mL should be administered? _____

Equivalents:

Conversion Equation:

Does your answer make sense?

5. Order: Atropine sulfate gr 1/100

Label: Atropine sulfate gr 1/150 per mL

Question: How many mL should be administered? _____

Equivalents:

Conversion Equation:

Does your answer make sense?

6. Order: Chloral hydrate elixir 1 g

Label: Chloral hydrate elixir gr 7½ per 5 mL

Question: How many mL will equal this dose? _____

Equivalents:

Conversion Equation:

Does your answer make sense?

7. Order: Colace Syrup 10 mL

Label: Colace Syrup (docusate sodium) 20 mg per tsp

Question: How many mg will be contained in this dose? _____

Equivalents:

Conversion Equation:

Does your answer make sense?

8. Order: Augmentin 200 mg

Label: Augmentin (cefaclor) 125 mg per 5 mL

Question: How many mL must be administered? _____

Equivalents:

Conversion Equation:

Does your answer make sense?

PRACTICE

Solving Conversion Equations (Continued)

9. Order: Dilantin 30 Pediatric Suspension 75 mg

Label: Dilantin 30 (phenytoin sodium) Pediatric Suspension 30 mg per 5 mL

Question: How many mL should be administered? _____

Equivalents:

Conversion Equation:

Does your answer make sense?

10. Order: Phenobarbital 90 mg

Label: Phenobarbital gr 1½ per tab

Question: How many tablets should be given? _____

Equivalents:

Conversion Equation:

Does your answer make sense?

(**Note:** See Appendix G for answer key.)

ACCURACY AND ACCOUNT- ABILITY

The learner is cautioned against blind reliance on any formula, particularly when its use has become familiar and automatic. The application of common sense and reasonable prudence will help prevent medication errors due to either carelessness or inaccuracy in determining equivalents and solving conversion equations.

Although the level of arithmetic required to solve nearly all dimensional analysis problems is almost elementary, math errors do occur. This means that it is essential to double-check the computation, even if a calculator is used.

To this end, the learner should develop the habit of carefully inspecting the information given in every problem and seeking simple benchmarks relative to the anticipated answer. For example, should it be less than or more than one tablet, grain, or milliliter? What is a typical and reasonable amount of solution for an intravenous, an intramuscular, or an oral medication? Extremely large numbers should be suspect: answers such as 12 tablets PO, 850 gtt per min IV, 16 mL IM should be questioned as *illogical* and *unreasonable.* Typical or average amounts of medication to be administered via various routes are utilized in the examples and practice sections throughout the text. With practice the learner will recognize excessive amounts. When there is any doubt as to the accuracy of a computation, a drug reference should be consulted to be sure the answer is consistent with the recommended range of dosage for that particular drug. An additional resource for verification is the registered pharmacist.

Medication errors constitute one of the greatest areas of risk for which healthcare providers can be vulnerable to negligence or malpractice litigation. Although it is hoped that the use of a single and consistent approach to calculating medication dosages will help prevent medication errors, it must be emphasized that any method or formula is only as safe as the individual using it.

REMEMBER

The final step in solving any problem, of course, is to ask whether the answer is reasonable. Common sense and common caution are prerequisites for using dimensional analysis in clinical calculations.

CHAPTER 2

The Metric System of Measurement

OBJECTIVES

Upon completion of this chapter, you should be able to:

- Identify the three basic units of measurement in the metric system: gram, liter, and meter.
- List metric abbreviations and prefixes commonly used in drug computations.
- Compare various metric units in relation to length, weight, and volume.
- Apply dimensional analysis to conversions within the metric system.

BASIC UNITS

The basic units of measurement in the metric system are the gram as the unit of weight, the liter as the unit of volume, and the meter as the unit of length. These basic units can be divided or multiplied into various related units, as seen in Table 2-1. The main feature of the metric system is that each of the basic units may be divided into decimal values or expanded into multiples of 10 by the use of standard prefixes, Table 2-2.

COMPARING METRIC UNITS

When converting metric values, make use of the obvious principle: "It takes many small units to equal a large unit." For example, in Table 2-3, it can be seen that a milligram is 0.001 gram and is a small unit. It would take 1000 milligrams to equal one gram, Figure 2-1. However, a kilogram is a large unit. It takes 1000 grams to equal one kilogram. Similarly, a milliliter is 0.001 L and is a small unit, Table 2-4. It takes 1000 mL to equal one liter, Figure 2-2. Finally, the small unit, millimeter, equals one one thousandth of a meter, Table 2-5. It takes 10 millimeters to equal 1 centimeter and 100 centimeters to equal 1 meter, Figure 2-3.

Obviously, there are many more divisions and multiples of the basic metric units possible. Tables 2-1 to 2-5 contain the quantities most frequently used in clinical calculations of dosages and measurements; these relationships should be memorized.

Table 2-1 Metric Units and Abbreviations

Unit	Abbreviations
weight	
gram	g
milligram	mg
microgram	mcg
kilogram	kg
volume	
liter	L
milliliter	mL
length	
meter	m
centimeter	cm
millimeter	mm

Table 2-2 Metric Prefixes

Small Units	Large Units
deci = 0.1	deka = 10
centi = 0.01	hecto = 100
milli = 0.001	kilo = 1,000
micro = 0.000001	mega = 1,000,000

Table 2-3 Metric Units of Weight

Many Small Units Equal One Large Unit
1 mg = 0.001 g; 1000 mg = 1 g
1 mcg = 0.000001 g; 1,000,000 mcg = 1 g
1 mcg = 0.000001 g; 1000 mcg = 1 mg
1 g = 0.001 kg; 1000 g = 1 kg

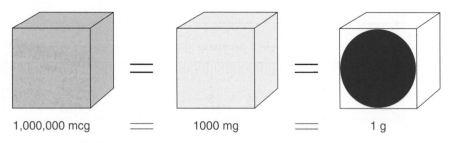

1,000,000 mcg === 1000 mg === 1 g

Figure 2-1 *Weight (metric)*

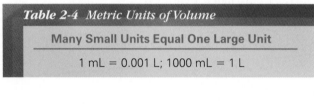

Table 2-4 Metric Units of Volume
Many Small Units Equal One Large Unit
1 mL = 0.001 L; 1000 mL = 1 L

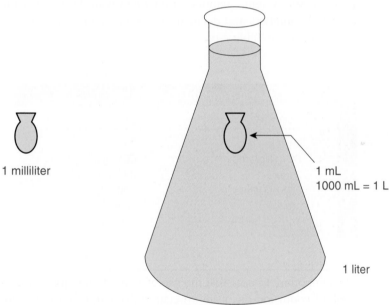

1 milliliter

1 mL
1000 mL = 1 L

1 liter

Figure 2-2 *Volume (metric)*

Table 2-5 Metric Units of Length
Many Small Units Equal One Large Unit
1 mm = 0.001 m; 1000 mm = 1 m
1 cm = 0.01 m; 100 cm = 1 m

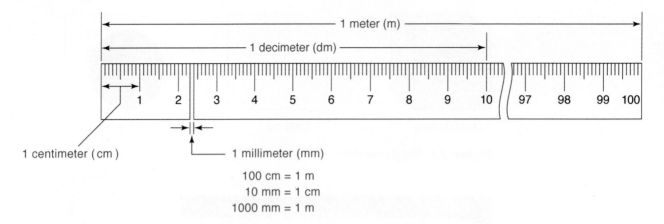

Figure 2-3 *Length (metric)*

METRIC NOTATION

In the metric system, quantities are written with the number preceding the unit. Arabic whole numbers and decimals are used rather than Roman numerals or fractions. See examples in Table 2-6.

Table 2-6 *Metric Notation*

Quantity	Notation
1 gram	1 g
60 milligrams	60 mg
3 liters	3 L
500 milliliters	500 mL
10 meters	10 m
150 centimeters	150 cm

It is important to note that the use of symbols and abbreviations always carries the risk of confusion or misinterpretation that can result in serious medication errors. To minimize the potential for error, the Joint Commission on Accreditation of Healthcare Organizations, as of this writing, has issued a strongly worded recommendation that use of certain abbreviations and symbols associated with medications should be avoided. Therefore, several abbreviations and symbols heretofore frequently used by health practitioners have been deleted from this text. These include U or u, cc, ss, qn, q.d. or QD, q.o.d. or QOD, o.d. or OD, SC or sub q, > and < , and symbols such as ℥, ℨ, ℳ, μg, and others. It may well be that some of the abbreviations included herein will soon be dropped from use in medical texts. The authors regret any confusion or inconvenience this may cause the learner.

CONVERTING UNITS WITHIN THE METRIC SYSTEM

Using the previously memorized prefixes and relationships as equivalent values, complete the practice problems following the steps used in the following examples. (Carry each answer to two decimal places and round to the nearest tenth.)

EXAMPLES   Convert 0.16 centimeter to millimeters.

Starting Factor   Answer Unit
0.16 cm   mm

Equivalents: 1 cm = 0.01 m; 1 mm = 0.001 m

Conversion Equation:

$$0.16 \text{ cm} \times \frac{0.01 \text{ m}}{1 \text{ cm}} \times \frac{1 \text{ mm}}{0.001 \text{ m}} = 1.6 \text{ mm}$$

EXAMPLE   Convert 240 micrograms to milligrams.

Starting Factor   Answer Unit
240 mcg   mg

Equivalents: 1 mg = 1000 mcg

Conversion Equation:

$$240 \text{ mcg} \times \frac{1 \text{ mg}}{1000 \text{ mcg}} = 0.2 \text{ mg}$$

EXAMPLE   Convert 375 milligrams to grams.

Equivalents: 1000 mg = 1 g; 1 mg = 0.001 g

Conversion Equation:

$$375 \text{ mg} \times \frac{1 \text{ g}}{1000 \text{ mg}} = 0.4 \text{ g}$$

OR

$$375 \text{ mg} \times \frac{0.001 \text{ g}}{1 \text{ mg}} = 0.4 \text{ g}$$

EXAMPLE   Convert 75 grams to kilograms.

Equivalents: 1000 g = 1 kg; 1 g = 0.001 kg

Conversion Equation:

$$75 \text{ g} \times \frac{1 \text{ kg}}{1000 \text{ g}} = 0.1 \text{ kg}$$

OR

$$75 \text{ g} \times \frac{0.001 \text{ kg}}{1 \text{ g}} = 0.1 \text{ kg}$$

PRACTICE

Convert within the Metric System

1. 3225 mL to L

2. 375 mg to g

3. 2000 g to kg

4. 5000 mcg to mg

5. 29 cm to m

6. 0.75 L to mL

7. 0.22 g to mg

8. 2.5 kg to g

9. 25 mm to cm

10. 12 mg to mcg

(*Note:* See Appendix G for answer key.)

CHAPTER 3

The Apothecaries System of Measurement

Upon completion of this chapter, you should be able to:

- Identify the four basic units of measurement in the apothecaries system: grain, minim, fluid dram, fluid ounce.
- List apothecaries abbreviations commonly used in drug computations.
- Compare various apothecaries units in relation to weight and volume.
- Apply dimensional analysis to conversions within the apothecaries system.

Although the apothecaries system of measurement is being replaced by the metric, the former system is still sometimes used in writing prescriptions and medication orders. Therefore, the nurse should be familiar with it, particularly its symbols and abbreviations, Table 3-1.

BASIC UNITS AND ABBREVIATIONS

In the apothecaries system, the grain is the basic unit of weight, and the minim, fluid dram, and fluid ounce are the basic units of volume. The latter two usually are shortened to dram and ounce. Although dry weights can be measured in drams and ounces, they are rarely so measured for medication computations. Therefore, when the terms *dram* and *ounce* are used in medication orders or calculations in this text, they refer to fluid volume. An exception to this rule is in the preparation of percentage solutions, which is illustrated in Appendix F. Additionally, the pint and quart are units of volume that are rarely used in the administration of medications.

When body weight is required for calculation of dosage, the pound unit is used. In the traditional apothecaries system, the pound consists of 12 (dry weight) ounces;

Table 3-1 *Basic Apothecaries Units*

Unit	Abbreviation
weight	
grain	gr
pound	lb
volume	
minim	(none)
dram	dr
ounce	oz
pint	pt
quart	qt

however, it is common practice in this country to employ the 16 ounce avoirdupois pound for dry weights. Therefore, any computation involving conversions of pound units in this text "implies" use of the 16 ounce pound.

APOTHECARIES NOTATION

When writing quantities in the apothecaries system, the number *follows* the unit, in contrast to the metric system. For small numbers up to 10, lowercase Roman numerals are used with a line drawn over the digits and a dot over each *i*. For numbers larger than 10, Arabic numbers may be substituted except for 20 (XX) and 30 (XXX).

Table 3-2 shows examples of traditional apothecaries notations. However, in the clinical setting, the practitioner frequently will encounter apothecaries notations written in the metric form, that is, Arabic numbers preceding the unit. The learner should become familiar with both methods of apothecaries notations; they are used interchangeably in this text.

Table 3-2 *Apothecaries Notation*

Quantity	Notation
$\frac{1}{10}$ grain	gr $\frac{1}{10}$
1 grain	gr i
1½ grains	gr 1½
7 grains	gr vii
10 grains	gr x
15 minims	minims 15
150 minims	minims 150
2½ ounces	oz 2½

COMPARING APOTHECARIES UNITS

In comparing apothecaries values, the learner should keep in mind, as with metric units, that many small units equal one large unit. For example, a minim is a small amount; it takes 60 minims to equal 1 dram, Figure 3-1. However, a quart is a large unit; it would take 256 drams to equal 1 quart, Table 3-3.

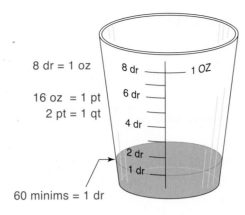

8 dr = 1 oz

16 oz = 1 pt

2 pt = 1 qt

60 minims = 1 dr

Figure 3-1 *Liquid relationships (apothecaries)*

Table 3-3 *Apothecaries Fluid Units*
60 minims = 1 dr
8 dr = 1 oz
16 oz = 1 pt
2 pt = 1 qt

PRACTICE

Write the Abbreviation for Each of the Following

1. dram = _____

2. grain = _____

3. pint = _____

4. pound = _____

5. ounce = _____

(***Note:*** See Appendix G for answer key.)

CONVERTING UNITS WITHIN THE APOTHECARIES SYSTEM

Using the apothecaries equivalents, complete the practice problems, following the steps used in the examples.

EXAMPLE Convert 30 minims to drams.

Starting Factor   Answer Unit

30 minims   dr

Equivalents: 60 minims = 1 dr

Conversion Equation: $30 \text{ minims} \times \dfrac{1 \text{ dr}}{60 \text{ minims}} = \frac{1}{2} \text{ dr}$

EXAMPLE   Convert 64 drams to pints.

$$\begin{array}{cc} \text{Starting Factor} & \text{Answer Unit} \\ 64 \text{ dr} & \text{pt} \end{array}$$

Equivalents: 8 dr = 1 oz, 16 oz = 1 pt

Conversion Equation: $64 \, \cancel{dr} \times \dfrac{1 \, \cancel{oz}}{8 \, \cancel{dr}} \times \dfrac{1 \text{ pt}}{16 \, \cancel{oz}} = \frac{1}{2} \text{ pt}$

EXAMPLE   Convert 55 ounces to quarts.

$$\begin{array}{cc} \text{Starting Factor} & \text{Answer Unit} \\ 55 \text{ oz} & \text{qt} \end{array}$$

Equivalents: 32 oz = 1 qt

Conversion Equation: $55 \, \cancel{oz} \times \dfrac{1 \text{ qt}}{32 \, \cancel{oz}} = 1\frac{7}{10} \text{ qt}$

EXAMPLE   Convert 4 drams to ounces.

$$\begin{array}{cc} \text{Starting Factor} & \text{Answer Unit} \\ 4 \text{ dr} & \text{oz} \end{array}$$

Equivalents: 8 dr = 1 oz

Conversion Equation: $4 \, \cancel{dr} \times \dfrac{1 \text{ oz}}{8 \, \cancel{dr}} = \frac{1}{2} \text{ oz}$

EXAMPLE   Convert pints 1½ to drams.

$$\begin{array}{cc} \text{Starting Factor} & \text{Answer Unit} \\ 1\frac{1}{2} \text{ pt} & \text{oz} \end{array}$$

Equivalents: 1 pt = 16 oz, 1 oz = 8 dr

Conversion Equation: $1\frac{1}{2} \, \cancel{pt} \times \dfrac{16 \, \cancel{oz}}{1 \, \cancel{pt}} \times \dfrac{8 \text{ dr}}{1 \, \cancel{oz}} = 192 \text{ dr}$

PRACTICE

Convert within the Apothecaries System

1. 55 oz to qt

2. 4 dr to oz

3. 1½ pt to oz

4. 30 minims to dr

5. 1½ dr to minims

6. 1¼ oz to dr

7. 120 minims to oz

8. 2 pts to dr

9. 3½ lb to oz

10. 62.4 oz to lb

(*Note:* See Appendix G for answer key.)

CHAPTER 4

The Household System of Measurement

OBJECTIVES

Upon completion of this chapter, you should be able to:

- Identify the units of measurement in the household system: drops, teaspoons, tablespoons, cups, and glasses.
- List household abbreviations commonly used in drug computations.
- Compare various household units in relation to volume.
- Apply dimensional analysis conversions within the household system.

HOUSEHOLD UNITS

The household system of measurement involves the use of drops, spoons, cups, and glasses, Table 4-1. These units, which are derived from household measuring utensils, are not very precise. For example, the size of a drop of fluid will vary depending on the temperature, the composition of the fluid, and the size of the opening from which the drop emerges. The use of cups and spoons as measuring apparatus cannot compare to the accuracy of graduates and syringes as used with the metric system.

Household units are used primarily in the administration of external preparations such as baths, soaks, gargles, enemas, compresses, and disinfectants. They also are used in measuring oral fluid intake where a high degree of accuracy is not necessary. These units and their approximate equivalents are listed in Table 4-2.

The more commonly used units should be memorized because of their frequency of use in the situations mentioned previously.

Table 4-1 *Household Units*

Unit	Abbreviation
volume	
drop	gtt
teaspoon	tsp or t
tablespoon	tbs, tbsp, or T
cup/glass	c/gl
pint	pt
quart	qt
gallon	gal
length	
inch	in
foot	ft

Table 4-2 *Household Equivalents*

60 gtt = 1 tsp
3 tsp = 1 tbs
2 tbs = 1 oz
6 oz = 1 teacup
8 oz = 1 glass or measuring cup
16 oz = 1 pt
2 pt = 1 qt
4 qt = 1 gal

HOUSEHOLD NOTATION

In the household system, quantities are written in the same manner as in the metric system; the number (quantity) precedes the unit and Arabic whole numbers are used. Fractions or decimals may be used for quantities that are portions of whole numbers, Table 4-3.

Table 4-3 *Household Notation*

Quantity	Notation
1 drop	1 gtt
3 teaspoons	3 tsp
8 ounces	8 oz
2 pints	2 pt

PRACTICE

Write the Abbreviations for Each of the Following

1. drop = _____

4. tablespoon = _____

2. gallon= _____

5. teaspoon   = _____

3. pint   = _____

(**Note:** See Appendix G for answer key.)

COMPARING HOUSEHOLD UNITS

Figure 4-1 illustrates the progression of the various units of volume in the household system of measurement.

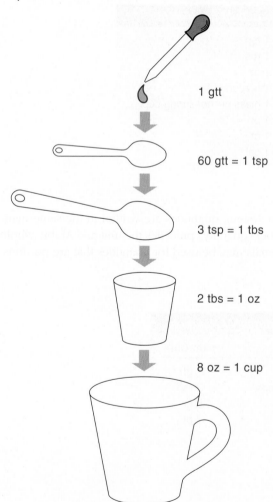

1 gtt

60 gtt = 1 tsp

3 tsp = 1 tbs

2 tbs = 1 oz

8 oz = 1 cup

Figure 4-1
Liquid
relationships
(household)

CONVERTING UNITS WITHIN THE HOUSEHOLD SYSTEM

Using the relationships given as equivalent values, complete the practice problems, following the steps used in the examples. (Carry each answer to two decimal places and round to nearest tenth.)

EXAMPLE   Convert 16 tablespoons to cups.

$$\text{Starting Factor} \qquad \text{Answer Unit}$$
$$16 \text{ tbs} \qquad\qquad \text{cup}$$

Equivalents: 2 tbs = 1 oz; 8 oz = 1 cup

Conversion Equation: $16 \text{ tbs} \times \dfrac{1 \text{ oz}}{2 \text{ tbs}} \times \dfrac{1 \text{ cup}}{8 \text{ oz}} = 1 \text{ cup}$

EXAMPLE   Convert 5 ounces to teaspoons.

$$\text{Starting Factor} \qquad \text{Answer Unit}$$
$$5 \text{ oz} \qquad\qquad \text{tsp}$$

Equivalents: 1 oz = 6 tsp

Conversion Equation: $5 \text{ oz} \times \dfrac{6 \text{ tsp}}{1 \text{ oz}} = 30 \text{ tsp}$

PRACTICE

Convert within the Household System

1. 1 glass to tsp

2. 2 gal to oz

3. 4 qt to cups

4. 68 in to ft

5. 4 tbs to oz

6. 6 tbs to tsp

7. 22 pts to gal

8. ½ measuring cup to tbs

9. 50 tsp to oz

10. 1 teacup to tbs

(*Note:* See Appendix G for answer key.)

CHAPTER 5

Conversion of Metric, Apothecaries, and Household Units

Upon completion of this chapter, you should be able to:

- List approximate equivalent values among the three systems of measurement: metric, apothecaries, and household.

- Apply dimensional analysis to conversions among these systems of measurement.

It is essential that nurses be able to convert accurately among the various systems of measurement, because medication orders often are written in one system and dispensed in another.

Having memorized the basic units and relationships within the metric, apothecaries, and household systems, the learner is now ready to apply dimensional analysis to conversions among these systems. Table 5-1 illustrates the equivalent relationships among the metric, apothecaries, and household systems. Also study Figures 5-1, 5-2, and 5-3 to visualize these relationships.

Table 5-1 *Approximate Equivalents among Metric, Apothecaries, and Household Systems*

Metric		Apothecaries		Household
Dry				
60 mg	=	1 gr		
1 g	=	15 gr		
15 g	=	4 dr	=	1 tbs (3 tsp)
30 g	=	1 oz (8 dr)	=	1 oz (2 tbs)
		16 oz	=	1 lb
1 kg			=	2.2 lb
Liquid				
1 mL	=	15–16 minims	=	15 gtt
4 mL	=	1 dr		
5 mL	=	75 minims	=	1 tsp
15 mL	=	4 dr	=	1 tbs (3 tsp)
30 mL	=	1 oz (8 dr)	=	1 oz (2 tbs)
500 mL	=	16 oz (1 pt)	=	16 oz (1 pt or 2 cups)
1000 mL	=	32 oz (1 qt)	=	32 oz (1 qt)
Length				
2.5 cm			=	1 in
1 m			=	39.4 in

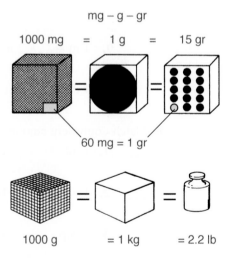

Figure 5-1 *Weight conversions*

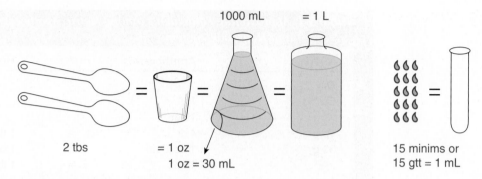

1000 mL   = 1 L

2 tbs   = 1 oz
               1 oz = 30 mL

15 minims or
15 gtt = 1 mL

Figure 5-2 *Volume conversions*

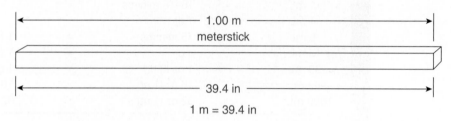

1.00 m
meterstick

39.4 in
1 m = 39.4 in

Figure 5-3 *Length conversions*

PRACTICE

Equivalents

A. Fill in the blanks

1. 60 mg = _____ gr

2. 15 gr = _____ g

3. 1 g = _____ mg

4. 1 kg = _____ g

5. 1 kg = _____ lb

6. 1 minim = _____ gtt

7. 1 L = _____ mL

8. 1 in = _____ cm

9. 1 m = _____ in

10. 1 tbs = _____ oz

B. Match equivalent amounts

_____ **1.** 1 mL   **a.** 1 oz

_____ **2.** 1 tsp   **b.** 4 dr

_____ **3.** 1 cup   **c.** 5 mL

_____ **4.** 15 mL   **d.** 15 minim

_____ **5.** 30 mL   **e.** 250 mL

                         f. 500 mL

(***Note:*** See Appendix G for answer key.)

CONVERSION FROM ONE SYSTEM TO ANOTHER

EXAMPLE   Convert 5 g to gr.

Starting Factor   Answer Unit
5 g   gr

Equivalents: 1 g = gr 15

Conversion Equation: $5 \cancel{g} \times \dfrac{\text{gr } 15}{1 \cancel{g}} = \text{gr } 75$

EXAMPLE   Convert 5.4 lb to kg.

Starting Factor   Answer Unit
5.4 lb   kg

Equivalents: kg = 2.2 lb

Conversion Equation: $5.4 \cancel{\text{lb}} \times \dfrac{1 \text{ kg}}{2.2 \cancel{\text{lb}}} = 2.5 \text{ kg}$

EXAMPLE   Convert gr 45 to g.

Starting Factor   Answer Unit
gr 45   g

Equivalents: gr 15 = 1 g

Conversion Equation: $\cancel{\text{gr}}\ 45 \times \dfrac{1 \text{ g}}{\cancel{\text{gr}}\ 15} = 3 \text{ g}$

EXAMPLE   Convert 54 kg to lb.

Starting Factor   Answer Unit
54 kg   lb

Equivalents: 2.2 lb = 1 kg

Conversion Equation: $54 \cancel{\text{kg}} \times \dfrac{2.2 \text{ lb}}{1 \cancel{\text{kg}}} = 118.8 \text{ lb}$

EXAMPLE   Convert 16 mL to dr.

Starting Factor   Answer Unit
16 mL   dr

Equivalents: 4 mL = 1 dr

Conversion Equation: $16 \cancel{\text{mL}} \times \dfrac{1 \text{ dr}}{4 \cancel{\text{mL}}} = 4 \text{ dr}$

EXAMPLE   Convert 8 oz to mL.

Starting Factor   Answer Unit
8 oz   mL

Equivalents: 1 oz = 30 mL

Conversion Equation: $8 \cancel{\text{oz}} \times \dfrac{30 \text{ mL}}{1 \cancel{\text{oz}}} = 240 \text{ mL}$

EXAMPLE Convert 480 mL to oz.

Starting Factor   Answer Unit
480 mL   oz

Equivalents: 30 mL = 1 oz

Conversion Equation: $480 \text{ mL} \times \dfrac{1 \text{ oz}}{30 \text{ mL}} = 16 \text{ oz}$

EXAMPLE Convert gr $2\frac{1}{2}$ to mg.

Starting Factor   Answer Unit
gr $2\frac{1}{2}$ mg

Equivalents: gr 1 = 60 mg

Conversion Equation: $\text{gr } 2\frac{1}{2} \times \dfrac{60 \text{ mg}}{\text{gr } 1} = 150 \text{ mg}$

EXAMPLE Convert 300 mg to gr.

Starting Factor   Answer Unit
300 mg   gr

Equivalents: 60 mg = gr 1

Conversion Equation: $300 \text{ mg} \times \dfrac{\text{gr } 1}{60 \text{ mg}} = \text{gr } 5$

EXAMPLE Convert 10 mL to tsp.

Starting Factor   Answer Unit
10 mL   tsp

Equivalents: 5 mL = 1 tsp

Conversion Equation: $10 \text{ mL} \times \dfrac{1 \text{ tsp}}{5 \text{ mL}} = 2 \text{ tsp}$

PRACTICE

Carry Each Answer to Two Decimal Places and Round to the Nearest Tenth

1. 2.5 pt to mL

2. 40 kg to lb

3. 600 mL to cups

4. 2 tsp to mL

5. gr $\frac{1}{2}$ to mg

6. oz 50 to kg

7. minims xx to mL

8. oz iv to tbs

9. 0.6 L to oz

10. 2 g to gr

PRACTICE

Carry Each Answer to Two Decimal Places and Round to the Nearest Tenth (Continued)

11. dr $1\frac{1}{2}$ to gtt

12. 5 mL to minims

13. 120 mg to gr

14. 10 gtt to mL

15. 12.5 mL to tsp

16. $1\frac{1}{2}$ tbs to mL

17. 2 cups to mL

18. 6 tsp to dr

19. 120 gr to g

20. 157 lb to kg

21. gr 3 to mg

22. 3 mL to minims

23. 5.2 kg to lb

24. 120 mm to cm

25. 60 cm to in

26. 0.5 pt to dr

27. 90 mg to gr

28. 5.5 g to gr

29. 60 mL to tbs

30. 5 gr to mg

(*Note:* See Appendix G for answer key.)

CHAPTER 6

Calculation of Oral Medications

OBJECTIVES

Upon completion of this chapter, you should be able to:

- Identify various forms of oral medications.
- Read dosage calibrations on a medicine cup, dropper, and syringe.
- Read drug labels to obtain information about specific drugs administered orally.
- Demonstrate knowledge of the appropriate method of rounding off doses when administering oral medications.
- Apply dimensional analysis to clinical calculations involving oral medications.

ORAL MEDICATIONS

Medications that are administered by mouth and absorbed via the gastrointestinal tract are known as PO (by mouth or orally) drugs. It is necessary to become familiar with this abbreviation to administer these drugs by the correct route, which should be designated as PO in the medication order.

A variation of the oral route is called the *sublingual route,* whereby medication is placed under the tongue for absorption via the mucous membrane into the circulatory system. This route is designated by the abbreviation sL in the medication order. When medication is ordered to be administered via the *buccal* route, it is placed between the cheek and gum for similar absorption. Neither sublingual nor buccal medications should be chewed or swallowed whole and, as a rule, are not followed by water.

It is necessary to recognize the various forms in which oral medications are dispensed and to understand how to read labels of medication containers, as well as calibrations on equipment used to dispense liquid medications.

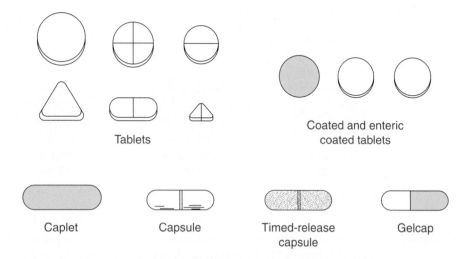

Figure 6-1 *Oral medication forms*

Figure 6-1 illustrates a variety of oral medication forms:

- Tablets—contain a powdered drug compressed into a tablet. Tablets come in various shapes and may be half-scored or quarter-scored. They may be broken or crushed and placed in food for clients who have difficulty swallowing.
- Coated tablets—covered with a flavored coating to facilitate swallowing and disguise taste. They cannot be divided and should not be crushed.
- Enteric coated—covered with a coating that delays dissolution and absorption until the tablet reaches the small intestine. They cannot be divided and should not be crushed.
- Capsules—contain a drug enclosed in a gelatin container to conceal taste. They may be opened and contents placed in food, unless this is contraindicated by desired action of the drug.
- Caplet—tablet shaped like a capsule. Caplets may be coated and should not be broken.
- Sustained-release capsules or tablets—drug granules coated to dissolve at different times to provide for continuous release of drug over an extended time period (also called timed-release capsules, spansules, tempules, or caplets). They must never be opened or broken apart before administering.
- Liquids—dispensed as elixirs, syrups, suspensions, or solutions.

THE MEDICINE CUP

The most common type of container used for dispensing fluid drugs is the medicine cup, made of glass or plastic, Figure 6-2. It usually is calibrated in one or more of the three measuring systems: metric, apothecaries, and household.

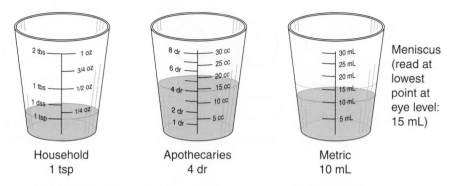

Figure 6-2 *Medicine cup*

When a solution is poured into a medicine cup, capillary attraction causes the fluid in contact with the cup to be drawn upward and the surface of the solution becomes concave. The curved surface is called the *meniscus* and the reading of the dose must be made at its lowest point. The medicine cup should be set on a flat surface to ensure accurate reading at eye level.

Note that the smallest amounts for which most medicine cups are calibrated are 1 dram, 1 teaspoon, or 5 milliliters. When measuring smaller amounts, it is recommended that the medication be drawn up into a syringe, which facilitates a more accurate measurement. Some liquid medications are premeasured for oral administration in a single-dose syringe.

When pills, tablets, or capsules are being dispensed from a prescription container, single doses may be placed in a plastic medicine cup or in a small paper (souffle) cup, depending on hospital policy. Many such medications are wrapped in individual doses and should be opened at the bedside just prior to administration. This provides one more opportunity to check for the correct drug and dose.

PRACTICE

Shade the Following Dosages on the Medicine Cups

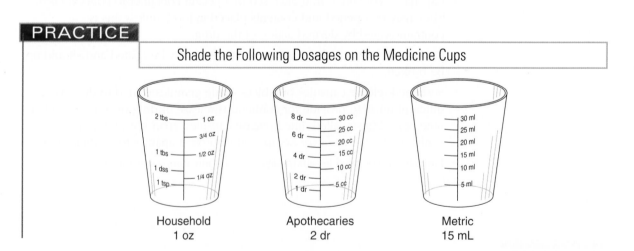

PRACTICE

Shade the Following Dosages on the Medicine Cups (Continued)

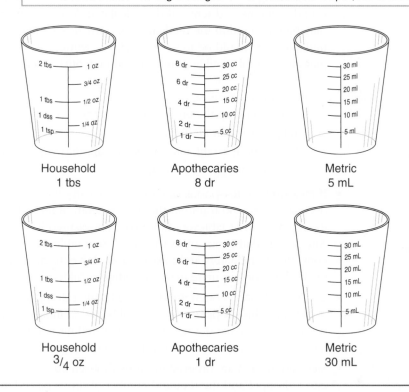

Household
1 tbs

Apothecaries
8 dr

Metric
5 mL

Household
3/4 oz

Apothecaries
1 dr

Metric
30 mL

ROUNDING OFF When Administering Tablets

- Tablets scored in halves or quarters may be broken in half or quarters in order to obtain as exact a dose as possible, Figure 6-1.

EXAMPLE If calculated dose is 1.5 tablets, give $1\frac{1}{2}$ tablets.

1.25 tablets, give $1\frac{1}{4}$ tablets

1.75 tablets, give $1\frac{3}{4}$ tablets

- If tablets are not scored, a pill splitter may be used if hospital policy permits. Because this can be a very inaccurate method, it should be used only when an alternative form (e.g., liquid) of the medication is not available. Check with the pharmacist regarding alternative dosage forms.

- Capsules, spansules, and enteric coated tablets cannot be divided. If the calculated dose is not a whole number, consult with the pharmacist or provider in regard to rounding.

When Administering Oral Liquids

- If measuring in milliliters, carry the calculation to two decimal places and round to the nearest tenth. If the calculated dose is an even multiple of 5, it may be measured in the medicine cup. Any dosage that is not an even multiple of 5 should be measured using a syringe, as this permits accurate measurement of small amounts, including tenths of milliliters, Figure 6-3.

EXAMPLE If calculated dose is:

2.3 mL, draw up the entire amount in the syringe

5 mL, measure in medicine cup

12.7 mL, pour 10 mL into medicine cup, draw up 2.7 mL into syringe, and add to medication in cup

- If measuring in teaspoons or tablespoons, carry the calculation to two decimal places and round to the nearest tenth. If the calculated dose is an exact teaspoon or tablespoon, it may be measured in the medicine cup. Any dosage that is not an exact teaspoon or tablespoon should be converted to milliliters and measured as above, using a syringe. This method is more accurate than converting milliliters to drops.

- Liquid medications often are dispensed with a dropper attached to the bottle cap. This dropper usually is calibrated in milliliters (e.g., 0.1 mL, 0.2 mL) or by actual dosage (e.g., 75 mg, 100 mg), thus facilitating accurate measurement of the medication, Figure 6-3.

- Medications that are ordered in drops (household system) can be drawn up into a dropper and the required number of drops placed in a spoon or medicine cup for administration, Figure 6-3.

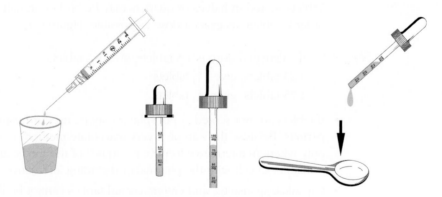

Figure 6-3 *Measuring liquids*

READING LABELS AND CALCULATING DOSAGE

All medication containers are labeled as to their contents and directions for use. Individuals administering medications must be able to read and understand the information given on the label. This information includes:

- Name of drug: Trade name—the brand name; the registered trademark assigned by the manufacturer; usually followed by ®. Generic name (by law this must appear on all drug labels)—the official name assigned to a drug; the name under which it is licensed. Drugs that have been in use for many years may thereafter be manufactured and sold under the generic name, eliminating the need for a brand name. Therefore, if only one name appears on a drug label, it is the generic name.

- Dosage strength: Amount or concentration of the drug—per mL, tablet, capsule, etc. This may be written in more than one system of measurement (e.g., metric, apothecaries).

- Name of manufacturer

- Form: Liquid—mL, oz, etc. Solid—tablet, capsule, powder, etc. (not always indicated on the label)

- Expiration date: How long the medication will remain stable or potent.

- Lot number: A number assigned by the manufacturer that can be used for identification in the event that a particular batch of drug must be traced or recalled. The lot number, along with the expiration date, is documented whenever any biological preparations (e.g., vaccines, serums, or immune globulins) are administered.

- Total amount per container: Total volume, if liquid; total number, if solid. It is important not to confuse this number or quantity with the dosage strength of the drug.

- Directions for administering (or storing): Mixing, reconstituting, shaking, refrigerating, etc.

- Bar code: Matching bar codes on the medication container and the client's wristband reveal the prescribed medication and dosing. Prior to administration, both bar codes are scanned for accuracy. In the event of any error, the scanning device beeps.

Reading Labels

EXAMPLE   Figure 6-4

1. Trade Name: Glucotrol
2. Generic Name: glipizide
3. Dosage Strength: 5 mg per tablet
4. Form: Tablet

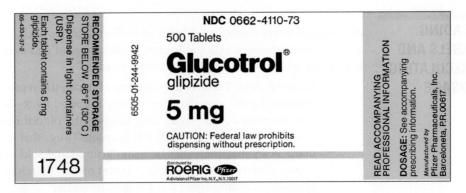

Figure 6-4 *(Label reproduced with permission of Pfizer, Inc.)*

5. Manufacturer's Name: Roerig Pfizer
6. Directions for Storage: Store below 86°F (30°C)
7. Total Amount per Container: 500 tablets
8. *Order:* Glucotrol 10 mg PO

How many tablets should the client receive?

   Starting Factor   Answer Unit
        10 mg   tab
   Equivalent: 5 mg = 1 tab

Conversion Equation: $10 \ \cancel{mg} \times \dfrac{1 \ tab}{5 \ \cancel{mg}} = 2 \ tab$

EXAMPLE   Figure 6-5

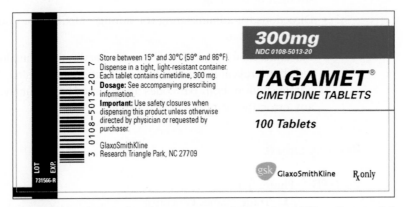

Figure 6-5 *(Printed with permission of GlaxoSmithKline Group of Companies, all rights reserved)*

1. Trade Name: Tagamet
2. Generic Name: Cimetidine
3. Dosage Strength: 200 mg per tablet
4. Form: tablets
5. Manufacturer's Name: SmithKline Beecham

6. *Order:* Tagamet 400 mg PO

How many tablets should the client receive?

   Starting Factor   Answer Unit
       400 mg   tab

Equivalent: 200 mg = 1 tab

Conversion Equation: $400 \text{ mg} \times \dfrac{1 \text{ tab}}{200 \text{ mg}} = 2 \text{ tab}$

PRACTICE

Reading Labels

A. Figure 6-6

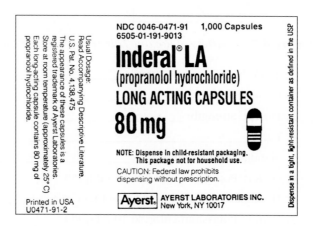

Figure 6-6 *(Courtesy of Wyeth-Ayerst Pharmaceuticals, New York, NY)*

1. Trade Name:_____

2. Generic Name: _____

3. Dosage Strength: _____

4. Form: _____

5. Manufacturer's Name: _____

6. *Order:* Inderal LA 80 mg PO

How many capsules should be administered? _____

7. *Order:* Inderal LA 160 mg PO

How many capsules should be administered? _____

Reading Labels (Continued)

B. Figure 6-7

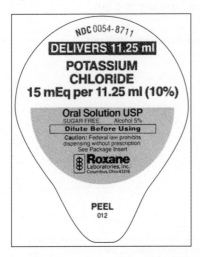

Figure 6-7 *(Courtesy of Roxane Laboratories, Inc., Columbus, OH)*

1. Trade Name: _____

2. Generic Name: _____

3. Dosage Strength: _____

4. Form: _____

5. Manufacturer's Name: _____

6. *Order:* Potassium chloride 15 mEq PO

How many mL should the client receive? _____

7. *Order:* Potassium chloride 10 mEq PO

How many mL should the client receive? _____

C. Figure 6-8

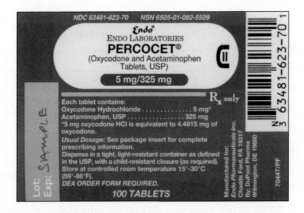

Figure 6-8 *(Courtesy of Endo Pharmaceuticals, Inc., Chadds Ford, PA)*

PRACTICE

Reading Labels (Continued)

1. Trade Name: _____

2. Generic Name: _____

3. Dosage Strength: _____

4. Form: _____

5. Manufacturer's Name: _____

D. Figure 6-9

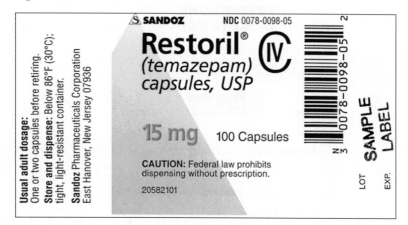

Figure 6-9   *(Used with the permission of Novartis Pharmaceuticals Corporation)*

1. Trade Name: _____

2. Generic Name: _____

3. Dosage Strength: _____

4. Form: _____

5. Manufacturer's Name: _____

(*Note:* See Appendix G for answer keys.)

Reading Labels and Clinical Calculations Involving Medications
Administered by the Oral Route (PO)

1. Order: Prednisone 20 mg PO

   Label: Figure 6-10

   How many tablets should be administered? _____

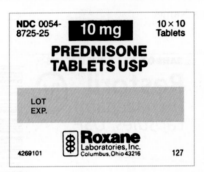

Figure 6-10 *(Courtesy of Roxane Laboratories, Inc., Columbus, OH)*

2. Order: Aldactone 0.05 g PO

   Label: Figure 6-11

   How many tablets should be administered? _____

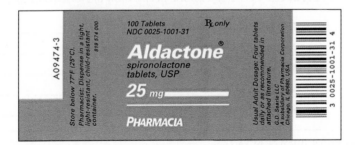

Figure 6-11 *(Courtesy of Pharmacia Corporation, Peapack, NJ)*

Reading Labels and Clinical Calculations Involving Medications
Administered by the Oral Route (PO) (Continued)

3. *Order:* Hydroxyzine pamoate 60 mg PO

Label: Figure 6-12

How many mL should be administered? _____

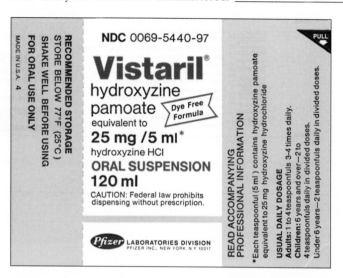

Figure 6-12 *(Courtesy of Pfizer Laboratories Division, Pfizer Inc., New York, NY)*

4. *Order:* Nilstat Suspension 1 tsp PO

Label: Figure 6-13. What is the generic name? _____

How many units should be administered? _____

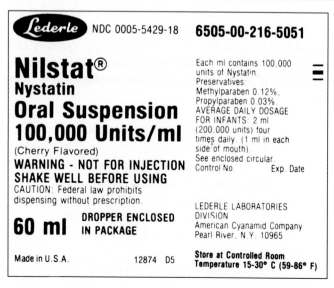

Figure 6-13 *(Courtesy of Lederle Laboratories, Pearl River, NY)*

Reading Labels and Clinical Calculations Involving Medications Administered by the Oral Route (PO) (Continued)

5. *Order:* Compazine 10 mg PO

Label: Figure 6-14. What is the generic name? _____

How many tablets should be administered? _____

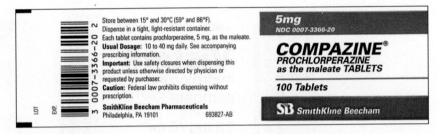

Store between 15° and 30°C (59° and 86°F).
Dispense in a tight, light-resistant container.
Each tablet contains prochlorperazine, 5 mg, as the maleate.
Usual Dosage: 10 to 40 mg daily. See accompanying prescribing information.
Important: Use safety closures when dispensing this product unless otherwise directed by physician or requested by purchaser.
Caution: Federal law prohibits dispensing without prescription.
SmithKline Beecham Pharmaceuticals
Philadelphia, PA 19101   693827-AB

NDC 0007-3366-20

5mg
NDC 0007-3366-20

COMPAZINE®
PROCHLORPERAZINE
as the maleate TABLETS

100 Tablets

SB SmithKline Beecham

Figure 6-14 (*Courtesy of SmithKline Beecham Pharmaceuticals, Philadelphia, PA*)

(***Note:*** See Appendix G for answer key.)

CALCULATIONS BASED ON BODY WEIGHT

Medications may be prescribed according to a designated amount of drug per kilogram or pound of body weight. Specific amounts of drug per unit of body weight are recommended by the drug manufacturer, and this information can be found in the product insert or in a drug reference publication. Medication orders may be written in amounts for individual doses or for total daily (24 hr) dosage, in which case the total calculated dosage must be divided by the specified number of doses to be given.

Because the amount of medication to be given is determined by the weight of the person, this weight and the calculated dosage can be considered an equivalent relationship. Our goal is to convert a particular quantity of weight to a corresponding quantity of medication. **Therefore, the starting factor is in *lb* or *kg* and the answer label is in whatever units the medication is dispensed (e.g., *mL, mg, tab,* etc.).**

EXAMPLE ***Order:*** Thiabendazole Suspension 25 /per kg /24 hr PO to an adult weighing 148 lb

Label: Thiabendazole Suspension 500 mg per 5 mL

How many mL should be administered?

Starting Factor	Answer Unit
148 lb	mL

Equivalents: 2.2 lb = 1 kg, 25 mg = 1 kg, 500 mg = 5 mL

Conversion Equation: $148 \text{ lb} \times \dfrac{1 \text{ kg}}{2.2 \text{ lb}} \times \dfrac{25 \text{ mg}}{1 \text{ kg}} \times \dfrac{5 \text{ mL}}{500 \text{ mg}} = 16.8 \text{ mL}$

In the first example, the total calculated dosage is administered in one dose. If the order specifies administering the medication in divided doses, it is necessary to divide the total calculated dosage by the number of doses prescribed so that the correct amount per dose will be administered.

EXAMPLE **Order:** Chloromycetin 50 mg/kg/day in four divided doses PO to an adult weighing 80 kg

Label: Chloromycetin (chloramphenicol) 250 mg per cap

How many capsules should be administered *per dose?*

Starting Factor   Answer Unit
80 kg   cap

Equivalents: 50 mg = 1 kg, 1 cap = 250 mg

Conversion Equation:

$$80 \text{ kg} \times \frac{50 \text{ mg}}{1 \text{ kg}} \times \frac{1 \text{ cap}}{250 \text{ mg}} = \frac{16 \text{ cap}}{4 \text{ doses}} = 4 \text{ cap per dose}$$

EXAMPLE **Order:** Ancobon 50 mg/kg/day in four divided doses PO to an adult weighing 135 lb

Label: Ancobon (flucytosine) 250 mg per cap

How many capsules should be administered *per dose?*

Starting Factor   Answer Unit
135 lb   cap

Equivalents: 1 kg = 2.2 lb, 50 mg = 1 kg, 1 cap = 250 mg

Conversion Equation:

$$135 \text{ lb} \times \frac{1 \text{ kg}}{2.2 \text{ lb}} \times \frac{50 \text{ mg}}{1 \text{ kg}} \times \frac{1 \text{ cap}}{250 \text{ mg}} = \frac{12.2 \text{ cap}}{4 \text{ doses}} = 3 \text{ cap per dose}$$

REMEMBER

It is critically important to perform this final step, dividing by number of doses, in computations based on body weight. Consistency in this regard helps avoid errors when medication is to be given in divided doses. If this step is omitted, it is easy to forget to divide the total daily dose into the prescribed number of doses, thus greatly increasing the risk of administering an overdosage.

Although all of the examples in this chapter and Chapters 8 and 10 illustrate calculations of *adult* dosages based on body weight, the same method is used to calculate *pediatric* dosages also based on body weight.

PRACTICE

Oral Dosage Based on Body Weight

1. **Order:** Ethambutol 15 mg/kg/24 hr PO to an adult weighing 130 lb

   Label: Ethambutol 400 mg per tab

   How many tablets should be administered per dose? _____

2. **Order:** Flucytosine 50 mg/kg/day PO in four divided doses to an adult weighing 69.4 kg

   Label: Flucytosine 250 mg per cap

   How many capsules should be administered per dose? _____

3. **Order:** Antiminth Oral Suspension 11 mg per kg PO, one dose only, to an adult weighing 146 lb

   Label: Antiminth (pyrantel pamoate) Oral Suspension 50 mg per mL

   How many mL should be administered? _____

4. **Order:** Myambutol 25 mg/kg/24 hr PO to an adult weighing 72.7 kg

   Label: Myambutol (ethambutol hydrochloride) 400 mg per tab (scored)

   How many tablets should be administered per dose? _____

5. **Order:** Isoniazid Tablets 5 mg per kg PO in two divided doses to an adult weighing 175 lb

   Label: Isoniazid Tablets 100 mg per tab

   How many tablets should be administered per dose? _____

PRACTICE

Clinical Calculations Involving Medications Administered by the Oral Route (PO)

A. Use dimensional analysis and calculate the correct amount to be administered per dose.

  1. *Order:* Amoxil Capsule 500 mg PO

  Label: Figure 6-15

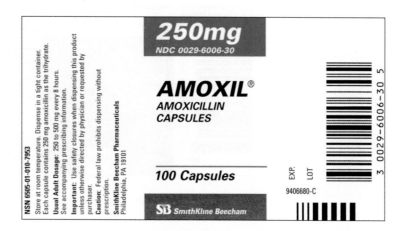

Figure 6-15 *(Courtesy of SmithKline Beecham Pharmaceuticals, Philadelphia, PA)*

  2. *Order:* Aldactone 100 mg PO

  Label: Figure 6-16

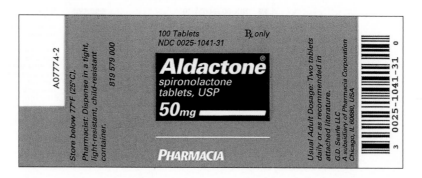

Figure 6-16 *(Courtesy of Pharmacia Corporation, Peapack, NJ)*

Clinical Calculations Involving Medications Administered by the Oral
Route (PO) (Continued)

3. *Order:* Ranitidine hydrochloride 300 mg PO

Label: Figure 6-17

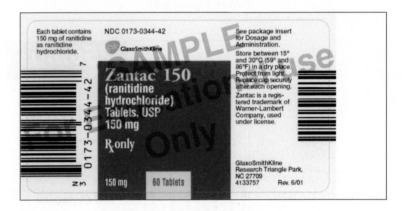

Figure 6-17 *(Courtesy of GlaxoSmithKline, Research Triangle Park, NC)*

4. *Order:* DiaBeta 7.5 mg PO

Label: Figure 6-18

Figure 6-18 *(Courtesy of Aventis Pharmaceuticals, Kansas City, MO)*

PRACTICE

Clinical Calculations Involving Medications Administered by the Oral Route (PO) (Continued)

5. *Order:* Keflex 1 g PO

Label: Figure 6-19

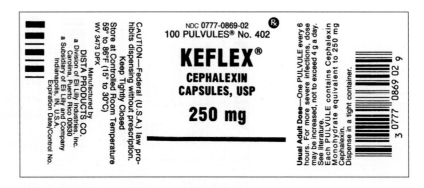

Figure 6-19 *(Courtesy of Eli Lilly Pharmaceuticals, Indianapolis, IN)*

6. *Order:* Cipro 750 mg PO

Label: Figure 6-20

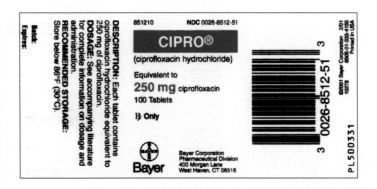

Figure 6-20 *(Courtesy of Bayer Corporation, West Haven, CT)*

Clinical Calculations Involving Medications Administered by the Oral
Route (PO) (Continued)

7. *Order:* Ampicillin 0.5 g PO

Label: Figure 6-21

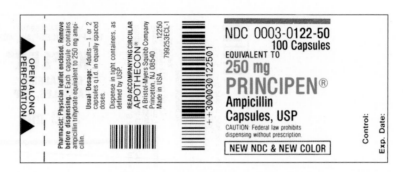

Figure 6-21 *(Courtesy of Apothecon Bristol Myers Squibb, Princeton, NJ)*

8. *Order:* Meclofenamate sodium 0.1 g PO

Label: Figure 6-22

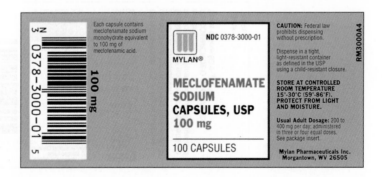

Figure 6-22 *(Courtesy of Mylan Pharmaceuticals Inc.,
Morgantown, WV)*

Clinical Calculations Involving Medications Administered by the Oral
Route (PO) (Continued)

9. *Order:* Augmentin 200 mg PO

   Label: Figure 6-23

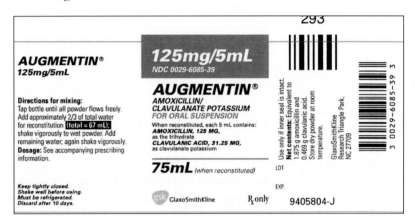

Figure 6-23 *(Reprinted with permission of GlaxoSmithKline Group of
Companies, all rights reserved)*

10. *Order:* Methadone hydrochloride Tablets 0.0025 g PO

   Label: Figure 6-24

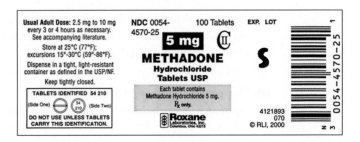

Figure 6-24 *(Used with permission of Roxane Laboratories Inc.,
Columbus, OH)*

PRACTICE

Clinical Calculations Involving Medications Administered by the Oral
Route (PO) (Continued)

11. The provider ordered Celestone 1.8 mg PO. The drug container label states:
    Celestone (beta-methasone) 0.6 mg per tablet. How many tablets should the
    client receive?

12. The provider ordered Erythromycin 150 mg PO. The label states: Ery-
    thromycin 0.75 g per fluid ounce. How many milliliters should be adminis-
    tered?

13. Aspirin gr 10 PO is ordered for the client. The strength on hand is Aspirin
    0.3 g per tablet. How many tablets should be administered?

14. Digoxin Elixir Pediatric 0.12 mg is ordered PO. The drug container label states:
    Digoxin 0.05 mg per mL. How many milliliters should the client receive?

15. The provider ordered Coumadin gr $\frac{1}{6}$ PO. How many tablets should the
    client receive if the label states: Coumadin (warfarin sodium) 5 mg per tablet?

16. Prolixin 0.125 mg is ordered PO. The strength on hand is Prolixin
    (fluphenazine) 0.25 mg per tablet (scored). How many tablets should be
    administered?

17. The client is to receive Penicillin G Potassium 250,000 units PO. The drug la-
    bel states: Penicillin G Potassium 500,000 units per tablet (scored). How
    many tablets should be administered?

18. The provider ordered Chloral Hydrate gr 15 PO hs. The label states: Chloral
    hydrate 500 mg per dram. How many drams should the client receive?

19. Nembutal Elixir 60 mg PO is ordered. The label states: Nembutal (pentobar-
    bital) Elixir 20 mg per 5 mL. How many milliliters should the client receive?

20. *Order:* Slo-phyllin 75 mg PO
    Label: Slo-phyllin (theophylline) 80 mg per 15 mL
    How many mL should be administered?

PRACTICE

Clinical Calculations Involving Medications Administered by the Oral Route (PO) (Continued)

21. **Order:** Aminophylline 300 mg PO

    Label: Aminophylline 0.1 g per tab

    How many tablets should the client receive?

22. **Order:** Azulfidine 1.5 g PO

    Label: Azulfidine (sulfasalazine) 500 mg per tab

    How many tablets should be administered?

23. **Order:** Chloromycetin 0.5 g PO

    Label: Chloromycetin (chloramphenicol) capsule 250 mg

    How many capsules should the client receive?

24. **Order:** Feosol Elixir 300 mg PO

    Label: Feosol (ferrous sulfate) Elixir 220 mg per 5 mL

    How many milliliters should be administered?

25. **Order:** Terramycin 500 mg PO

    Label: Terramycin (tetracycline hydrochloride) 50 mg per mL

    How many milliliters should be administered?

26. **Order:** Haldol 1.5 mg PO

    Label: Haldol (haloperidol) 0.5 mg per tab

    How many tablets should be administered?

27. **Order:** Sulfisoxazole 0.25 g PO

    Label: Sulfisoxazole 500 mg per tab (scored)

    How many tablets should be administered?

28. **Order:** Aldomet 250 mg PO

    Label: Aldomet (methyldopa) 1 g per tab (scored in quarters)

    How many tablets should be administered?

29. **Order:** Vibramycin 100 mg PO

    Label: Vibramycin (doxycycline) 50 mg per cap

    How many capsules should be administered?

Clinical Calculations Involving Medications Administered by the Oral Route (PO) (Continued)

B. Calculate the correct amount per dose.

30. *Order:* Potassium chloride 10 mEq PO

Label: Figure 6-25

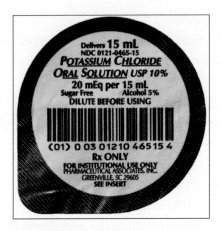

Figure 6-25 *(Courtesy of Roxane Laboratories Inc., Columbus, OH)*

31. *Order:* Cephalexin Capsule 0.5 g PO

Label: Figure 6-26

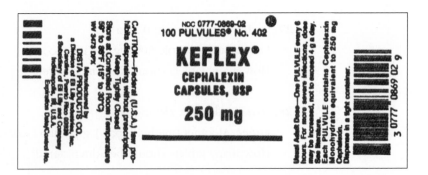

Figure 6-26 *(Courtesy of Eli Lilly Pharmaceuticals, Indianapolis, IN)*

Clinical Calculations Involving Medications Administered by the Oral Route (PO) (Continued)

32. *Order:* Codeine sulfate gr $\frac{1}{2}$ PO

    Label: Figure 6-27

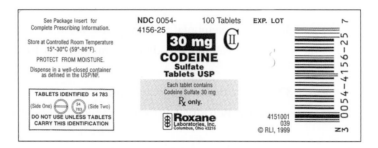

Figure 6-27   *(Courtesy of Roxane Laboratories Inc., Columbus, OH)*

33. *Order:* Phenobarbital gr $\frac{1}{4}$ PO

    Label: Figure 6-28

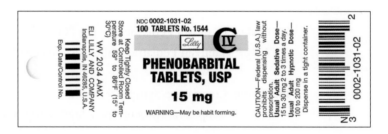

Figure 6-28   *(Courtesy of Eli Lilly Pharmaceuticals, Indianapolis, IN)*

34. *Order:* Seconal Sodium gr $1\frac{1}{2}$ PO

    Label: Figure 6-29

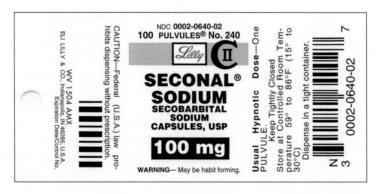

Figure 6-29   *(Courtesy of Eli Lilly Pharmaceuticals, Indianapolis, IN)*

Clinical Calculations Involving Medications Administered by the Oral
Route (PO) (Continued)

35. *Order:* Tylenol Elixir 60 mg PO

   Label: Tylenol (acetaminophen) Elixir 120 mg per 5 mL

36. *Order:* Nembutal Sodium gr $1\frac{1}{2}$ PO

   Label: Nembutal Sodium (pentobarbital) 100 mg per cap

37. *Order:* Benadryl Elixir 20 mg PO

   Label: Benadryl (diphenhydramine hydrochloride) Elixir 2.5 mg per mL

38. *Order:* Phenergan 0.05 g PO

   Label: Phenergan (promethazine hydrochloride) 12.5 mg per tab

39. *Order:* Prolixin 1 mg PO

   Label: Prolixin (fluphenazine) 2 mg per tab (scored)

40. *Order:* Gantrisin Pediatric 750 mg PO

   Label: Gantrisin Pediatric (sulfisoxazole acetyl) 500 mg per 5 mL

41. *Order:* Compazine Syrup 2.5 mg PO

   Label: Compazine (prochlorperazine) Syrup 5 mg per 5 mL

42. *Order:* Ascorbic Acid 0.1 g PO

   Label: Ascorbic Acid 50 mg per tab

43. *Order:* Dilantin Elixir 100 mg PO

   Label: Dilantin (phenytoin sodium) Elixir 125 mg per 5 mL

44. *Order:* Dilaudid Cough Syrup 3 mg PO

   Label: Dilaudid (dilaudid with guaifenesin) Cough Syrup 1 mg per 5 mL
   (Give _____ tsp)

45. *Order:* Mysoline Suspension 125 mg PO

   Label: Mysoline (primidone) Suspension 250 mg per 5 mL

PRACTICE

> ### Clinical Calculations Involving Medications Administered by the Oral Route (PO) (Continued)

46. *Order:* Aldomet Oral Suspension 400 mg PO

    Label: Aldomet (methyldopa) Oral Suspension 250 mg per 5 mL

47. *Order:* Mylicon 80 mg PO

    Label: Mylicon (simethicone) 40 mg per 0.6 mL

48. *Order:* Mycostatin 1,000,000 Units PO

    Label: Mycostatin (nystatin) 500,000 Units per tab

49. *Order:* Cleocin 150 mg PO

    Label: Cleocin (clindamycin) 75 mg per cap

50. *Order:* Synthroid 0.2 mg PO

    Label: Synthroid (levothyroxine sodium) 200 mcg per tab

51. *Order:* Minetezol Suspension 25 mg/kg/dose PO to an adult weighing 110 lb

    Label: Minetezol (thiabendazole) Suspension 500 mg per 5 mL

52. *Order:* Myambutol 25 mg/kg/day to an adult weighing 137 lb

    Label: Myambutol (ethambutol hydrochloride) 400 mg per tab

53. *Order:* Nydrazid 5 mg per kg in two divided doses to an adult weighing 115 lb

    Label: Nydrazid (nystatin) 100 mg per tab

54. *Order:* Trimethoprim 20 mg/kg/24 hr PO in four divided doses to an adult weighing 70 kg

    Label: Trimethoprim 160 mg per tab

55. *Order:* Sulfamethoxazole 100 mg/kg/24 hr PO in four divided doses to an adult weighing 154 lb

    Label: Sulfamethoxazole 800 mg per tab

    How many tablets should be administered per dose?

(*Note:* See Appendix G for answer key.)

CHAPTER 7

Administration of Oral Medications

OBJECTIVES

Upon completion of this chapter, you should be able to:

- Interpret and follow a medication order for the purpose of administering oral medications.
- List the standard abbreviations used in prescribing and administering medications.
- Identify various routes for administering medications.
- List the general rules for safe administration of oral medications: pouring, administering, and recording.
- Identify performance criteria related to administering oral medications.
- Perform a simulated administration of oral medications.

MEDICATION ORDER

A written order, signed by a physician, physician's assistant, or nurse practitioner, is required for medications administered by nurses. Any of these individuals authorized to write orders will hereinafter be designated as *provider*. Hospital policies and procedures for medication orders vary, but in most agencies these orders are written on a special form that is a part of the client's permanent record. The nurse should be sure that a written and signed order exists for any medication given. The only exception to this rule would be under special circumstances, such as emergencies, where a provider may give a verbal order, either directly or by phone. The registered nurse may write the order; the provider must later sign it.

The written order (Figure 7-1) consists of the following:

1. Client's name
2. Date and time the order is written

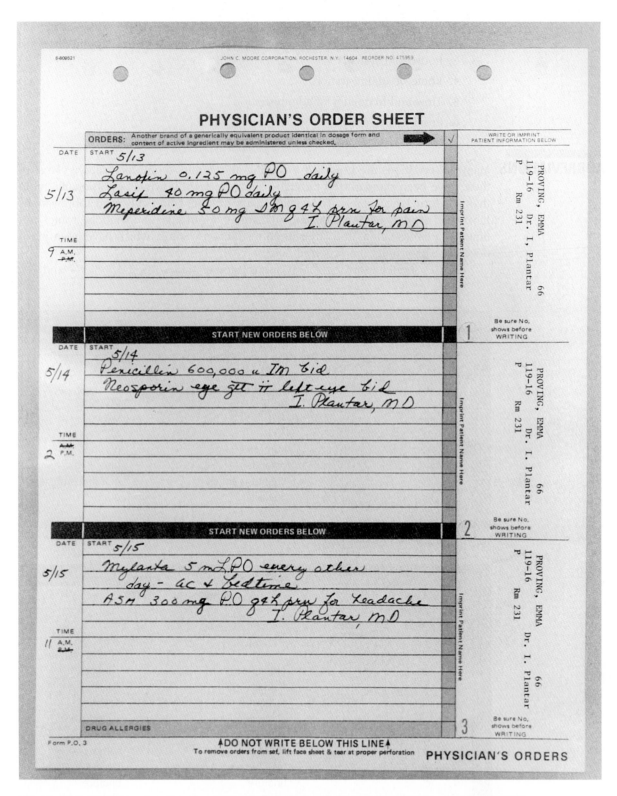

Figure 7-1 *Physician's order sheet (Courtesy of John C. Moore Corporation, Rochester, NY)*

3. Name and dosage of the medication (**Note:** Name may be written as generic or brand (trade), and dosage may be written in metric, apothecaries, or household systems.)

4. Route of administration

5. Time and frequency of administration

6. Provider's signature

ABBREVIATIONS

Many abbreviations are used in prescribing and administering medications. Most of these have been standardized through common usage; however, occasionally, more than one form is acceptable. To facilitate memorization, commonly used abbreviations have been divided into those dealing with amount or dosage, preparations, routes and times of administration, and any special instructions. Some, which have been introduced in earlier units, are repeated here.

Nurses should know the abbreviations listed in Tables 7-1, 7-2, 7-3, 7-4, and 7-5.

Table 7-1   Amount/Dosage

Abbreviation	Latin Derivation	English
g	gramma	gram
gr	granum	grain
gtt	gutta	drop
lb	libra	pound
mL		milliliter
no	numerus	number
pt	octarius	pint
qs	quantum sifficit	quantity sufficient
dr	dracama	dram
oz	uncia	ounce

Table 7-2   Preparations

Abbreviation	Latin Derivation	English
cap	capsula	capsule
elix	elixir	elixir
EC		enteric coated
ext	extractum	extract
fl	fluidus	fluid
sol	solutio	solution
supp	suppositorium	suppository
susp		suspension
syr	syrupus	syrup
tab	tabella	tablet
tr	tincture	tincture
ung	unguentum	ointment

Table 7-3 Routes

Abbreviation	Latin Derivation	English
ID		intradermal
IM		intramuscular
IV		intravenous
IVPB		intravenous piggyback
OD	oculus dexter	right eye
OS	oculus sinister	left eye
OU	oculo utro	both eyes
AD	auricula dexter	right ear
AS	auricula sinister	left ear
PO	per os	by mouth
subcut	sub cutis	subcutaneous
SL	sub lingual	sublingual
GT		gastrostomy
NG		nasogastric
NJ		nasojejunal

Table 7-4 Times

Abbreviation	Latin Derivation	English
a	ante	before
ac	ante cibum	before meals
am	ante meridian	before noon
bid	bis in die	*twice a day
h	hora	hour
hs	hora somni	hour of sleep or at bedtime
noct	noctis	night
oh	omni hora	every hour
p	post	after
pc	post cibum	after meals
pm	post meridian	after noon
prn	pro re nata	whenever necessary
q	quaque	every
qh (q3h, etc.)	quaque hora	*every hour (every 3 hours, etc.)
qid	quater in die	*four times a day
sos	si opus sit	if necessary (one dose only)
tid	ter in die	three times a day

*Note: Medications ordered q2h, q3h, q4h, etc., are given "around the clock" (i.e., throughout a 24-hour period). It is important not to confuse these abbreviations with bid, which means to administer twice a day (not every 2 hours), and qid, which means to administer 4 times a day (not every 4 hours).

Table 7-5 *Special Instructions*

Abbreviation	Latin Derivation	English
aa	ana (Gr.)	of each
ad lib	ad libitum	as desired
$\bar{c}$	cum	with
dil	dilutus	dilute
per	per	through or by
Rx	recipe	take (or prescription)
$\bar{s}$	sine	without
stat	statim	immediately

SELF-QUIZ— ABBREVIATIONS

A. Match the abbreviations with the correct meaning.

_____ **1.** gtt

_____ **2.** dr

_____ **3.** sos

_____ **4.** qh

_____ **5.** ad lib

_____ **6.** bid

_____ **7.** ext

_____ **8.** $\bar{c}$

_____ **9.** stat

_____ **10.** q

A. as desired

B. dram

C. drop

D. every

E. every hour

F. extract

G. fluid

H. immediately

I. one dose only

J. ounce

K. three times a day

L. twice a day

M. whenever necessary

N. with

B. Write the term.

1. ac = _____

2. cap = _____

3. g = _____

4. pc = _____

5. q3h = _____

6. $\bar{s}$ = _____

7. elix = _____

8. prn = _____

9. qid = _____

10. mL = _____

C. Identify the route.

1. IM   = _____

2. IV   = _____

3. subcut = _____

4. OS   = _____

5. OD   = _____

6. OU   = _____

7. PO   = _____

8. SL   = _____

9. ID   = _____

(***Note:*** See Appendix G for answer key.)

ROUTES FOR ADMINISTERING MEDICATIONS

The common routes by which medications are administered are:

- mouth—PO
- gastrointestinal—GI
- injection (parenteral)
  - subcutaneous—subcut
  - intramuscular—IM
  - intradermal—ID
  - intravenous—IV
  - intrathecal (into the spinal canal) ⎫
  - intracardial (into the heart)   ⎬ Less common parenteral routes
  - intra-articular (into a joint)   ⎭
- inhalation—respiratory tract
- topical—placing on skin, mucous membrane, or in body cavity
  - sublingual (under the tongue)
  - instillation (dropping liquid into a cavity: eye drops)
  - inunction (rubbing ointment on skin)
  - irrigation (into a wound or body cavity)
  - suppository (vaginal, rectal, urethral)
  - transdermal patch (applied to the skin, with medication absorbed through the skin)

MEDICATION ADMINISTRA-TION RECORD (MAR)

Safe nursing practice requires the use of some type of medication administration record (MAR) or guide to which the nurse can refer when administering medications. Usually this is in the form of a special Kardex, sometimes called a Medex, on which all medication orders for individual clients are reproduced on separate cards or pages. Figure 7-2 is a sample MAR.

COMMUNITY HOSPITAL

NURSE'S SIGNATURE	INIT.	NURSE'S SIGNATURE	INIT.	NURSE'S SIGNATURE	INIT.
Marilyn Cuve RN	MC				
A Donald Insley R.N.	ASI				
Rosemary Winckler RN	RF				
M Kathleen Wickwirth RN	MD				
Joan Perretta, RN	JP				
Teresa Jerical SN	TJ				

RA-Right Arm RB-Right Buttocks RL-Right Leg LA-Left Arm LB-Left Buttocks LL-Left Leg

ROUTINE MEDICATION ORDERS

ORD DATE	EXP DATE	Medication Frequency	Dosage Route	Shift	HOUR	5/13 INIT.	5/14 INIT.	5/15 INIT.	5/16 INIT.	5/17 INIT.	5/18 INIT.	5/19 INIT.
5/13		LANOXIN daily	0.125mg PO	11-7								
				7-3	9	MC	MC	ASI	TJ			
				3-11		P74	P72	P77	P68			
5/13		LASIX daily	40mg PO	11-7								
				7-3	9	MC	MC	ASI	TJ			
				3-11								
5/14		PENICILLIN G bid	600000u IM	11-7								
				7-3	9		MC/LL ASI/LB TJ/LL					
				3-11	9		RF/RB RF/RB TJ/RL					
5/14		NEOSPORIN cye gtt ii bid	OS	11-7								
				7-3	10		MC	ASI	TJ			
				3-11	6		RF	RF	JP			
5/15		MYLANTA every other day (AC & HS)	5mL PO	11-7								
				7-3	7=11			ASI/ ASI TJ/TJ				
				3-11	4=9			RF/RF JP/JP				
				11-7								
				7-3								
				3-11								

PRN MEDICATIONS
DOCUMENT PRN INJECTION SITE IN NURSE'S NOTES

ORD DATE	EXP DATE	Medication Frequency	Dosage Route		Doses Given
5/13	5/15	Meperidine, 50mg IM q4h PRN for pain		Date	5/13 5/14 5/15
				Time	12 9 2:3
				INIT	MC ASI MD
5/15		ASA 300mg PO q3h PRN FOR HEADACHE		Date	5/15 5/16
				Time	4 12
				INIT	ASI MD
				Date	
				Time	
				INIT	
				Date	
				Time	
				INIT	

Room No.: 231	Name: EMMA PROVING	Hosp. No.: 119-16	Age: 66	Physician: I PLANTAR, M.D

Allergies: NKA

Figure 7-2 Medication administration record (MAR)

Note that the client's name and room number appear on the MAR, along with all pertinent information relating to the order: drug, dose, route, date, and time of administration. As a rule, space for recording each dose given also appears on the record. If pertinent, start and stop dates and special instructions or precautions are included. The presence or absence of allergies should be noted by listing any substance to which the client is allergic or by using some notation such as NKA (no known allergies). As the MAR is filled up or discontinued, it becomes part of the client's permanent record.

A nurse should never give a medication without referring to this reproduction of the medication order or, if there is any question, to the original order in the client's medical record. It is essential that the MAR be up to date and that any delayed or temporarily omitted medication (e.g., client fasting for test or on call for surgery, etc.) be identified appropriately so it is not administered inadvertently. Hospital policy should specify the procedure for recording or reporting omitted or delayed medications.

RECORDING MEDICATIONS

All medications given must be recorded immediately on the client's MAR, according to the policy of the institution. Only the nurse who administered the medications should sign for them. Usually initials are used for recording, with a place for the full signature somewhere on the sheet or card. Refer to Figure 7-2 for an example of such documentation.

In some situations, medication order processing and documentation may be computerized; for example, ordering from pharmacy, billing via business office, recording administration or omission, safety factors such as drug allergies or incompatibilities. Refer to Figure 7-3 for an example of computerized documentation.

There is usually some method for indicating that a medication has been omitted. Whenever this occurs, the reason for the omission should be recorded in the nurse's notes. All narcotics and other controlled drugs must be accounted for on a special record (e.g., narcotic log), again according to the policy of the institution.

The importance of accurate recording of medications cannot be overemphasized.

DRUG DISTRIBUTION SYSTEM

The provider may order a drug by either its generic name or a brand name. This is the name that will be transcribed to the MAR. Because of the price differences that may exist between generic and brand name products, many hospital pharmacies are currently dispensing generic drugs, insofar as possible. Therefore, the nurse frequently may find a drug labeled by the generic name, rather than the name under which it was ordered. It is essential to verify that the correct drug is being given; a comparison handbook, the *Physicians' Desk Reference,* a pharmacist, or some other source should be available for this purpose. The importance of this verification cannot be overemphasized.

The unit dose system is being used more frequently as a method of dispensing drugs. With this method, premeasured drugs are packaged individually and usually are not opened until the time of administration. This method reduces the chance of error, as well as the time spent in preparing and pouring medications. In many instances, the necessity for computation is eliminated, because the drug is dispensed in the same dosage strength as the ordered dose. The nurse still must verify that the correct medication and dose are being administered. Some agencies still may be dispensing medications from labeled containers, rather than unit doses, in which case the nurse has greater responsibility for obtaining and verifying the correct dose.

PATIENT

ACCT #:	V008	**UNIT #:**
AGE/SEX:	84/F	**REG DATE:**
STATUS:	ADM IN	**DIS DATE:**

LOCATION: SNF
ROOM: 123
BED: B

ADM DX:

HEIGHT: 4 FT 9 IN 145 CM   **WEIGHT:** 121 LB 0Z 54.88 KG   **BSA** 1.50   **MAR DATE:**   **TO:**

ALLERGIES: NO KNOWN DRUG ALLERGIES

MEDICATION		04/29	04/30	05/01	05/02	05/03	05/04	05/05	05/06	05/07	05/08	05/09	05/10	05/11	05/12	05/13
AMLODIPINE BESYLATE 2.5 MG TAB (NORVASC) (None) QD@0730 RX: MC008831 CMTS: 2.5MG PO DAILY TO CONTROL HYPERTENSION	PO SCH	0730/ ℓs	/ ℐ.D	/	/	/	/	/	/	/	/	/	/	/	/	/
POTASSIUM CHLORIDE SOLN 10% 20 MEQ/15 ML (KAOCHLOR SF) (None) 0730 RX: 194819 CMTS: 20MEQ = 15ML POTASSIUM SUPPLEMENT DOSE = 7.5ML (10MEQ) DAILY IN JUICE	PO SCH	0730/ ℓs	/ ℐ.D	/	/	/	/	/	/	/	/	/	/	/	/	/
LANSOPRAZOLE 30 MG CAP (PREVACID) 30 MG (1 CAP) QD@0730 RX: 195816 CMTS: 30 MG PO DAILY TO CONTROL REFLUX ACID - DO NOT CRUSH IF NECESSARY. CAPSULES MAY BE OPENED AND PUT IN APPLESCAUCE	PO SCH	0730/ ℓs	/ ℐ.D	/	/	/	/	/	/	/	/	/	/	/	/	/
TIMOLOL MALEATE OPTH SOLN 0.5% 2.5 ML SO (TIMOPTIC-XE) (None) HS RX: 199969 CMTS: 1 GTT BOTH EYES AT BEDTIME FOR GLAUCOMA. TIMOPTIC XE	OP SCH	2200/ ℓs	/ ℐ.D	/	/	/	/	/	/	/	/	/	/	/	/	/

SIGNATURE	INIT.	SIGNATURE	INIT.	SIGNATURE	INIT.	SIGNATURE	INIT.	SIGNATURE	INIT.
Loretta Smith, R.N.	ℓs								
Jeanne Daniels, R.N.	ℐ.D								

PAGE 2

Figure 7-3 *Computerized medication order documentation (Reprinted with permission of Medical Information Technology, Inc., Westwood, MA)*

ACCOUNTABILITY

The nurse is accountable for safe practice in administering medications. This includes questioning and verifying any provider's order that is outside the normal dosage range, as recommended by the drug manufacturer's product insert or a drug reference manual. The nurse should question any medication order that might be contraindicated due to the client's current condition or that may appear to be having an adverse effect. Moreover, the nurse must be alert for drug allergies, incompatibilities, or interactions and must have knowledge of appropriate nursing implications and interventions relative to the drugs being administered.

GENERAL RULES FOR ADMINISTRATION OF MEDICATIONS

In the administration of medications, regardless of the route used, the nurse should do the following:

1. Always have a provider's order for medications administered.
2. Wash hands before pouring any medication.
3. Concentrate entirely on preparing and administering medications. Do not allow distractions to interfere with this procedure.
4. Refer to a medication administration record (MAR) for every medication administered, one that corresponds exactly with the provider's order.
5. Check for any known drug allergies the client might have.
6. If the unit dose system is employed, check the prepackaged unit label against the MAR when obtaining any prepackaged medications from the client's storage area.
7. If a stock or client supply system is employed, read the label of the medication three times and check with the MAR:
   a. when obtaining the container
   b. just before pouring the medication
   c. immediately after pouring the dose
8. Obtain medications only from legibly labeled containers.
9. Check to be sure the medication is not outdated or has an abnormal appearance.
10. Check the MAR for the time of the most recent administration of a prn medication and to be sure that the total daily maximum dosage has not been exceeded.
11. Record controlled drugs on the appropriate control sheet when the medication is removed from a locked cupboard.
12. Do not administer medications that have been poured or prepared by another person. **Exception:** If the unit dose system is employed, individual doses will have been dispensed by the pharmacist. The nurse must still verify that the correct medication and dose are administered.
13. Ascertain pertinent information about medications being administered: action, results expected, untoward effects, usual dose, and special nursing considerations.

14. Keep the medication cart or tray within sight at all times.

15. Before administering the medication, use at least two methods for identification of client, for example:
    - Ask or state the client's name.
    - Examine the wristband.
    - Compare the information on the wristband to the MAR.
    - Sensor-check the client and medication bar codes for matching.

16. If the client questions or expresses concern about a medication, withhold the medication long enough to recheck the order, the medication, and the dose.

17. If the client refuses a medication, attempt to ascertain the reason and report and record this information appropriately.

18. Before administering a medication, perform any pertinent assessment relative to the medication; check pulse, blood pressure, respiration, reflexes, pupillary size, etc.

19. Remain with the client until the medication is taken. Never leave the medication at the client's bedside without an order from the provider.

20. Maintain an aseptic (clean) technique throughout the procedure.

21. Record the medication immediately after administering it. Observe the client for desired or undesired effects and report and document any pertinent information.

22. Remember the SIX RIGHTS. Administer:
    - the right medication.
    - to the right client.
    - at the right time.
    - in the right amount.
    - by the right route.
    - with the right documentation.

ADMINISTERING ORAL MEDICATIONS

In administration of oral medications, it is important to keep in mind the following:

- Check to determine if:

    the dose should be withheld (NPO, nausea, etc.).

    a previously delayed dose that is given once daily may now be administered (test completed, etc.).

    a previously delayed dose that is given several times a day may now be administered according to daily schedule.

- When dispensing prepackaged doses, open the packets at bedside just prior to administration.
- When dispensing pills, tablets, or capsules that are not wrapped, use the cap of the container to transfer the medication into the medicine cup. If possible, the fingers should not come into contact with the drugs.
- If tablets are scored, they may be broken into halves or quarters if necessary. In many agencies, this is done in the pharmacy prior to dispensing.
- If several tablets, pills, or capsules are to be given at one time, they may be poured into the same cup, with the exception of any medications that require assessment prior to administration (e.g., checking pulse, BP, or reflex). These should be poured separately as a reminder or because they may have to be omitted.
- Use a medicine dropper to measure medications ordered in drops.
- When pouring liquid medications, place the thumbnail on the medicine glass marking the correct dose and pour at eye level with the glass on a flat surface. (Palm label to pour and wipe off lip of bottle, as necessary.)
- The measure of liquid medicine is read at the lowest point of the meniscus.
- Liquid medications may or may not need to be diluted with water or another liquid. Check specific instructions.
- Crush, dissolve, and mix medications with a small amount of food or liquid as necessary. **Exceptions:** capsules, enteric-coated tablets, or timed-release drugs.
- Assist clients to take their medications:

  Elevate head of bed.

  Assess swallowing ability.

  Have water available at bedside.

  If several tablets are to be taken, offer them one at a time.

  Give sips of water after each tablet to increase fluid intake.

  Make sure the client has swallowed all medications.

  Medications administered sublingually, chewables, or medications that should not be followed by water should be given last.
- Record the amount of liquid given on the Fluid Balance Sheet, if indicated.

The learner is referred to Performance Criteria: Administration of Oral Medications checklist (Appendix H) to use as a guide in the administration of oral medications.

PRACTICE

Simulated Medication Administration Using MAR

The labels in Figure 7-4 represent medications found in a client's medication storage area. Figure 7-5 is the MAR for this client.

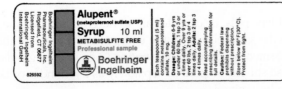

Figure 7-4a   *(Courtesy of Boehringer Ingelheim Pharmaceuticals, Inc., Ridgefield, CT)*

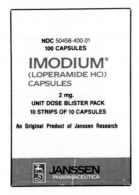

Figure 7-4b
(Courtesy of Janssen Pharmaceuticals Inc.)

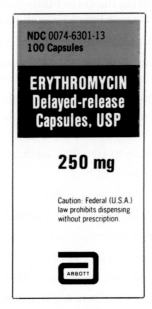

Figure 7-4c   *(Courtesy of Abbott Laboratories, North Chicago, IL)*

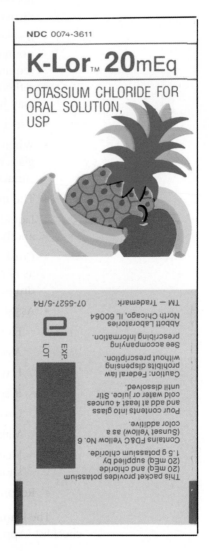

Figure 7-4d   *(Courtesy of Abbott Laboratories, North Chicago, IL)*

Simulated Medication Administration Using MAR (Continued)

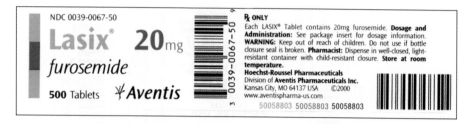

Figure 7-4e *(Courtesy of Aventis Pharmaceuticals)*

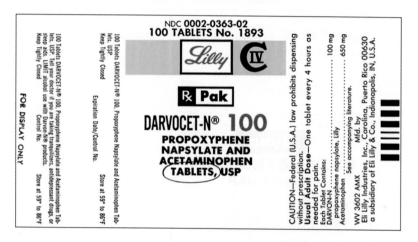

Figure 7-4f *(Courtesy of Eli Lilly & Co., Indianapolis, IN)*

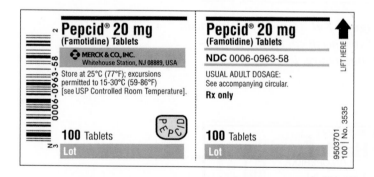

Figure 7-4g *(Used with permission from Merck & Co., Inc., West Point, PA)*

PRACTICE

Simulated Medication Administration Using MAR (Continued)

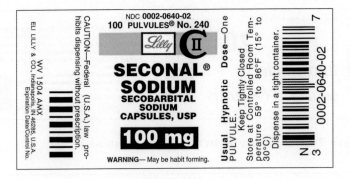

Figure 7-4b   (*Courtesy of Eli Lilly Pharmaceuticals, Indianapolis, IN*)

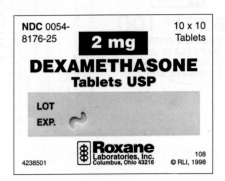

Figure 7-4i   (*Courtesy of American Pharmaceutical Partners, Inc., Schaumburg, IL*)

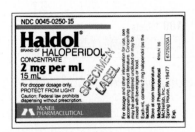

Figure 7-4j   (*Courtesy of McNeilab Inc., Spring House, PA*)

PRACTICE

Simulated Medication Administration Using MAR (Continued)

COMMUNITY HOSPITAL

NURSE'S SIGNATURE	INIT.	NURSE'S SIGNATURE	INIT.	NURSE'S SIGNATURE	INIT.

RA–Right Arm RB–Right Buttocks RL–Right Leg LA–Left Arm LB–Left Buttocks LL–Left Leg

ROUTINE MEDICATION ORDERS

Ord Date	Exp Date	Medication Frequency	Dosage Route	Shift	Date→ ↓Hour	6/22 Init.	6/23 Init.	6/24 Init.	6/25 Init.	6/26 Init.	6/27 Init.	6/28 Init.
6/22		Dexamethasone daily	2 mg PO	11–7 7–3 3–11	9							
6/22		Lasix daily	80 mg PO	11–7 7–3 3–11	7:30							
6/22		K Lor tid pc Dissolve in 4 oz water or juice	20 mEq PO	11–7 7–3 3–11	9-1 6							
6/22		Pepcid bid-ac	20 mg PO	11–7 7–3 3–11	7:30 4:30							
6/22		Alupent Syrup every other day	1.5 tsp PO	11–7 7–3 3–11	9-1 5-9							
6/22		Erythromycin D-R Cap bid	500 mg PO	11–7 7–3 3–11	9 9							
6/22		HALDOL tid	1.5 mg PO	11–7 7–3 3–11	9-1 6							
6/22	6/05	Seconal Sodium hs	100 mg PO	11–7 7–3 3–11	9							

PRN MEDICATION ORDERS

Ord. Date	Exp. Date	Medication Frequency	Dosage Route		Doses Given
6/22		Imodium following each unformed stool	† PO	Date Time INIT	
6/22		Darvocet N-100 q 4h prn for pain	† PO	Date Time INIT	

MEDICATION	AMOUNT TO BE GIVEN

Figure 7-5 Medication administration record

PRACTICE

Simulated Medication Administration Using MAR (Continued)

1. Assume you are to administer the 9:00 A.M. oral medications. In the chart in Figure 7-5, record the quantity (mL, capsules, tablets, etc.) of each medication you would administer. In some instances no computation is necessary, because it can be determined by inspection of the label or by simple mental arithmetic. When it is necessary to calculate, *use dimensional analysis.*

2. The Lasix is ordered ac breakfast. How many tablets should the client receive, and when? _____

3. The K-Lor must be dissolved in liquid prior to administration.
   • What liquids can be used? _____
   • How many mL would you record on the fluid intake record? _____

4. What is the dosage strength of the Pepcid? _____
   • How many tablets should be administered at 7:30 A.M.? _____

5. You administered 1.5 tsp of Alupent. Using dimensional analysis, calculate the following:
   • How many mL did the client receive? _____
   • How many mg did the client receive? _____
   • The usual adult dose is 20 mg 3–4 times a day. Did this client receive a safe dose? _____

6. How many mL does the Haldol bottle contain? _____
   • What is the total number of 1.5 mg doses available from this amount? ___

7. What is the dosage strength of the secobarbital capsules? _____
   • How many capsules will the client receive at bedtime? _____

8. The original medication order for Imodium was written: Give 2 capsules stat and 1 capsule following each unformed stool.
   • How many mg were administered stat? _____
   • How many mg are to be administered following each unformed stool? ___

9. If the client is complaining of pain, what medication may be administered?
   _____
   • How often may the client receive this medication? _____
   • How many tablets would be administered per dose? _____

(*Note:* See Appendix G for answer key.)

Calculation of Parenteral Medications

Upon completion of this chapter, you should be able to:

- Identify appropriate equipment used in the administration of parenteral medications, including types of syringes and the length and gauge of needles.
- Demonstrate the ability to accurately read calibrations on various types of syringes.
- Demonstrate knowledge of the appropriate method for rounding off doses when administering parenteral medications.
- Identify various forms of parenteral medications.
- Read drug labels to obtain information about specific parenteral drugs, including reconstitution.
- Apply dimensional analysis to clinical calculations involving drugs administered by subcutaneous and intramuscular routes.

PARENTERAL MEDICATIONS

Medications that are administered via injection into dermal, subcutaneous, or intramuscular tissues or directly into a vein are called parenteral medications, because they are administered by routes outside the gastrointestinal tract.

Parenteral routes include:

1. Intradermal (ID)
2. Subcutaneous (subcut)
3. Intramuscular (IM)
4. Intravenous (IV)
5. Intrathecal

6. Intracardial

7. Intra-articular

This chapter focuses on medications administered by intradermal, subcutaneous, and intramuscular routes. Intravenous medications are the subject of Chapters 10 and 11. Intrathecal, intracardial, and intra-articular injections are excluded, because these medication routes require specialized knowledge and training and are beyond the scope of this text.

In this chapter you will learn about the equipment used in administering parenteral medications, the various forms of these medications, and how to read labels and calculate dosages.

THE SYRINGE AND NEEDLE

The Syringe

Figure 8-1 illustrates the three parts of a syringe: the barrel holds the medication, is calibrated in tenths (0.1 mL) to measure the quantity to be given, and can range from 0.5 to 50 mL in size. The plunger is made of clouded or colored glass or plastic and is operated to fill or empty the barrel. The lower end of the syringe terminates in a hub to which the needle is attached. It is essential that all parts of the syringe that contact the medication be kept free of contamination. This includes the needle, the outer edge of the hub, the plunger, and the inside of the barrel.

There are various types of syringes available, most of which, at present, are single-use disposable units with attached needles. The needle usually can be detached and replaced. These syringes are made of plastic and are prepackaged in sterile packets. Reusable glass syringes are available, but their use is limited due to the increasing utilization of disposable equipment. Most syringes are equipped with some type of protective device to reduce the risk of needle-stick injuries. This is usually a plastic guard or sheath that slips over the needle after an injection is administered, Figure 8-2. Another protective type of syringe is designed to retract the contaminated needle into the barrel after use, Figure 8-3.

The syringe of choice depends on the route, action, and volume of medication to be administered.

The Tuberculin Syringe
The tuberculin syringe measures a total of 1 mL, and is calibrated in hundredths (0.01 mL) and also in minims (16 minims per mL). This syringe is used when very small quantities of medication must be measured (i.e., less than 1 mL). It usually is prepackaged with a ⅝″ long needle, Figure 8-4.

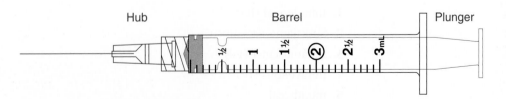

Figure 8-1   *3 mL syringe*

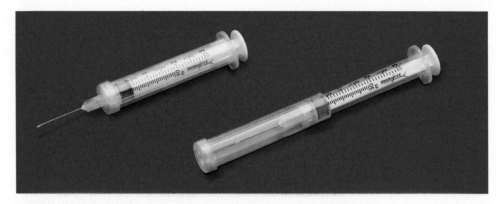

Figure 8-2 Kendall "Monojet Safety Syringe" contains a protective sheath, which can be used to protect its sterility for transport for injection and be locked into place to provide a permanent shield for disposal following injection. (Monojet is a proprietary trademark of Sherwood Services AG, a Tyco Healthcare Group affiliate.)

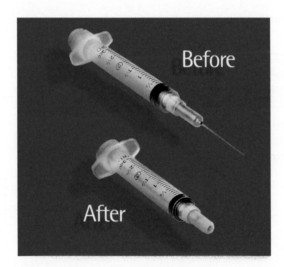

Figure 8-3 Retractable Technologies "VanishPoint" needle automatically retracts into the syringe barrel after injection. (Courtesy of Retractable Technologies)

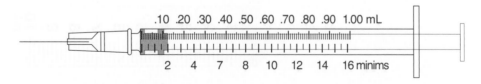

Figure 8-4 Tuberculin syringe

The Insulin Syringe The insulin syringe is calibrated in units and should be used exclusively in the administration of insulin because it will give the most accurate measurement. This syringe is available in 0.3 mL, 0.5 mL, and 1 mL sizes. When very small quantities of insulin are ordered, it is also possible to measure the dosage using a tuberculin syringe, in which case the dosage must be converted to mL or minims, Figures 8-5a and b.

The 0.5, 3, 6, 10, 12, and 35 mL Syringes The 0.5 mL and 3 mL syringes are calibrated in tenths (0.1 mL) and also in minims. Note that on the mL side, each calibration line measures 0.1 mL.

Ten or 12 mL syringes may be used when a large volume of medication is to be measured or administered. It is important to note that on these syringes each calibration line measures 0.2 mL, Figure 8-6.

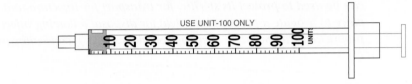

Figure 8-5a Insulin syringe

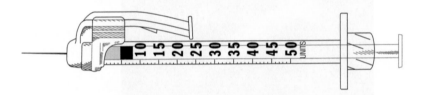

Figure 8-5b Insulin syringe with safety shield

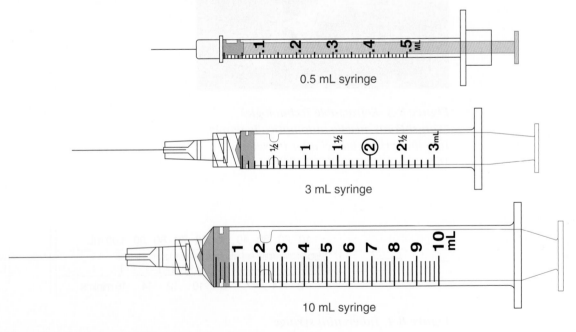

0.5 mL syringe

3 mL syringe

10 mL syringe

Figure 8-6 Syringe calibrations

The Needle

The choice of needle depends on the route and site of administration, the size and obesity of the client, and the viscosity of the medication. Needles vary in length from $\frac{1}{4}''$ to 3″. Shorter needles ($\frac{1}{4}''$–1″) are used for intradermal or subcutaneous injections and small or thin clients; longer needles (1″–2″) are used for intramuscular injections, irritating medications, and larger or obese clients.

The diameter of the needle is indicated by a gauge number. Gauge number runs from 14 to 27; the larger the number, the smaller the diameter of the needle. Fine needles are used for aqueous solutions and heavier needles for suspensions and oils. The widened portion of the needle, called the hub, attaches to the syringe. The angled point, which is called the bevel, increases the sharpness of the needle. A protective cap is provided to maintain sterility. Most needles are now disposable and are destroyed after a single use, Figure 8-7. Whenever possible, needles should be used with syringes or systems designed to protect from needle-stick injuries.

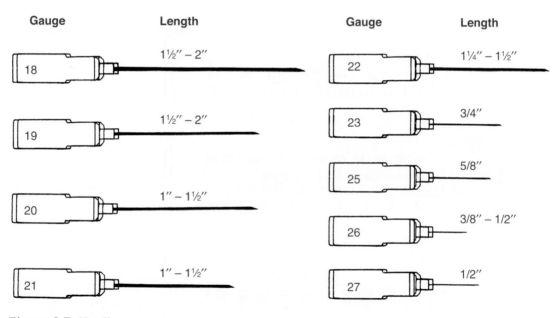

Figure 8-7 Needles

READING THE SYRINGE

On most single-use syringes the plunger has a rubber tip that has two rings in contact with the barrel, Figure 8-8. Measurement must be made at the top ring—the one closest to the tip—in order to have an accurate dose. Refer to Figure 8-9.

1. The 3 mL syringe contains 1.2 mL of solution.
2. The tuberculin syringe contains 0.74 mL of solution.
3. The insulin syringe contains 30 units of solution.

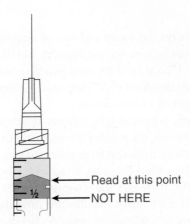

Figure 8-8 *Reading the syringe*

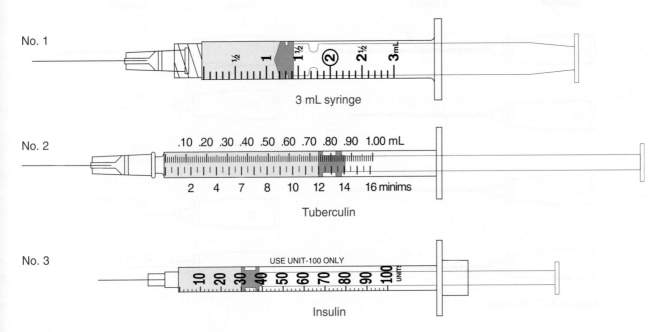

Figure 8-9 *Reading of three syringes*

Shade in the dosage on the following syringes: Refer to Figure 8-10.

1. 0.6 mL

2. 0.52 mL

3. 64 units

(**Note:** See Appendix G for answer key.)

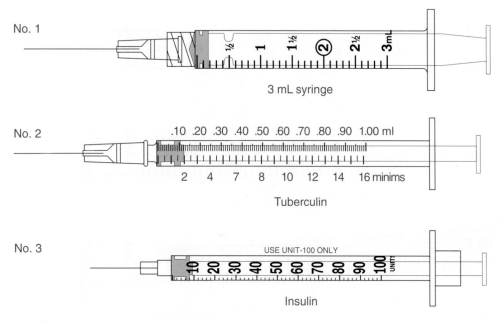

Figure 8-10 *Reading of three syringes*

ROUNDING OFF Because clinical calculations do not always result in dosages of whole numbers, it is necessary to use the correct procedure for rounding off these values.

- When the calculated dose is obtained in exact tenths of milliliters, the solution may be accurately measured in a 0.5 or 3 milliliter syringe calibrated in tenths; refer to Figure 8-11.
  1. 0.8 mL
  2. 1.3 mL
  3. 2.2 mL

- When the calculated dosage does not result in exact tenths of milliliters, the decimal result is carried to hundredths and rounded in the following manner:

  If the digit in the hundredths place is less than 5, this digit is dropped.

  If the digit in the hundredths place is 5 or greater, the tenths digit is increased by 1.

These dosages can be administered in a syringe of suitable capacity, calibrated in tenths of milliliters. For example:

1. 2.31 mL; give 2.3 mL

2. 1.87 mL; give 1.9 mL

3. 1.25 mL; give 1.3 mL

If a tuberculin syringe is used, it is possible to measure hundredths of a milliliter. Therefore, the computation should be carried to thousandths and then rounded to hundredths.

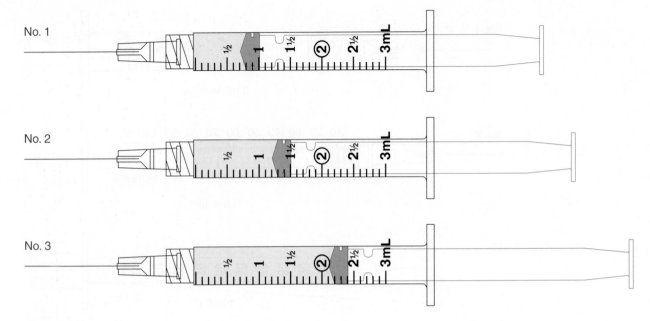

No. 1

No. 2

No. 3

Figure 8-11 *3 mL syringe*

PARENTERAL MEDICATION FORMS

Drugs for parenteral administration are available in a variety of forms. Some come in powder or frozen form and must be reconstituted to a liquid, whereas others are in solution and are dispensed in ampules, vials, or cartridges.

Single-Dose Ampules

Most ampules have a constricted stem that facilitates snapping them open. For protection, a piece of gauze or alcohol wipe may be wrapped around the stem before it is broken (Figure 8-12). Any medication in the stem should be shaken down into the ampule before opening. A metal file or an ampule opener can be used to ensure an even break if the ampule is not prescored.

A filter needle is used to remove the medication from the ampule in order to prevent inadvertent aspiration of glass particles. Another safeguard is the use of a filter straw. This is a device inserted into the opened ampule and to which a syringe is attached for withdrawing the solution. In either case, the device is removed and a sterile needle is then attached to the syringe for administration. Another use of the filter needle is for withdrawal of liquid from a vial to prevent aspiration of rubber particles.

Single- and Multiple-Dose Vials

Some drugs are dispensed in single-dose vials, whereas others are in vials containing several doses. The vial is entered through the rubber diaphragm, which should be cleansed first with an antiseptic. An amount of air comparable to the amount of drug to be withdrawn is injected. The solution can then be withdrawn easily, because

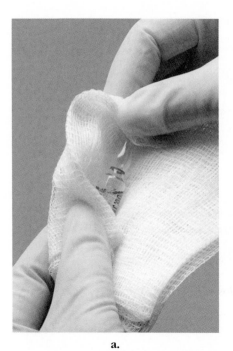
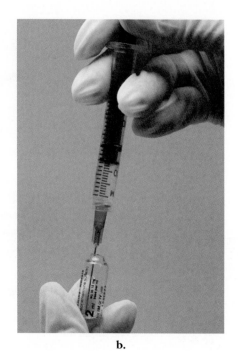

a.   b.

Figure 8-12a, b *Obtaining medication from an ampule*

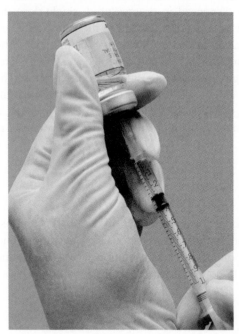

Figure 8-13 *Obtaining medication from a vial*

fluids move from an area of greater pressure to that of a lesser pressure. It is essential that there be no air bubbles present in the measured quantity in order to have an accurate dose (Figure 8-13).

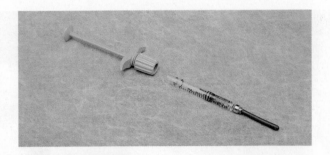

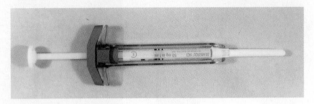

Figure 8-14 Prefilled closed injection systems

Prefilled Cartridges

Some medications are dispensed in premeasured, single-dose disposable cartridges. There may or may not be a needle attached to the cartridge. The prefilled unit is advantageous as a time-saver and reduced risk of contamination. The unit is placed into a cartridge holder or injector, which functions like a syringe. Excess air must be expelled from the cartridge prior to administering the medication. The cartridge holder is reusable; the cartridge and needles are discarded after the medication is administered.

To lessen the risk of needle-stick injuries, the newer injectors are designed to eliminate the need for handling or manipulating the used cartridge or needle, Figure 8-14.

READING LABELS

The manufacturer's product insert describes, in detail, the composition of the drug, its actions, indications and contraindications for use, precautions and adverse reactions, dosage, directions for dilution or reconstitution, if necessary, and directions for administration. Figure 8-15 contains excerpts from a manufacturer's product insert.

TICAR®
brand of
sterile ticarcillin disodium
for Intramuscular or Intravenous Administration

TR:L4IV

PRESCRIBING
INFORMATION

9608600

DESCRIPTION
Ticar is a semisynthetic injectable penicillin derived from the penicillin nucleus, 6-aminopenicillanic acid. Chemically, it is *N*-(2-Carboxy-3,3-dimethyl-7-oxo-4-thia-1-azabicyclo[3.2.0]hept-6-yl)-3-thiophenemalonamic acid disodium salt.

It is supplied as a white to pale yellow powder for reconstitution. The reconstituted solution is clear, colorless or pale yellow, having a pH of 6.0 to 8.0. Ticarcillin is very soluble in water; its solubility is greater than 600 mg/mL.

ACTIONS
Pharmacology
Ticarcillin is not absorbed orally; therefore, it must be given intravenously or intramuscularly. Following intramuscular administration, peak serum concentrations occur within 1/2 to 1 hour. Somewhat higher and more prolonged serum levels can be achieved with the concurrent administration of probenecid.

The minimum inhibitory concentrations (MICs) for many strains of *Pseudomonas* are relatively high by usual standards; serum levels of 60 mcg/mL or greater are required. However, the low degree of toxicity of ticarcillin permits the use of doses large enough to achieve inhibitory levels for these strains in serum or tissues. Other susceptible organisms usually require serum levels in the 10 to 25 mcg/mL range.

TICARCILLIN SERUM LEVELS
mcg/mL

Dosage	Route	1/4 hr.	1/2 hr.	1 hr.	2 hr.	3 hr.	4 hr.	6 hr.
Adults:								
500 mg	I.M.	–	7.7	8.6	6.0	4.0	–	2.9
1 gram	I.M.	–	31.0	18.7	15.7	9.7	–	3.4
2 grams	I.M.	–	63.6	39.7	32.3	18.9	–	3.4
3 grams	I.V.	190.0	140.0	107.0	52.2	31.3	13.8	4.2
5 grams	I.V.	327.0	280.0	175.0	106.0	63.0	28.5	9.6
3 grams +	I.V.							
1 gram probenecid	Oral	223.0	166.0	123.0	78.0	54.0	35.4	17.1

		1/2 hr.	1 hr.	1 1/2 hr.	2 hr.	4 hr.	8 hr.
Neonates:							
50 mg/kg	I.M.	64.0	70.7	63.7	60.1	33.2	11.6

As with other penicillins, ticarcillin is eliminated by glomerular filtration and tubular secretion. It is not highly bound to serum protein (approximately 45%) and is excreted unchanged in high concentrations in the urine. After the administration of a 1 to 2 gram I.M. dose, a urine concentration of 2000 to 4000 mcg/mL may be obtained in patients with normal renal function. The serum half-life of ticarcillin in normal individuals is approximately 70 minutes.

An inverse relationship exists between serum half-life and creatinine clearance, but the dosage of *Ticar* need only be adjusted in cases of severe renal impairment (see DOSAGE AND ADMINISTRATION). The administered ticarcillin may be removed from patients undergoing dialysis; the actual amount removed depends on the duration and type of dialysis.

Ticarcillin can be detected in tissues and interstitial fluid following parenteral administration. Penetration into the cerebrospinal fluid, bile and pleural fluid has been demonstrated.

Microbiology
Ticarcillin is bactericidal and demonstrates substantial *in vitro* activity against both gram-positive and gram-negative organisms. Many strains of the following organisms were found to be susceptible to ticarcillin *in vitro*:

Pseudomonas aeruginosa
  (and other species)
Escherichia coli
Proteus mirabilis
Morganella morganii (formerly *Proteus morganii*)
Providencia rettgeri (formerly *Proteus rettgeri*)
Proteus vulgaris
Enterobacter species
Haemophilus influenzae
Neisseria species

Salmonella species
Staphylococcus aureus
  (non-penicillinase
  producing)
Staphylococcus epidermidis
Beta-hemolytic streptococci
  (Group A)
Streptococcus faecalis
  (*Enterococcus*)
Streptococcus pneumoniae

Anaerobic bacteria,
  including:
Bacteroides species
  including *B. fragilis*
Fusobacterium species
Veillonella species
Clostridium species
Eubacterium species
Peptococcus species
Peptostreptococcus species

In vitro synergism between ticarcillin and gentamicin sulfate, tobramycin sulfate or amikacin sulfate against certain strains of *Pseudomonas aeruginosa* has been demonstrated.

Some strains of such microorganisms as *Mima-Herellea* (*Acinetobacter*), *Citrobacter* and *Serratia* have shown susceptibility. Ticarcillin is not stable in the presence of penicillinase.

Figure 8-15 *Manufacturer's product insert (Courtesy of SmithKline Beecham Pharmaceuticals, Pittsburgh, PA) (continues)*

Some strains of *Pseudomonas* have developed resistance fairly rapidly.

DISK SUSCEPTIBILITY TESTS

Susceptibility Tests: Ticarcillin disks or powders should be used for testing susceptibility to ticarcillin. However, organisms reportedly susceptible to carbenicillin are susceptible to ticarcillin.

Diffusion Techniques: For the disk diffusion method of susceptibility testing a 75 mcg *Ticar* disk should be used. The method for this test is the one outlined in NCCLS publication M2-A3* with the following interpretative criteria:

Culture	Susceptible	Intermediate	Resistant
P. aeruginosa and Enterobacteriaceae	≥15 mm	12 to 14 mm	≤11 mm

The MIC correlates are: Resistant >128 mcg/mL
Susceptible ≤64 mcg/mL

Dilution Techniques: Dilution techniques for determining the MIC (minimum inhibitory concentration) are published by NCCLS for the broth and agar dilution procedures. The MIC data should be interpreted in light of the concentrations present in serum, tissue and body fluids. Organisms with MIC ≤64 are considered susceptible when they are in tissue but organisms with MIC ≤128 would be susceptible in urine where the *Ticar* concentrations are much greater. At present, only dilution methods can be recommended for testing antibiotic susceptibility of obligate anaerobes.

Susceptibility testing methods require the use of control organisms. The 75 mcg ticarcillin disk should give zone diameters between 22 and 28 mm for *P. aeruginosa* ATCC 27853 and 24 and 30 mm for *E. coli* ATCC 25922. Reference strains are available for dilution testing of ticarcillin. 95% of the MICs should fall within the following MIC ranges and the majority of MICs should be at values close to the center of the pertinent range (reference NCCLS publication M7-A†).

S. aureus ATCC 29213, 2.0 to 8.0 mcg/mL; *S. faecalis* ATCC 29212, 16 to 64 mcg/mL; *E. coli* ATCC 25922, 2.0 to 8.0 mcg/mL; *P. aeruginosa* ATCC 27853, 8.0 to 32 mcg/mL.

*Performance Standards for Antimicrobial Disc Susceptibility Tests, National Committee for Clinical Laboratory Standards, Vol. 4, No. 16, pp. 369-402, 1984.

†Methods for Dilution Antimicrobial Susceptibility Tests for Bacteria That Grow Aerobically, Vol. 5, No. 22, pp. 579-618, 1985.

INDICATIONS

Ticar is indicated for the treatment of the following infections:

Bacterial septicemia‡

Skin and soft-tissue infections‡

Acute and chronic respiratory tract infections‡§

‡Caused by susceptible strains of *Pseudomonas aeruginosa, Proteus* species (both indole-positive and indole-negative) and *Escherichia coli.*

§Though clinical improvement has been shown, bacteriological cures cannot be expected in patients with chronic respiratory disease or cystic fibrosis.

Genitourinary tract infections (complicated and uncomplicated) due to susceptible strains of *Pseudomonas aeruginosa, Proteus* species (both indole-positive and indole-negative), *Escherichia coli, Enterobacter* and *Streptococcus faecalis* (enterococcus).

Ticarcillin is also indicated in the treatment of the following infections due to susceptible anaerobic bacteria:

1. Bacterial septicemia.
2. Lower respiratory tract infections such as empyema, anaerobic pneumonitis and lung abscess.
3. Intra-abdominal infections such as peritonitis and intra-abdominal abscess (typically resulting from anaerobic organisms resident in the normal gastrointestinal tract).
4. Infections of the female pelvis and genital tract, such as endometritis, pelvic inflammatory disease, pelvic abscess and salpingitis.
5. Skin and soft-tissue infections.

Although ticarcillin is primarily indicated in gram-negative infections, its *in vitro* activity against gram-positive organisms should be considered in treating infections caused by both gram-negative and gram-positive organisms (see Microbiology).

Based on the *in vitro* synergism between ticarcillin and gentamicin sulfate, tobramycin sulfate or amikacin sulfate against certain strains of *Pseudomonas aeruginosa,* combined therapy has been successful, using full therapeutic dosages. (For additional prescribing information, see the gentamicin sulfate, tobramycin sulfate and amikacin sulfate package inserts.)

NOTE: Culturing and susceptibility testing should be performed initially and during treatment to monitor the effectiveness of therapy and the susceptibility of the bacteria.

CONTRAINDICATIONS

A history of allergic reaction to any of the penicillins is a contraindication.

WARNINGS

Serious and occasionally fatal hypersensitivity (anaphylactoid) reactions have been reported in patients receiving penicillin. These reactions are more likely to occur in persons with a history of sensitivity to multiple allergens.

There are reports of patients with a history of penicillin hypersensitivity reactions who experience severe hypersensitivity reactions when treated with a cephalosporin. Before therapy with a penicillin, careful inquiry should be made about previous hypersensitivity reactions to penicillins, cephalosporins and other allergens. If a reaction occurs, the drug should be discontinued unless, in the opinion of the physician, the condition being treated is life-threatening and amenable only to ticarcillin therapy. **Serious anaphylactoid reactions require immediate emergency treatment with epinephrine. Oxygen, intravenous steroids and airway management, including intubation, should also be administered as indicated.**

Some patients receiving high doses of ticarcillin may develop hemorrhagic manifestations associated with abnormalities of coagulation tests, such as bleeding time and platelet aggregation. On withdrawal of the drug, the bleeding should cease and coagulation abnormalities revert to normal. Other causes of abnormal bleeding should also be considered. Patients with renal impairment, in whom excretion of ticarcillin is delayed, should be observed for bleeding manifestations. Such patients should be dosed strictly according to recommendations (see DOSAGE AND ADMINISTRATION). If bleeding manifestations appear, ticarcillin treatment should be discontinued and appropriate therapy instituted.

Pseudomembranous colitis has been reported with nearly all antibacterial agents, including *Ticar*, and has ranged in severity from mild to life-threatening. Therefore, it is important to consider this diagnosis in patients who present with diarrhea subsequent to the administration of antibacterial agents.

Treatment with antibacterial agents alters the normal flora of the colon and may permit overgrowth of clostridia. Studies indicate that a toxin produced by *Clostridium difficile* is 1 primary cause of "antibiotic-associated colitis."

Mild cases of pseudomembranous colitis usually respond to drug discontinuation alone. In moderate to severe cases, consideration should be given to management with fluids and electrolytes, protein supplementation and treatment with an antibacterial drug effective against *C. difficile.*

PRECAUTIONS

Although *Ticar* exhibits the characteristic low toxicity of the penicillins, as with any other potent agent, it is advisable to check periodically for organ system dysfunction (including renal, hepatic and hematopoietic) during prolonged treatment. If overgrowth of resistant organisms occurs, the appropriate therapy should be initiated.

Since the theoretical sodium content is 5.2 mEq (120 mg) per gram of ticarcillin, and the actual vial content can be as high as 6.5 mEq/gram, electrolyte and cardiac status should be monitored carefully.

(continued on other side)

Figure 8-15 *(Continued)*

PRACTICE

Reading Labels

1. Figure 8-16—Circle the generic name and answer the following questions.
   a. What is the total amount of drug in the container? _____
   b. How many mL of diluting solution should be added to the vial for injection? _____
   c. What is the dosage strength of the prepared solution? _____

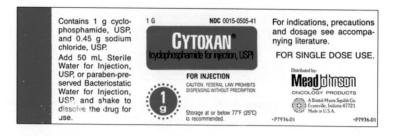

Figure 8-16 (*Courtesy of Bristol Myers Squibb, Evansville, IN*)

2. Figure 8-17—Circle the number of dosette ampuls in the package and answer the following questions.
   a. By what route(s) can this medication be given? _____
   b. How is the solution protected from light? _____
   c. List the drug companies involved in the manufacture of this medication. _____

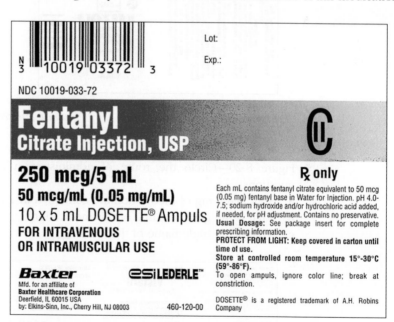

Figure 8-17 (*Courtesy of Baxter Healthcare Corporation, New Providence, NJ*)

Reading Labels (Continued)

3. Figure 8-18—Circle the total amount of drug in the vial and answer the following questions.
   a. What is the dosage strength of the solution? _____
   b. What is the generic name? _____
   c. Who is the manufacturer? _____

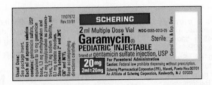

Figure 8-18 *(Courtesy of Schering Pharmaceutical Corporation, Kenilworth, NJ)*

4. Figure 8-19—Circle the generic name and answer the following questions.
   a. How many mL of diluting solution should be added to the vial? _____
   b. What is the dosage strength of the prepared solution? _____
   c. After reconstitution, where should the solution be stored? _____

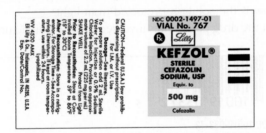

Figure 8-19 *(Courtesy of Eli Lilly Pharmaceuticals, Indianapolis, IN)*

5. Figure 8-20—Circle the route of administration and answer the following questions.
   a. How many mg of medication are contained in 2 mL? _____
   b. What is the generic name of this medication? _____
   c. What is the trade name of this drug? _____

Figure 8-20 *(Reproduced with permission of Pfizer, Inc.)*

Reading Labels (Continued)

6. Figure 8-21—Circle the dosage strength of this medication and answer the following questions.
   a. How much solution is contained in each dosette ampul? _____
   b. By what routes can this medication be given? _____
   c. Where do you find information about the usual dosage of this medication? _____

NDC 10019-039-68

Naloxone
HCl Injection, USP

400 mcg/mL (0.4 mg/mL)   ℞ only
10 x 1 mL DOSETTE® Ampuls
FOR INTRAMUSCULAR, SUBCUTANEOUS OR INTRAVENOUS USE
Each mL contains naloxone hydrochloride 400 mcg, sodium chloride
8.6 mg, methylparaben 1.8 mg and propylparaben 0.2 mg in Water
for Injection. pH 3.0-4.5; hydrochloric acid and/or sodium hydroxide
used, if needed, for pH adjustment.
Usual Dosage: See package insert for complete prescribing
information.
PROTECT FROM LIGHT: Keep covered in carton until time of use.
Store at controlled room temperature 15°-30°C (59°-86°F).
Avoid freezing.
To open ampuls, ignore color line; break at constriction.
Baxter   e**Si**LEDERLE™
Mfd. for an affiliate of Baxter Healthcare Corporation
Deerfield, IL 60015 USA
by: Elkins-Sinn, Cherry Hill, NJ 08003
DOSETTE® is a registered trademark of A.H. Robins Company.   400-797-01

Figure 8-21 *(Courtesy of Baxter Healthcare Corporation, New Providence, NJ)*

7. Figure 8-22—Circle the generic name and answer the following questions.(Note: this is an oral medication.)
   a. Is this a single- or multiple-dose container? _____
   b. At what temperature should this medication be stored? _____
   c. What is the dosage strength of this medication? _____

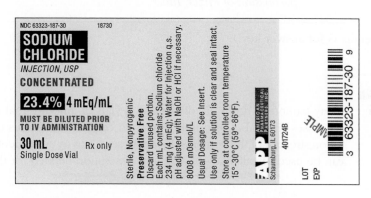

Figure 8-22 *(Courtesy of American Pharmaceutical Partners)*

PRACTICE

Reading Labels (Continued)

8. Figure 8-23—Circle the total amount contained in the vial and answer the following questions.
   a. What is the dosage strength of this medication? _____
   b. What is the generic name? _____
   c. Who manufactures this product? _____

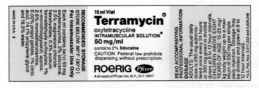

Figure 8-23 *(Reproduced with permission of Pfizer, Inc.)*

9. Figure 8-24—Circle the generic name and answer the following questions.
   a. By what route *only* can the medication be given? _____
   b. Can the reconstituted solution be stored at room temperature? _____
   c. What is the total amount (volume) of solution in the vial? _____

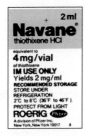

Figure 8-24 *(Reproduced with permission of Pfizer, Inc.)*

(**Note:** See Appendix G for answer key.)

CALCULATING DOSAGES OBTAINED FROM PREMIXED SOLUTIONS

Many parenteral drugs are dispensed in vials or ampules that contain single or multiple doses. The label or printing on each container indicates the amount and the solution strength of the contents. Using these values as equivalents, dimensional analysis can be used to calculate the quantity of solution needed for the required dosage.

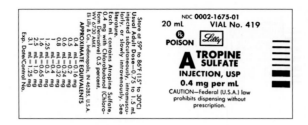

Figure 8-25 *(Courtesy of Eli Lilly Pharmaceuticals, Indianapolis, IN)*

EXAMPLE   A prescription order states: Atropine Sulfate gr $^1/_{150}$ IM. The vial of atropine (Figure 8-25) is labeled: Atropine Sulfate 0.4 mg per mL. How much solution will be administered?

Equivalents:gr 1 = 60 mg, 1 mL = 0.4 mg

Conversion Equation: $gr \ 1/150 \times \dfrac{60 \ mg}{gr \ 1} \times \dfrac{1 \ mL}{0.4 \ mg} = 1 \ mL$

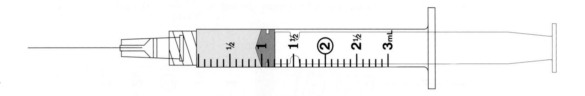

OR

$gr \ 0.007 \times \dfrac{60 \ mg}{gr \ 1} \times \dfrac{1 \ mL}{0.4 \ mg} = 1.05 = 1.1 \ mL$

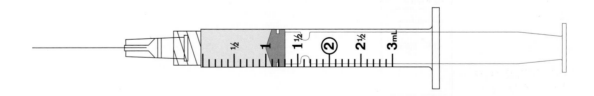

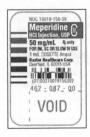

Figure 8-26 *(Courtesy of Baxter Healthcare Corporation, New Providence, NJ)*

EXAMPLE The provider orders Demerol 20 mg IM. The medication is dispensed under the label Meperidine 50 mg per mL (Figure 8-26). Find the quantity of solution to be administered.

1. First: Consult a drug reference source to determine that Demerol is a brand name for the generic drug meperidine.
2. Equivalents: 1 mL = 50 mg

Conversion Equation: $20 \text{ mg} \times \dfrac{1 \text{ mL}}{50 \text{ mg}} = 0.4 \text{ mL}$

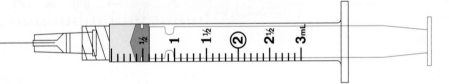

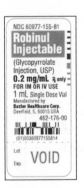

Figure 8-27 *(Courtesy of Baxter Healthcare Corporation, New Providence, NJ)*

EXAMPLE Robinul 0.15 mg IM is ordered for the client. On hand is a vial labeled: Robinul, (glycopyrrolate) 0.2 mg per mL (Figure 8-27). How many mL should be administered?

Equivalents: 0.2 mg = 1 mL

Conversion Equation: $0.15 \text{ mg} \times \dfrac{1 \text{ mL}}{0.2 \text{ mg}} = 0.8 \text{ mL}$

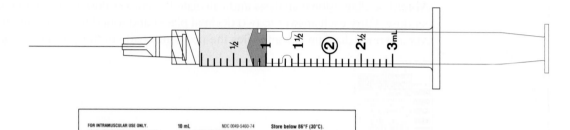

FOR INTRAMUSCULAR USE ONLY.

USUAL ADULT DOSE: Intramuscularly: 25 -
100 mg stat; repeat every 4 to 6 hours,
as needed.

See accompanying prescribing information.

Each mL contains **50 mg** of hydroxyzine
hydrochloride, 0.9% benzyl alcohol and
sodium hydroxide to adjust to optimum pH.

To avoid discoloration, protect from prolonged exposure to light.

Rx only

10 mL   NDC 0049-5460-74

Vistaril®
(hydroxyzine hydrochloride)

Intramuscular Solution

50 mg/mL

Pfizer Roerig
Division of Pfizer Inc, NY, NY 10017

Store below 86°F (30°C).

PROTECT FROM FREEZING.

PATIENT: _____

ROOM NO.: _____

05-1111-32-4
MADE IN USA   9249

Figure 8-28   *(Reproduced with permission of Pfizer, Inc.)*

EXAMPLE   A client is to receive Vistaril 35 mg IM. The medication comes in a vial labeled: Vistaril (hydroxyzine hydrochloride) 50 mg per mL (Figure 8-28). Equivalents: 50 mg = 1 mL

Conversion Equation: $35 \text{ mg} \times \dfrac{1 \text{ mL}}{50 \text{ mg}} = 0.7 \text{ mL}$

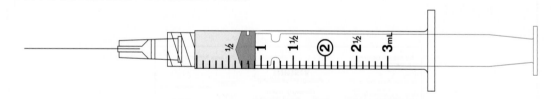

Calculating Dosages from Premixed Solutions

(*Note:* Use dimensional analysis and calculate the correct dosage to be administered per dose. Carry each answer to two decimal places and round to nearest tenth. Wherever a syringe diagram accompanies the problem, shade in the correct dosage.)

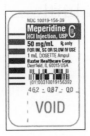

Figure 8-29 *(Courtesy of Baxter Healthcare Corporation, New Providence, NJ)*

1. ***Order:*** Meperidine 30 mg IM

    Label: Figure 8-29

    How many milliliters should be administered?

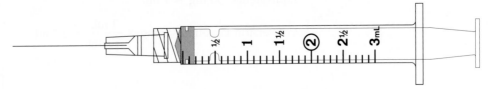

Figure 8-30 *(Reproduced with permission of Pfizer, Inc.)*

2. ***Order:*** Vistaril 75 mg IM

    Label: Figure 8-30. What is the generic name? _____

    How many milliliters should be administered?

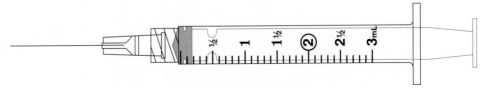

PRACTICE

Calculating Dosages from Premixed Solutions (Continued)

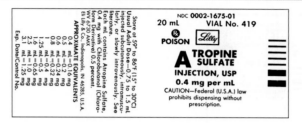

Figure 8-31   *(Courtesy of Eli Lilly Pharmaceuticals, Indianapolis, IN)*

3. Order: Atropine Sulfate gr $^1/_{100}$ IM

   Label: Figure 8-31

   How many milliliters should be administered?

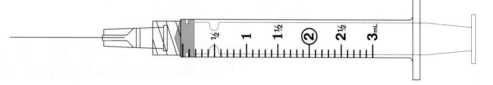

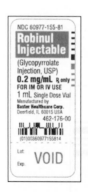

Figure 8-32   *(Courtesy of Baxter Healthcare Corporation, New Providence, NJ)*

4. Order: Robinul 0.1 mg IM

   Label: Figure 8-32. What is the generic name? _____

   How many milliliters should be administered?

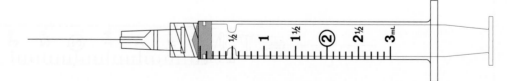

PRACTICE

Calculating Dosages from Premixed Solutions (Continued)

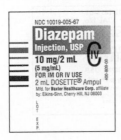

Figure 8-33 *(Courtesy of Baxter Healthcare Corporation, New Providence, NJ)*

5. Order: Diazepam Injection 7.5 mg IM

Label: Figure 8-33.

How many milliliters should be administered?

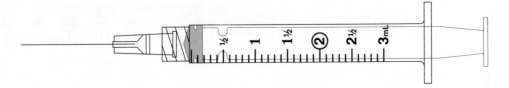

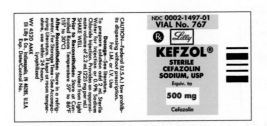

Figure 8-34 *(Courtesy of Eli Lilly Pharmaceuticals, Indianapolis, IN)*

6. Order: Kefzol 135 mg IM

Label: Figure 8-34. What is the generic name? _____

How many milliliters should be administered?

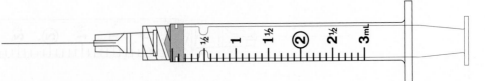

PRACTICE

Calculating Dosages from Premixed Solutions (Continued)

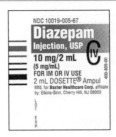

Figure 8-35 *(Courtesy of Baxter Healthcare Corporation, New Providence, NJ)*

7. **Order:** Diazepam 2 mg IM

   Label: Figure 8-35. By what other route can this medication be administered? _____

   How many milliliters should be administered?

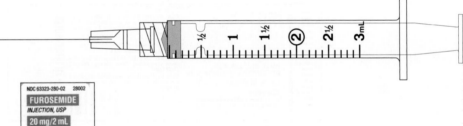

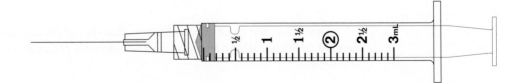

Figure 8-36 *(Courtesy of American Pharmaceutical Partners, Inc., Schaumberg, IL)*

8. **Order:** Furosemide 5 mg IM

   Label: Figure 8-36. Who is the manufacturer? _____

   How many milliliters should be administered?

PRACTICE

Calculating Dosages from Premixed Solutions (Continued)

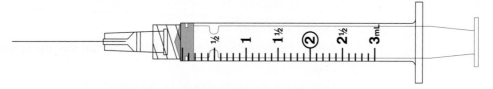

Figure 8-37 *(Reproduced with permission of Pfizer, Inc.)*

9. ***Order:*** Vistaril 25 mg IM

   Label: Figure 8-37. What is the generic name? _____

   How many milliliters should be administered?

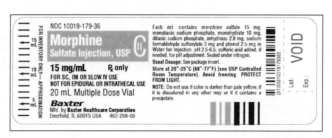

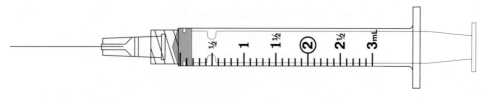

Figure 8-38 *(Courtesy of Baxter Healthcare Corporation, New Providence, NJ)*

10. ***Order:*** Morphine Sulfate gr 1/8 subcut

    Label: Figure 8-38

    How many milliliters should be administered?

Determine the number of milliliters that should be administered in the following problems. (Carry all answers to two decimal places and round to the nearest tenth.)

PRACTICE

Calculating Dosages from Premixed Solutions (Continued)

11. *Order:* Phenobarbital Sodium 100 mg IM

    Label: Phenobarbital Sodium 125 mg per 2 mL

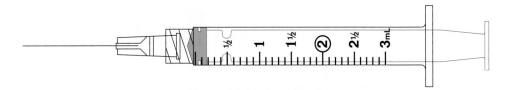

12. *Order:* Compazine 8 mg IM

    Label: Compazine (prochlorperazine) 10 mg per 2 mL

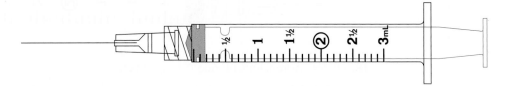

13. *Order:* Valium 4 mg IM

    Label: Valium (diazepam) 5 mg per mL

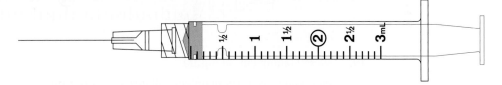

14. *Order:* Vitamin K 20 mg IM

    Label: Vitamin K 25 mg per 2.5 mL

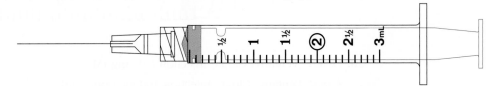

15. *Order:* Lanoxin 0.25 mg IM

    Label: Lanoxin (digoxin) 500 mcg per 2 mL

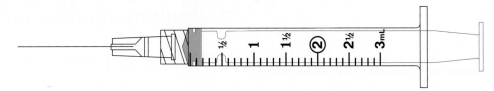

| Calculating Dosages from Premixed Solutions (Continued) |

16. *Order:* Solu-Medrol 225 mg IM

Label: Solu-Medrol (methylprednisolone sodium succinate) 500 mg per 4 mL

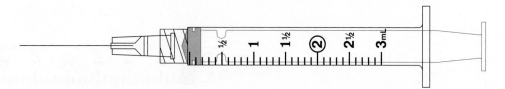

17. *Order:* Phenergan 40 mg IM

Label: Phenergan (promethazine) 50 mg per mL

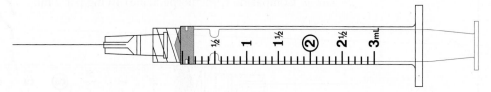

18. *Order:* Adrenalin Chloride 0.4 mg subcut

Label: Adrenalin Chloride (epinephrine hydrochloride) 1 mg per 2 mL

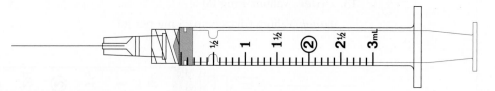

19. *Order:* Garamycin 60 mg IM

Label: Garamycin (gentamicin sulfate) 40 mg per mL

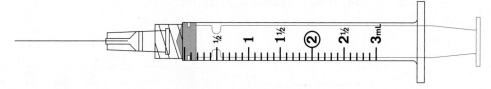

20. *Order:* Fentanyl Citrate Injection 0.05 mg IM

Label: Fentanyl Citrate Injection 100 mcg per 2 mL

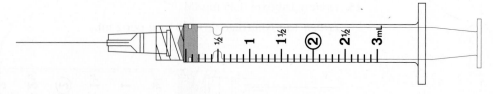

(***Note:*** See Appendix G for answer key.)

CALCULATIONS BASED ON BODY WEIGHT

The method of calculating oral dosages based on body weight is described in Chapter 6. The method for calculating parenteral dosages is identical.

EXAMPLE **Order:** Isoniazid Injection 5 mg/kg/day IM to an adult weighing 58 kg

Label: Isoniazid Injection 100 mg per mL

How many mL should be administered per dose?

$$58 \text{ kg} \times \frac{5 \text{ mg}}{1 \text{ kg}} \times \frac{1 \text{ mL}}{100 \text{ mg}} = 2.9 \text{ mL}$$

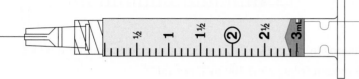

EXAMPLE **Order:** Amikin 15 mg/kg/day IM in three divided doses to an adult weighing 155 lb

Label: Amikin (amikacin) 500 mg per 2 mL

How many mL should be administered per dose?

$$155 \text{ lb} \times \frac{1 \text{ kg}}{2.2 \text{ lb}} \times \frac{15 \text{ mg}}{1 \text{ kg}} \times \frac{2 \text{ mL}}{500 \text{ mg}} = \frac{4.2 \text{ mL}}{3 \text{ doses}} = 1.4 \text{ mL per dose}$$

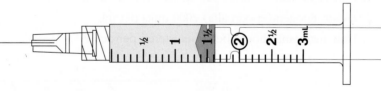

PRACTICE

IM Calculations Based on Body Weight

1. Order: Gentamicin Sulfate 3 mg/kg/24 hr IM in three divided doses to an adult weighing 77 kg

Label: Gentamicin Sulfate 40 mg per mL

How many mL should be administered per dose?

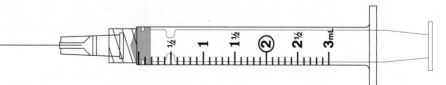

PRACTICE

IM Calculations Based on Body Weight (Continued)

2. *Order:* Streptomycin Sulfate 15 mg/kg/dose IM to an adult weighing 120 lb

Label: Streptomycin Sulfate 1 g per 2.5 mL

How many mL should be administered per dose?

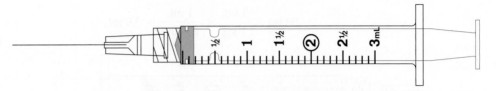

3. *Order:* Neupogen 5 mcg/kg/24 hr subcut to an adult weighing 60 kg

Label: Neupogen (filgrastim) 300 mcg per mL

How many mL should be administered per dose?

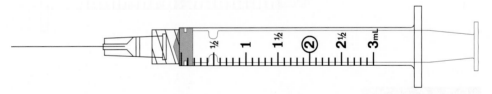

4. *Order:* Epogen 75 units per kg subcut to an adult weighing 140 lb

Label: Epogen (epotin alfa) 2000 units per mL

How many mL should be administered per dose?

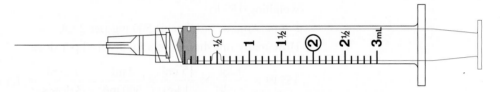

5. *Order:* Nebcin 3 mg/kg/day IM in three divided doses to an adult weighing 80 kg

Label: Nebcin (tobramycin sulfate) 80 mg per 2 mL

How many mL should be administered per dose?

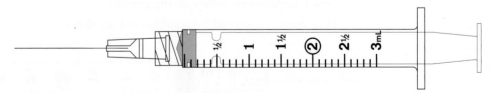

PRACTICE

IM Calculations Based on Body Weight (Continued)

6. *Order:* Pronestyl 50 mg per kg IM in four divided doses to an adult weighing 152 lb

   Label: Pronestyl (procainamide hydrochloride) 500 mg per mL

   How many mL should be administered per dose?

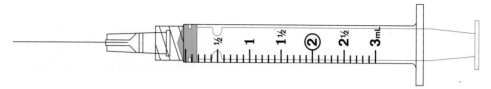

7. *Order:* Amikacin Sulfate 15 mg/kg/day IM in two divided doses to an adult weighing 81.8 kg

   Label: Amikacin sulfate 500 mg per 2 mL

   How many mL should be administered per dose?

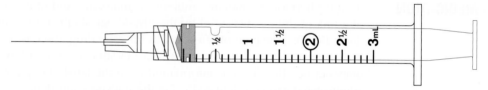

8. *Order:* Kantrex Injection 15 mg/kg/day IM in four divided doses to an adult weighing 159 lb

   Label: Kantrex (kanamycin sulfate) Injection 1 g per 3 mL

   How many mL should be administered per dose?

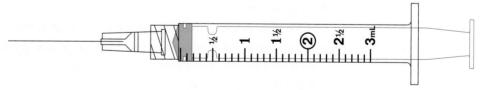

9. *Order:* Humatrope 0.18 mg per kg IM to a child weighing 11 kg

   Label: Humatrope (somatropin) 5 mg per 1.5 mL

   How many mL should be administered per dose?

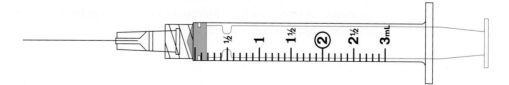

PRACTICE

IM Calculations Based on Body Weight (Continued)

10. *Order:* Oxytetracycline 15 mg per kg IM in four divided doses to a child whose weight is 60 lb

Label: Terramycin (oxytetracycline) 100 mg per 2 mL

How many mL should be administered per dose?

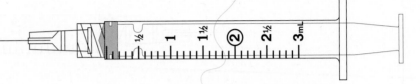

(*Note:* See Appendix G for answer key.)

UNITS OF MEDICATION

Some drugs are measured in quantities called **units.** Unit quantities are frequently used for hormones, vitamins, antibiotics, antitoxins, and other biologicals. The value of a unit of drug is measured by the physiological effect a certain quantity will produce. Because the type of effect varies for each drug, there is no common definition for a unit. Vials of these drugs may vary in strength from a few units to millions of units per mL. Because this information is on the label, the quantity of solution to be administered can be calculated using these given equivalents.

Because many of the drugs dispensed in units are extremely potent, dosages are often very small, requiring use of special syringes that can measure small doses. For example, the tuberculin syringe can measure quantities as small as 0.01 mL. Clinical calculations involving medications that will be measured in a tuberculin syringe should be carried to three decimal places and rounded to the nearest hundredth in the following manner:

- If the digit in the thousandths place is less than 5, this digit is dropped.
- If the digit in the thousandths place is 5 or greater, the hundredths digit is increased by one. For example:

  0.256 mL; give 0.26 mL

  0.382 mL; give 0.38 mL

  0.615 mL; give 0.62 mL

The learner is reminded that insulin, which also is dispensed in units, should be measured only in an insulin syringe. Other medications that are ordered in larger quantities of units can be administered using a regular 2–3 mL syringe. Dimensional analysis is used to convert units to milliliters.

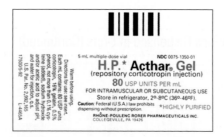

Figure 8-39 (*Courtesy of Rhône-Poulenc Rorer Pharmaceuticals, Inc.*)

EXAMPLE   *Order:* H.P. Acthar Gel 50 units IM

Label: Figure 8-39

Dosage Strength: 80 units per/mL

Conversion Equation: $50 \text{ units} \times \dfrac{1 \text{ mL}}{80 \text{ units}} = 0.63 \text{ mL}$

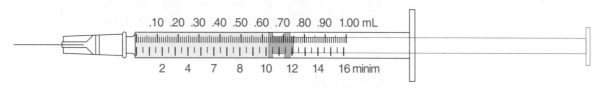

PRACTICE

Medications Dispensed in Units

Determine the number of milliliters that should be administered in the following problems.

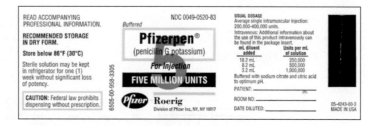

Figure 8-40 (*Reproduced with permission of Pfizer, Inc.*)

1. *Order:* Pfizerpen 400,000 units IM

Label: Figure 8-40. Reconstitute with 8.2 mL diluent.

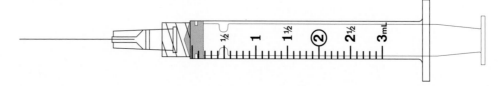

PRACTICE

Medications Dispensed in Units (Continued)

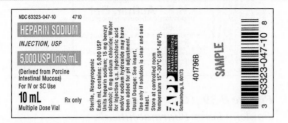

Figure 8-41 *(Courtesy of American Pharmaceutical Partners)*

2. *Order:* Heparin Sodium Injection 3500 units subcut

**   *Label:*** Figure 8-41

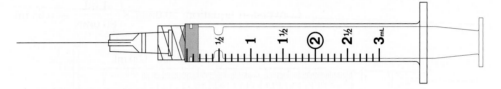

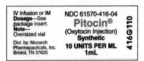

Figure 8-42
(Courtesy of King Pharmaceuticals, Inc., Bristol, TN 37620)

3. *Order:* Pitocin 7 units IM

**   *Label:*** Figure 8-42

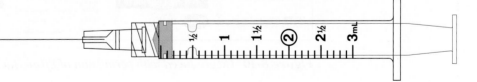

Medications Dispensed in Units (Continued)

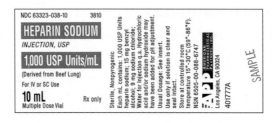

NDC 63323-038-10   3810
HEPARIN SODIUM
INJECTION, USP
1,000 USP Units/mL
(Derived from Beef Lung)
For IV or SC Use
10 mL   Rx only
Multiple Dose Vial

Sterile, Nonpyrogenic
Each mL contains: 1,000 USP Units
heparin sodium; 15 mg benzyl
alcohol; 9 mg sodium chloride;
Water for Injection q.s. Hydrochloric
acid and/or sodium hydroxide may
have been added for pH adjustment.
Usual Dosage: See insert.
Use only if solution is clear and
seal intact.
Store at controlled room
temperature 15°-30°C (59°-86°F).
NSN 6505-00-088-6747

Los Angeles, CA 90024
4017777A

SAMPLE

Figure 8-43 *(Courtesy of American
Pharmaceutical Partners)*

4. ***Order:*** Heparin 800 units subcut
   Label: Figure 8-43

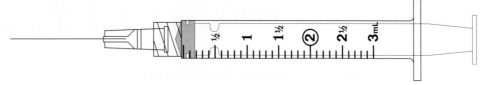

5. ***Order:*** Tetanus Immune Globulin 200 units IM
   Label: Tetanus Immune Globulin 250 units per mL

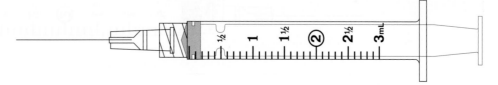

6. ***Order:*** Wycillin 450,000 units IM
   Label: Wycillin (penicillin G procaine) 600,000 units per mL

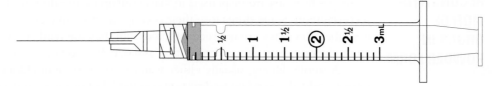

7. ***Order:*** Varicella-Zoster Immune Globulin 100 units IM
   Label: Varicella-Zoster Immune Globulin 125 units per 2.5 mL

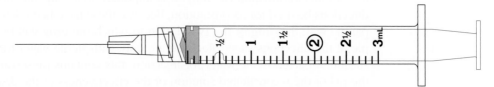

PRACTICE

Medications Dispensed in Units (Continued)

8. *Order:* A.C.T.H. "80" Injectable 90 units IM

    Label: A.C.T.H. "80" (corticotropin) Injectable 400 units per 5 mL

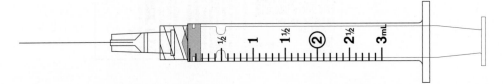

9. *Order:* BCG Vaccine 800,000 units ID

    Label: BCG Vaccine 8,000,000 units per mL

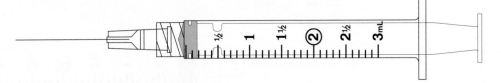

10. *Order:* Vitamin A 15,000 units IM

    Label: Vitamin A 50,000 units per mL

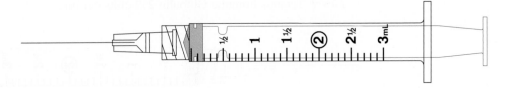

(*Note:* See Appendix G for answer key.)

RECONSTITUTION OF DRUGS IN POWDER FORM

Some medications are dispensed in vials containing the drug in dry powder form for reconstitution. Some drugs lose their potency a short time after being placed in solution; therefore, they are not reconstituted until they are ready to be used. Other drugs retain their potency after reconstitution and may be used over a period of several days.

A sterile diluent, usually either water or 0.9% sodium chloride (normal saline), must be added according to directions on the label or the manufacturer's package insert. This diluent must be labeled *"Injection"* or *"For Injection,"* Figure 8-44. Because other diluents may be specified on the label or accompanying circular (insert), be sure to read this information carefully. It is important that only diluents designated in the directions be used for reconstitution, because these have been determined to be compatible with the drug or the IV solution to which the drug will be added. For example, if the directions state, "Reconstitute only with sterile water for injection," do *not* substitute bacteriostatic water for injection; this contains preservatives that may alter the pH of the reconstituted solution or the effectiveness of the drug.

STERILE WATER FOR INJECTION, USP For Drug Diluent Use Only	0.9% SODIUM CHLORIDE INJECTION, USP For Drug Diluent Use Only

Figure 8-44 *Examples of labels for sterile diluents used for reconstitution.*

After the diluent is added, the vial must be shaken to dissolve the powdered drug, which can then be drawn up into a syringe and administered. In some instances, the dissolved drug will expand the total resulting volume of solution. This must be taken into account when identifying equivalents; for example, the addition of 2 mL of diluent to a measured amount of dry drug may result in a total volume exceeding 2 mL. Therefore, it is necessary to refer to either the label or the package insert to ascertain the correct volume containing the desired dosage strength or concentration of the reconstituted solution and to use the correct volume in your calculation.

The drug label or accompanying instructions state the amount of diluent that should be added to the container to result in a specific concentration of drug. In preparing a solution for intramuscular injection for adults or children, select the dilution that would provide the ordered dose in an amount not excessive for the site being injected. If a dose exceeds the maximum recommended volume, it should be divided and administered in two injections.

If the total amount of reconstituted medication is to be administered immediately (single dose vial), the expiration date need not be filled in, because the empty vial will be discarded. If the total amount of reconstituted medication is not to be administered immediately (multiple dose vial), the label or product insert will state how long the medication can be stored. This expiration date or time, or both, should then be written on the label, along with the initials of the person who reconstituted the drug.

A Control (Lot) Number is stamped on the vial by the manufacturer. This refers to information regarding production and distribution of the drug.

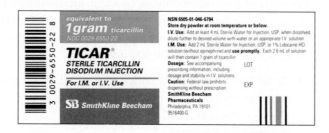

Figure 8-45 *(Courtesy of SmithKline Beecham Pharmaceuticals, Pittsburgh, PA)*

EXAMPLE *Order:* Ticar (ticarcillin disodium) 500 mg IM
        Label: Figure 8-45

    1. What diluent(s) should be used? *Sterile Water for Injection USP* or
        1% Lidocaine HCl Solution (without Epinephrine)
    2. How many mL should be added to the vial? <u>2 mL</u>

3. What is the dosage strength of the prepared solution? <u>2.6 mL = 1 g</u>
4. How many mL should the client receive?

$$500 \text{ mg} \times \frac{1 \text{ g}}{1000 \text{ mg}} \times \frac{2.6 \text{ mL}}{1 \text{ g}} = 1.3 \text{ mL}$$

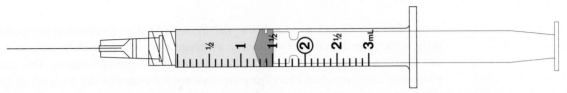

Some drug labels will indicate that various amounts of diluent can be added to the vial to yield various concentrations of solution, Figure 8-46. After the drug has been reconstituted, the strength of the resulting solution should be indicated on the label (check, underscore, circle, or write in the appropriate dilution). In addition, the expiration date should be noted and initialed so that the drug will not be used beyond its expiration date.

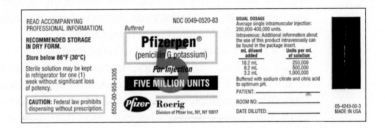

Figure 8-46 *(Reproduced with permission of Pfizer, Inc.)*

EXAMPLE For each of the concentrations (dosage strength) listed on the label (Figure 8-46), how much diluent should be added to the vial and how much of the resulting solution would be administered to the client if the order states "administer 600,000 units IM"?

1. If 18.2 mL of diluent is added to the vial, the resulting solution will contain 250,000 units per mL.
   Dosage Strength: 1 mL = 250,000 units
   Convertion Equation:

$$600,000 \text{ units} \times \frac{1 \text{ mL}}{250,000 \text{ units}} = 2.4 \text{ mL}$$

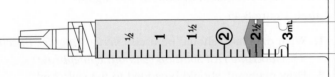

2. If 8.2 mL of diluent is added to the vial, the resulting solution will contain 500,000 units per mL.

Dosage Strength: 1 mL = 500,000 units

Convertion Equation:

$$600{,}000 \text{ units} \times \frac{1 \text{ mL}}{500{,}000 \text{ units}} = 1.2 \text{ mL}$$

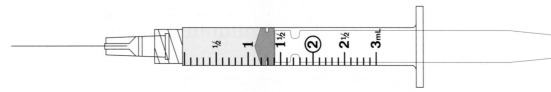

3. If 3.2 mL of diluent is added to the vial, the resulting solution will contain 1,000,000 units per mL.

Dosage Strength: 1 mL = 1,000,000 units

Convertion Equation:

$$600{,}000 \text{ units} \times \frac{1 \text{ mL}}{1{,}000{,}000 \text{ units}} = 0.6 \text{ mL}$$

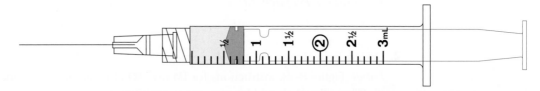

4. How long may the reconstituted solution be stored? <u>1 week</u>

5. Where should it be stored? <u>Refrigerator</u>

PRACTICE

Reconstitution of Drugs in Powder Form

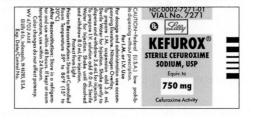

NDC 0002-7271-01
VIAL No. 7271
℞ *Lilly*

KEFUROX®
STERILE CEFUROXIME
SODIUM, USP

Equiv. to

750 mg

Cefuroxime Activity

Figure 8-47 *(Courtesy of Eli Lilly Pharmaceuticals, Indianapolis, IN)*

1. ***Order:*** Kefurox 500 mg IM

Label: Figure 8-47; instructions for IM use. What is the generic name? _____

a. How many mL should be added to the vial? _____

b. How will you know what diluent to add? _____

Reconstitution of Drugs in Powder Form (Continued)

c. What is the dosage strength of the resulting solution? _____
d. How many mL should the client receive? _____

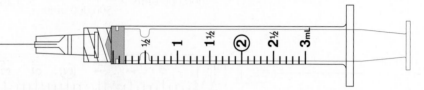

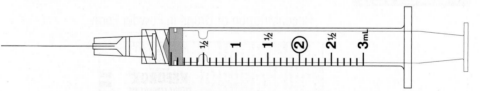

R only
NDC 0009-0758-01
4—125 mg doses

See package insert for complete product
information. Store at controlled room
temperature 20° to 25°C (68° to 77°F) [see
USPI. Protect from light. Reconstitute with
8 mL Bacteriostatic Water for Injection with
Benzyl Alcohol. **When reconstituted as
directed each 8 mL contains:**
*Methylprednisolone sodium succinate
equivalent to 500 mg methylprednisolone
(62.5 mg per mL). Store solution at
controlled room temperature 20° to 25°C
(68° to 77°F) [see USP] and use within 48
hours after mixing. Lyophilized in container.
Protect from light.
Reconstituted: _____

Solu-Medrol®
methylprednisolone
sodium succinate for
injection, USP

500 mg*

For intramuscular or intravenous use

Figure 8-48 *(Courtesy of Pharmacia
Corporation, Peapack, NJ)*

2. *Order:* Solu-Medrol 80 mg IM

Label: Figure 8-48; instructions for IM use. What is the generic name? _____
a. What diluent should be used for reconstitution? _____
b. How much diluent should be added to the vial? _____
c. What is the dosage strength per mL of the prepared solution? _____
d. How many mL should the client receive? _____

e. Assume you reconstituted the drug at 10 A.M. on $9/16$. What is the expiration
time/date:? _____
f. At what temperature should the reconstituted solution be stored? _____

PRACTICE

Reconstitution of Drugs in Powder Form (Continued)

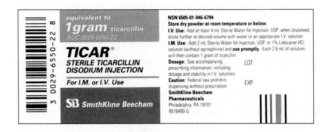

NSN 6505-01-046-6794
Store dry powder at room temperature or below.
I.V. Use: Add at least 4 mL Sterile Water for Injection, USP, when dissolved, dilute further to desired volume with water or an appropriate I.V. solution.
I.M. Use: Add 2 mL Sterile Water for Injection, USP, or 1% Lidocaine HCl solution (without epinephrine) and use promptly. Each 2.6 mL of solution will then contain 1 gram of ticarcillin.
Dosage: See accompanying prescribing information, including dosage and stability in I.V. solutions.
Caution: Federal law prohibits dispensing without prescription.
SmithKline Beecham Pharmaceuticals
Philadelphia, PA 19101
9516400-G

LOT

EXP

equivalent to
1gram ticarcillin
NDC 0029-6550-22
TICAR®
STERILE TICARCILLIN
DISODIUM INJECTION
For I.M. or I.V. Use
SB SmithKline Beecham

3 0029-6550-22 8

Figure 8-49 *(Courtesy of SmithKline Beecham Pharmaceuticals, Pittsburgh, PA)*

3. *Order:* Ticar 700 mg IM

Label: Figure 8-49; instructions for IM use. What is the generic name? _____
a. What diluent should be added to the vial? _____
b. Assume you added 2 mL of diluent; what is the resulting dosage strength? _____

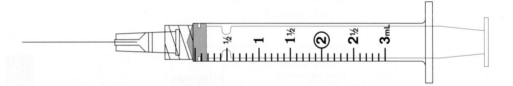

c. How many mL should the client receive? _____
d. What other route can be used? _____

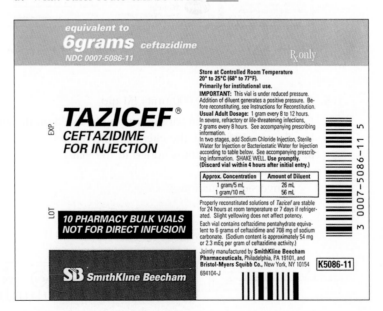

equivalent to
6grams ceftazidime
NDC 0007-5086-11   R̞only

Store at Controlled Room Temperature
20° to 25°C (68° to 77°F).
Primarily for institutional use.
IMPORTANT: This vial is under reduced pressure. Addition of diluent generates a positive pressure. Before reconstituting, see Instructions for Reconstitution.
Usual Adult Dosage: 1 gram every 8 to 12 hours. In severe, refractory or life-threatening infections, 2 grams every 8 hours. See accompanying prescribing information.
In two stages, add Sodium Chloride Injection, Sterile Water for Injection or Bacteriostatic Water for Injection according to table below. See accompanying prescribing information. SHAKE WELL. **Use promptly.**
(Discard vial within 4 hours after initial entry.)

TAZICEF®
CEFTAZIDIME
FOR INJECTION

Approx. Concentration	Amount of Diluent
1 gram/5 mL	26 mL
1 gram/10 mL	56 mL

Properly reconstituted solutions of *Tazicef* are stable for 24 hours at room temperature or 7 days if refrigerated. Slight yellowing does not affect potency.
Each vial contains ceftazidime pentahydrate equivalent to 6 grams of ceftazidime and 708 mg of sodium carbonate. (Sodium content is approximately 54 mg or 2.3 mEq per gram of ceftazidime activity.)
Jointly manufactured by **SmithKline Beecham Pharmaceuticals**, Philadelphia, PA 19101, and **Bristol-Myers Squibb Co.**, New York, NY 10154
694104-J

**10 PHARMACY BULK VIALS
NOT FOR DIRECT INFUSION**

SB SmithKline Beecham

K5086-11

3 0007-5086-11 5

Figure 8-50 *(Reprinted with permission from GlaxoSmithKline, Philadelphia, PA)*

> ### Reconstitution of Drugs in Powder Form (Continued)

4. *Order:* Tazicef 250 mg IM q 8 h

Label: Figure 8-50. What is the generic name? _____

a. What diluents may be used for reconstitution? _____

b. How much diluent should be added to the vial to obtain a dosage strength of 1 g per 5 mL? _____

c. How many mL should the client receive per dose? _____

d. How many g would this client receive over a 24 hr period? _____

e. What is the adult dose of this drug for a life-threatening infection? _____

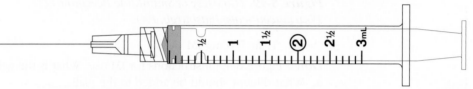

f. Assume you reconstituted the drug at 9 A.M. on 11/9. What is the expiration time/date if the solution is stored in the refrigerator? _____

g. How soon after reconstitution must the medication be administered if it is not refrigerated? _____

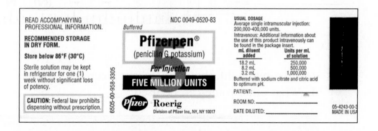

Figure 8-51   *(Reproduced with permission of Pfizer, Inc.)*

5. *Order:* Pfizerpen 400,000 units IM qid

For each concentration (dosage strength) listed on the label (Figure 8-51), calculate the number of mL the client should receive.

a. If 18.2 mL of diluent is added to the vial:

Dosage Strength:

Conversion Equation:

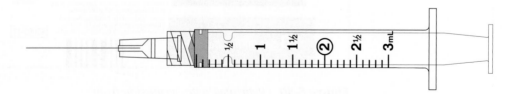

PRACTICE

Reconstitution of Drugs in Powder Form (Continued)

b. If 8.2 mL of diluent is added to the vial:
   Dosage Strength:

   Conversion Equation:

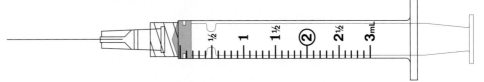

c. If 3.2 mL of diluent is added to the vial:
   Dosage Strength:

   Conversion Equation:

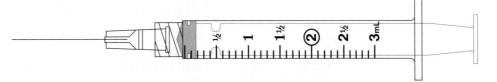

d. How long may the reconstituted solution be stored? _____
e. Where should the solution be stored? _____

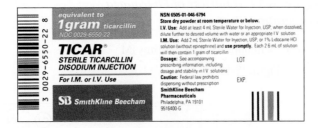

Figure 8-52 *(Courtesy of SmithKline Beecham Pharmaceuticals, Pittsburgh, PA)*

Determine the number of milliliters that should be administered in the following problems. (Carry all answers to two decimal places and round to the nearest tenth.)

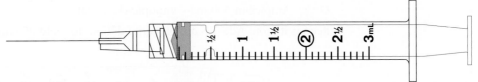

Reconstitution of Drugs in Powder Form (Continued)

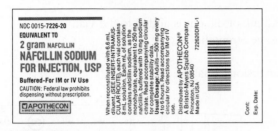

Figure 8-53 *(Courtesy of Apothecon Bristol-Myers Squibb Company, Princeton, NJ)*

6. **Order:** Ticar 600 mg IM

   Label: Figure 8-52

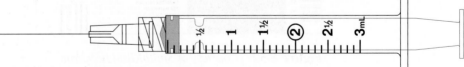

Figure 8-54 *(Courtesy of Pharmacia Corporation, Peapack, NJ)*

7. **Order:** Nafcillin Sodium 300 mg IM

   Label: Figure 8-53

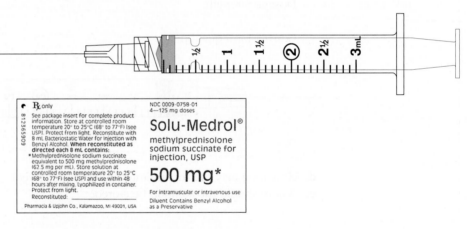

8. **Order:** Solu-Medrol 75 mg IM

   Label: Figure 8-54

9. **Order:** Ampicillin 150 mg IM

   Label: Ampicillin 500 mg—multiple-dose vial

   Reconstitution: Add 1.8 mL of sterile diluent to yield 250 mg per mL.

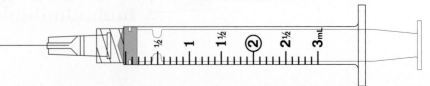

PRACTICE

Reconstitution of Drugs in Powder Form (Continued)

10. *Order:* Pipracil 800 mg IM

    Label: Pipracil (piperacillin sodium) 1 g powder form

    Reconstitution: Add 2 mL of sterile diluent to yield 1 g per 2.5 mL.

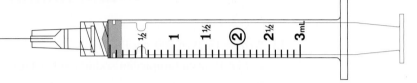

11. *Order:* Kefzol 500 mg IM

    Label: Kefzol (cefazolin) 1 g

    Reconstitution: Add 2.5 mL of sterile diluent to yield 330 mg per mL.

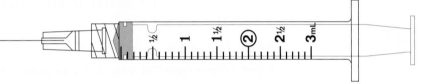

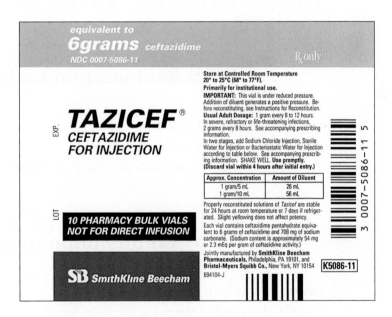

Figure 8-55 *(Reprinted with permission from GlaxoSmithKline, Philadelphia, PA)*

12. *Order:* Tazicef 150 mg IM

    Label: Figure 8-55

    Reconstitution: Add 56 mL of sterile diluent to yield _____

PRACTICE

Reconstitution of Drugs in Powder Form (Continued)

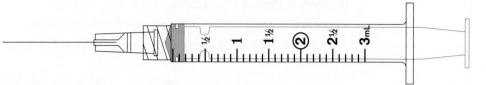

13. *Order:* Unasyn 500 mg IM

   Label: Unasyn (ampicillin sodium/sulbactam sodium) 3 g in dry form

   Reconstitution: Add 6.4 mL of sterile diluent to yield 3 g per 8 mL.

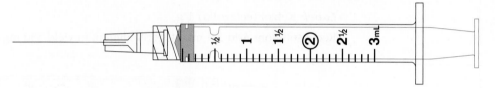

14. *Order:* Unipen 400 mg IM

   Label: Unipen (nafcillin sodium) 1 g in powder form

   Reconstitution: Add 3.4 mL sterile water for injection to yield 1 g per 4 mL

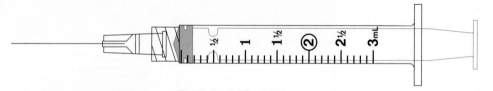

15. *Order:* Ampicillin 500 mg IM

   Label: Ampicillin 1 g per vial in dry form

   Reconstitution: Add 1.8 mL sterile water to yield 250 mg per mL.

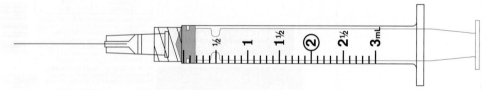

16. *Order:* Cefizox 0.5 g IM

   Label: Cefizox (ceftizoxime) 2 g vial in dry form

   Reconstitution: Add 6 mL of sterile diluent to yield 270 mg per mL.

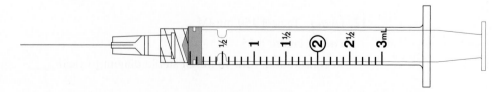

PRACTICE

Reconstitution of Drugs in Powder Form (Continued)

17. *Order:* Cefobid 0.75 g IM

   Label: Cefobid (cefoperazone sodium) 2 g in dry form

   Reconstitution: Add 3.8 mL of sterile water to yield 333 mg per mL.

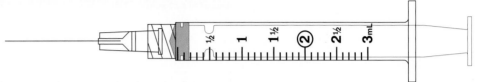

18. *Order:* Cefuroxime Sodium 350 mg IM

   Label: Kefurox (cefuroxime sodium) 1 g in dry form

   Reconstitution: Add 2.5 mL of sterile water to yield 330 mg per mL.

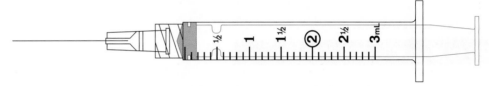

19. *Order:* Mandol 800 mg IM

   Label: Mandol (cefamandole nafate) 1 g per vial in dry form

   Reconstitution: Add 3 mL of sterile diluent to provide 1 g per 3 mL.

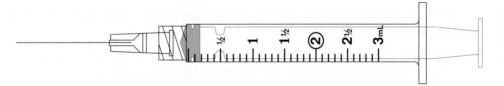

20. *Order:* Tazidine 0.75 g IM

   Label: Tazidine (ceftazidime) 1 g per vial in dry form

   Reconstitution: Add 3 mL of sterile water to yield 280 mg per mL.

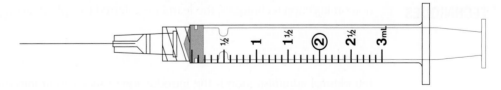

(*Note:* See Appendix G for answer key.)

CHAPTER 9

Administration of Parenteral Medications

OBJECTIVES

Upon completion of this chapter, you should be able to:

- Identify safe and suitable sites for intradermal, subcutaneous, and intramuscular injections, including boundaries and anatomical landmarks.

- Follow infection-control guidelines with respect to handling or manipulating needles and syringes.

- List the general rules for safe administration of parenteral medications: preparing, administering, and recording.

- Identify performance criteria related to administering drugs by subcutaneous and intramuscular routes, including variations when administering heparin and insulin.

- Read drug labels to differentiate various types of insulin.

INJECTION SITES AND TECHNIQUES

A descriptive overview of injection sites and procedures follows, along with recommended guidelines for administration of parenteral medications. For detailed instruction on injection techniques, the learner is referred to a pharmacology or nursing text.

Intradermal Injection

Intradermal administration is the introduction of medication into the dermal layers of the skin. The needle penetrates the epidermis and enters the dermis. A very small amount of drug is given, usually for the purpose of skin testing. A 1 mL tuberculin syringe is used with a fine (25–26) gauge, 1/4″–5/8″ needle. The medial surface of the forearm and the upper chest and back are the most commonly used sites, Figure 9-1. A very shallow angle of insertion, 10–15°, is used. The needle is inserted bevel up

FRONT **BACK**

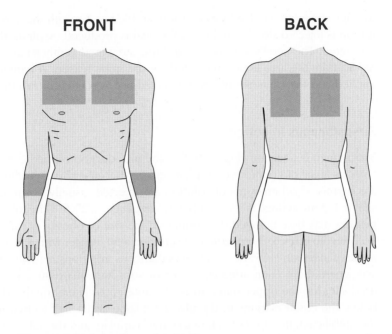

Figure 9-1 *Intradermal injections*

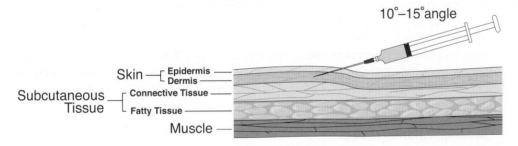

10°–15°angle

Skin — Epidermis
— Dermis

Subcutaneous — Connective Tissue
Tissue — Fatty Tissue

Muscle

Figure 9-1a *Needle insertion*

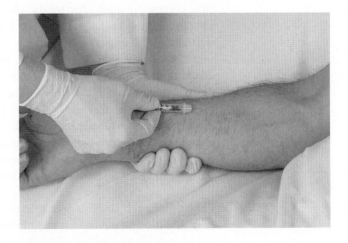

Figure 9-1b *Holding skin*

through the tautly held skin so that it is visible just beneath the surface and the medication is injected slowly until a small wheal is produced. Aspiration prior to injection is omitted. The needle is removed and the site wiped gently so as not to disperse the medication; the area is not massaged for the same reason. A bandage should not be applied and the client should be instructed not to scratch or rub the site.

Subcutaneous Injection

Subcutaneous injection (Figure 9-2) is the introduction of medication into the subcutaneous layer of connective and fatty tissue. Because this layer lies directly beneath the dermis, small amounts of solution are injected, usually not more than 2 mL in a site. A 1–3 mL syringe is used with a 25–28 gauge, 1/2″–5/8″ needle. Shorter or longer needles may be employed depending on the size or obesity of the recipient. When a 1/2″ needle is used, the needle is inserted at a 90° angle; with a 5/8″–3/4″ needle, the angle of insertion is 45° bevel up. Subcutaneous injections may be administered at any site where there is an adequate layer of subcutaneous tissue. The most commonly used sites are the upper outer arms, the anterior or lateral thighs, the abdomen from below the costal margins to the iliac crest (one and a half to two inches away from the umbilicus), the upper back below the scapulae, and the subcutaneous tissue over the dorsogluteal area. The areas over the deltoid and vastus lateralis or rectus femoris muscles often are used as long as the subcutaneous tissue can be bunched up so that the needle does not enter the muscle. When frequent subcutaneous injections are administered—such as daily insulin injections—a plan should be devised for rotating sites to promote absorption and avoid tissue fibrosis. When performing a subcutaneous injection, aspiration is omitted to lessen risk of tissue damage, such as hematoma or bruising. The likelihood of intravascular injections is small.

Intramuscular Injection

Intramuscular administration of medications is made through the skin and subcutaneous tissues into a muscle, Figure 9-3. Sites must be chosen with care to avoid damage to major nerves and blood vessels either by the needle or the medication. The most commonly used sites are the gluteal muscles. Also used are the deltoid, the vastus lateralis, and the rectus femoris. The sites should be rotated when the medication is irritating or repeated frequently.

The size of syringe and needle chosen depends on the amount and viscosity of medication to be given and the size or obesity of the recipient. For aqueous solutions, a 21 or 22 gauge, 1″–1 1/2″ needle is usually suitable. For viscous or oily solutions, a 20 or 21 gauge needle of appropriate length is used. For both a 90° angle of insertion is used.

It is necessary to aspirate prior to injection of the medication to avoid inadvertent intravenous injection. Following injection of most medications, the area is massaged gently to aid dispersion and absorption. The nurse always should ascertain the correct procedure regarding massage when intramuscular medications are administered.

Ventrogluteal Site This site utilizes the ventral area of the gluteal muscles, specifically, the gluteus medius and minimus muscles below the iliac crest. These muscles can absorb up to 3 mL of solution per injection for an adult and 1–2 mL for children

Figure 9-2 Subcutaneous Injections

FRONT   **BACK**

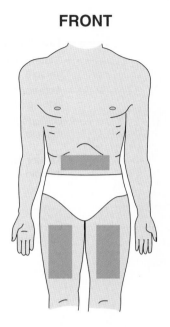
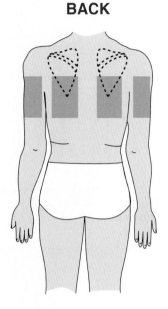

Figure 9-2a Subcutaneous sites

Angle of Insertion

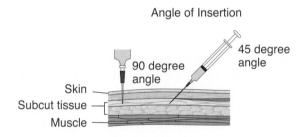

Figure 9-2b Angle of insertion

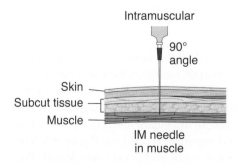

Figure 9-3 Intramuscular injection—
angle of insertion

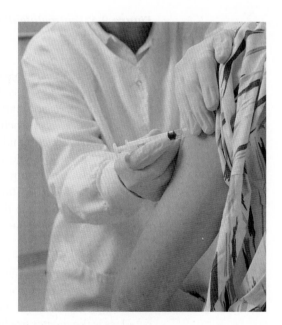

Figure 9-2c Bunch up tissue

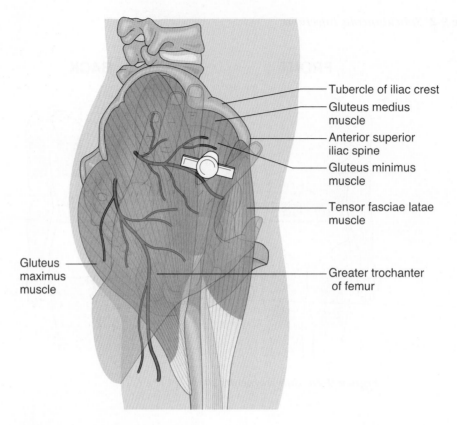

Tubercle of iliac crest

Gluteus medius
muscle

Anterior superior
iliac spine

Gluteus minimus
muscle

Tensor fasciae latae
muscle

Greater trochanter
of femur

Gluteus
maximus
muscle

Figure 9-4 Ventrogluteal site

over the age of 1 year. This versatile site can be used with the client in a lateral, supine, or prone position or—less desirable but possible—with the person standing or seated. Three anatomical landmarks are used to identify the site. The palm of the hand is placed on the greater trochanter of the femur, the index finger on the anterior superior iliac spine, and the middle finger abducted posteriorly along the iliac crest to form a V-shaped area. The injection site is in the center of the triangle between the index and middle fingers, Figure 9-4.

This is a safe injection site for both adults and for children over the age of 1 year. It is particularly useful in the case of small or emaciated persons, because the muscle layer is thick and easily accessible.

Dorsogluteal Site   The dorsogluteal site is located in the upper, outer quadrant of the buttock. Injection is made into the gluteus maximus muscle, which also can absorb up to 3 mL of solution for an adult. The client may be positioned on one side or the other or on the abdomen with the toes pointed inward. The posterior iliac spine is palpated, as is the greater trochanter of the femur, and an imaginary line is drawn between these two points. The injection site is lateral and superior to this line, Figure 9-5. The gluteal muscle is not used for infants, because it is small and poorly developed. The site may be used by the age of 3 years for children who have been walking at least a year, maximum volume 1–2 mL.

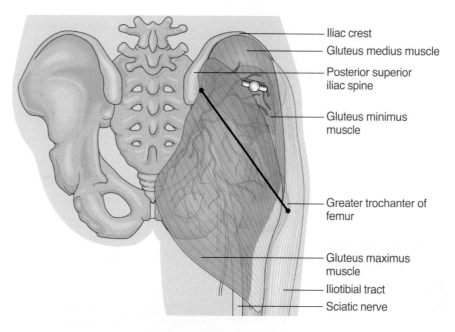

Iliac crest
Gluteus medius muscle
Posterior superior
iliac spine
Gluteus minimus
muscle
Greater trochanter of
femur
Gluteus maximus
muscle
Iliotibial tract
Sciatic nerve

Figure 9-5 Dorsogluteal site

Deltoid Site The recommended site of injection into the deltoid muscle is into the thicker midportion of the muscle. This area is relatively small and is used when small amounts of solution are to be given, not exceeding 2 mL in adults. Because the deltoid muscle is very thin in infants and children, it is used only when very small amounts, not exceeding 0.5 mL, are to be given. The client may be positioned on either side or sitting up. It is important that the arm hang loosely at the side when the client is seated because this keeps the muscle relaxed. Holding the arm away from the body tenses the muscle and increases discomfort as well as impeding dispersion of the medication. The anatomical landmarks for identification of the deltoid site include the acromion process of the scapula and the axillary fold. The site is located at the center of the triangular area bounded superiorly by the acromion process and inferiorly by a line extending from the axillary fold across the lateral aspect of the arm, Figure 9-6.

Vastus Lateralis Site The vastus lateralis muscle is a commonly used injection site, because it is usually thick and well developed in both adults and children. The site can absorb up to 3 mL of solution, depending on the size of the individual. Smaller amounts should be administered to children. The client may be in a lateral or supine position or sitting upright. The anatomical landmarks for identification of the site are the knee and the greater trochanter of the femur. Injection is made into the midportion of the muscle, located by measuring a hand's width above the knee and below the trochanter. The muscle extends from the midanterior to midlateral thigh between the two bony landmarks, Figure 9-7.

Rectus Femoris Site The rectus femoris muscle, on the anterior aspect of the thigh, can be used for intramuscular injections of up to 3 mL and is especially accessible for

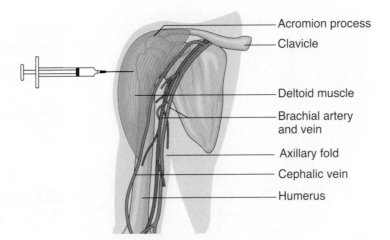

Figure 9-6 Deltoid site

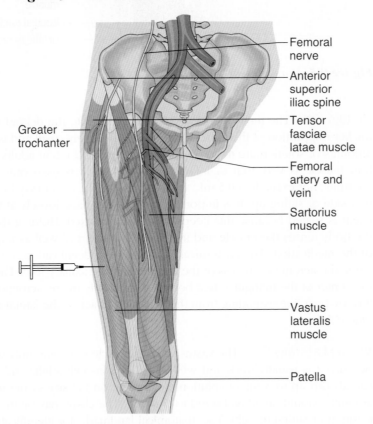

Figure 9-7 Vastus lateralis site

individuals who self-administer their injections. The client assumes a sitting or lying position and the injection site is in the lateral midportion of the anterior thigh. The medial aspect of the thigh should be avoided, Figure 9-8. This site may be used for children and infants, no more than 1–2 mL depending on age and size.

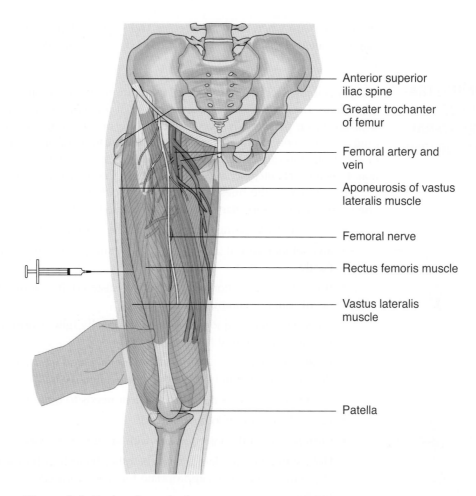

Anterior superior iliac spine

Greater trochanter of femur

Femoral artery and vein

Aponeurosis of vastus lateralis muscle

Femoral nerve

Rectus femoris muscle

Vastus lateralis muscle

Patella

Figure 9-8 Rectus femoris site

PRECAUTIONS IN HANDLING NEEDLES AND SYRINGES

Because of the risk associated with contacting blood contaminated with microorganisms, personnel must use special precautions when handling all used needles and syringes. It is recommended that a glove be placed on the nondominant hand (i.e., the hand that comes into contact with the client) when any injection is administered. In addition, because of the danger of needle-stick injuries, used needles should not be recapped, bent, or broken following injection. They should not be removed from disposable syringes or otherwise manipulated by hand. Insofar as possible, only needleless injection systems should be used, for example, syringes with protective devices such as retractable or safety sheath needles. If a safeguarded syringe is not available, the nurse may use a scoop technique for recapping a contaminated needle. (Place the needle cap on a level surface and insert the needle into the cap using one hand only. Secure the cap by pressing the covered needle against a firm surface.) All used needles and syringes should immediately be discarded into puncture-resistant containers. Personnel should ascertain agency policy with regard to handling and disposing of syringes and needles, and they should follow these guidelines meticulously. Any time gloves are worn when handling needles and syringes, hands should be washed thoroughly immediately after gloves are removed, even if the gloves appear to be intact.

ADMINISTRATION OF PARENTERAL MEDICATIONS

The general rules for administration of medications, which are listed in Chapter 7, also apply here. Because of the additional potential for harm to the client when medications are given parenterally, accuracy and care in preparing and administering these drugs assumes critical proportions. Precise identification of sites and proper techniques of administration cannot be overemphasized because of the danger of injury or infection. Principles of safety, comfort, and effective intervention are equally important.

In addition to the rules in Chapter 7, specific recommendations for administration of intradermal, subcutaneous, and intramuscular injections include:

- Select a sterile syringe and needle of the appropriate size and length.
- Mix solution in vial, if necessary, by rotating between palms or shaking gently.
- If irritating medications are being administered, it is desirable to change the needle after obtaining the correct dose.
- Carefully select and identify injection sites by fully exposing area and palpating anatomical landmarks.
- Rotate injection sites as appropriate for repeated injections. A chart or diagram for rotation of injection sites is often desirable.
- Obtain assistance as necessary if client needs to be restrained.
- Place glove on nondominant hand.
- Cleanse skin at the injection site with an antiseptic wipe.
- Hold syringe in one hand; with the other hand bunch or hold the skin taut at the injection site, as appropriate for type of injection and angle of insertion.
- Insert the needle about seven-eighths of its length, thus preventing complete disappearance in case of breakage.
- Aspirate for blood to avoid an accidental intravascular injection. If blood is aspirated, remove the needle, obtain a new needle, syringe, and dose and select a new site. Aspiration is omitted with intradermal and subcutaneous injections.
- Inject the medication into the tissue with slow, steady pressure.
- For IM injection, place the antiseptic wipe adjacent to the needle, apply reverse pressure, and quickly withdraw the needle, immediately making slight pressure over the site with the wipe.
- For subcutaneous injection: (5/8–3/4" needle, 45° angle, bevel up), lay the antiseptic wipe over the injection site without exerting pressure on the needle, quickly remove the needle, and then apply pressure over the site; 1/2" needle, 90° angle, proceed as in IM injection above.
- Gently massage the injection site with an antiseptic wipe to increase the rate of dispersion and absorption. Avoid massage with subcutaneous, intradermal, or Z-track injections.

- Perform needle coverage and safety capping per policy.
- Discard used syringe and needle into puncture-resistant container.

The learner is referred to Performance Criteria: Administration of Injections checklist (Appendix H) for use as a guide in the administration of injections.

VARIATION OF PARENTERAL INJECTION TECHNIQUES: IM

Z-Track

This is a method of administering a deep intramuscular injection to prevent seepage of medication along the needle track. The method is used when any medication that is irritating or a substance that stains such as iron is given, because it is more effective in sealing medication within the desired site than the customary (usual) intramuscular injection technique. Figure 9-9 illustrates the technique of Z-track injection.

It is important to select a deep site in a large muscle, preferably the dorsogluteal site. See Figure 9-9. **It is also important to apply a new needle after obtaining the desired dose to prevent depositing medication in the subcutaneous tissues as the needle is inserted into the muscle.** In addition, a 0.2–0.3 mL air lock is used to clear the needle of medication after injection and to help prevent leakage or tracking. Therefore, after the correct dosage is obtained, 0.2–0.3 mL of air is drawn into the syringe to provide the desired air lock following injection of the medication.

The learner is referred to Performance Criteria: Z-Track Method—Deep Intramuscular Injection checklist (Appendix H) for use as a guide in the administration of drugs to be administered by this route.

In the Z-track technique, the skin and subcutaneous tissues are displaced to one side, resulting in a shift of tissue layers out of normal alignment (see Figure 9-9). The needle is inserted directly into the muscle layer and the medication is injected slowly at a rate of 1 mL every 10 seconds while tissue displacement is maintained. It is therefore necessary to aspirate (5–10 seconds) and hold the syringe with the same hand.

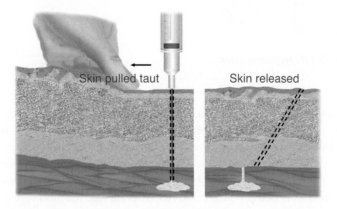

Skin pulled taut   Skin released

Figure 9-9 The Z-track technique for deep intramuscular injection (Courtesy of Reiss and Evans, Pharmacological Aspects of Nursing Care, *5th ed. Copyright 1996 by Thomson Delmar Learning, Clifton Park, NY)*

A period of 10 seconds is allowed to elapse before needle removal to ensure adequate dispersion. When the needle is removed, the tissues are quickly released and return to their normal position, leaving a Z-shaped channel that prevents seepage and tracking. The site is not massaged.

The checklist in Appendix H may be used as a guide for the Z-track variation.

VARIATION OF PARENTERAL INJECTION TECHNIQUES: SUBCUT

Heparin Injection

Subcutaneous injection of heparin requires special modifications in technique to cause as little trauma as possible to the tissues at the injection site. The purpose is to prevent or minimize bleeding caused by the anticoagulant properties of this drug. To avoid inadvertent intramuscular injection, it is important to select a short needle and a site with adequate subcutaneous tissue. Separate needles should be used for obtaining and injecting the heparin. Sites on the abdomen above the level of the anterior iliac spines are most commonly used, Figure 9-10. It is important to rotate sites and to select sites free from bruising or scarring and at least 2″ away from the umbilicus. Gentle cleansing of the skin helps prevent trauma, as does omission of aspiration and massage. The client also should be reminded not to rub the site. Application of an icebag following injection may prevent ecchymosis.

The learner is referred to Performance Criteria: Administration of Heparin checklist (Appendix H) for use as a guide in the administration of heparin.

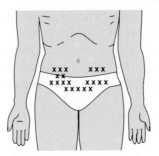

Figure 9-10 Heparin sites

INSULIN PREPARATIONS

Persons who have diabetes caused by insulin-secretion deficiency may be treated by one or more injections daily of manufactured insulin. Synthetic human insulin produced from recombinant DNA is most widely used in this country. In the past, other sources of manufactured insulin were pork pancreas and beef pancreas or a combination of the two. The use of beef pancreas has been discontinued, and the use of pork pancreas is being phased out. Because allergic reactions are possible, alternative forms of insulin may be prescribed. If the source is specified in the insulin order, it is essential that the correct bottle be selected.

Regular insulin is a *clear* solution designated by the letter R on the bottle. See Figure 9-11. While regular insulin is fast-acting, it is of short duration. It can be administered subcutaneously or intravenously. It is important to remember that regular insulin is the *only type of insulin* that can be administered intravenously.

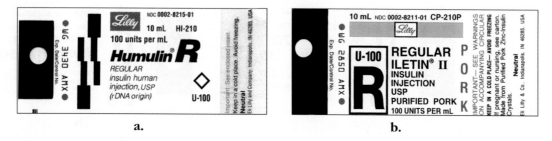

Figure 9-11a, b *Regular insulin (Courtesy of Eli Lilly Pharmaceuticals, Indianapolis, IN)*

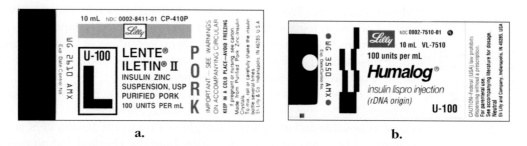

Figure 9-12a, b *Modified insulin (Courtesy of Eli Lilly Pharmaceuticals, Indianapolis, IN)*

Insulins differ as to time of onset, peak activity, and duration of action. These characteristics are controlled by adding zinc or protamine, or both, to regular (fast-acting) insulin to produce either intermediate or long-acting effects. These extended-action products are called *modified* insulins and are designated by the letters L, N, and U. Due to the suspension of zinc or protamine, modified insulin is cloudy and can only be administered subcutaneously. Figure 9-12 shows two examples.

A third type of insulin, called Lantus, is a long-acting synthetic human insulin that provides 24-hour coverage and is administered daily at bedtime. It should be given subcutaneously, never intravenously, nor should it ever be diluted with any other solution or type of insulin. The advantage of this insulin is its 24-hour effectiveness, which permits once-daily dosing.

An example of an insulin preparation that has both a rapid onset and a short duration is Humalog (insulin lispro). Because of its rapid onset, this insulin must be taken either immediately before or after eating. Because of its short duration, it also may be necessary to use a longer-acting insulin in conjunction.

A combination of regular and modified insulins is sometimes ordered to provide for both rapid and prolonged action. Such combinations can contain varying proportions of regular and modified insulins premixed, Figure 9-13.

These insulin mixtures are convenient to use when the prescribed dose is identical to the mixture available. However, in many instances this is not the case. If an identical combination is not available, the ordered insulin dosages may be administered separately or mixed in one syringe for administration. In mixing two different types of insulin in one syringe, it is important that no modified insulin be introduced into the bottle of regular insulin. Therefore, when mixing two types of insulin in one syringe, the regular insulin (clear) should be drawn up first and the modified insulin

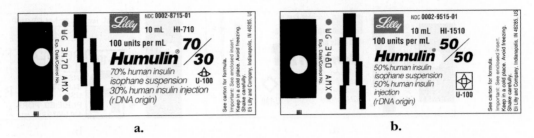

a.

b.

Figure 9-13a, b *Premixed insulin (Courtesy of Eli Lilly Pharmaceuticals, Indianapolis, IN)*

(cloudy) second. (See Procedure for Mixing Insulins, Appendix H, page 369.) Because mixtures of insulin remain stable for only a few minutes, it is important to administer these injections immediately after mixing them. Regardless of whether regular, modified, or mixed insulins are ordered, it is essential that the correct type be selected and that the exact prescribed amount be administered.

Insulin preparations should be stored in a cold place, preferably refrigerated, but not frozen. Insulin currently in use may be stored unrefrigerated, as long as it is kept as cool as possible and away from sunlight or direct heat. Insulin kept at room temperature will last a month or so. Label date should be checked and no insulin should be used beyond its expiration date.

PRACTICE

Reading Insulin Labels

From Figure 9-14, select the correct bottle (by letter) and answer the questions relating to the insulin order.

1. What is the concentration of each of the insulin preparations shown?

   _____

2. Identify the two manufacturers represented. _____

3. Select by letter:
   - All of the varieties of human (synthetic) insulin pictured. _____
   - All of the varieties of NPH insulin pictured. _____
   - A regular insulin prepared from pork. _____

4. What letter appears on the label for:
   - Regular Insulin _____
   - NPH Insulin _____
   - Lente Insulin _____
   - Ultralente Insulin _____

5. Prepare the following doses of insulin for administration. You have available a 1 mL, unit-100 syringe. Select (by letter) the correct medication label from Figure 9-14. Shade in the correct dose on the insulin syringe.

Reading Insulin Labels (Continued)

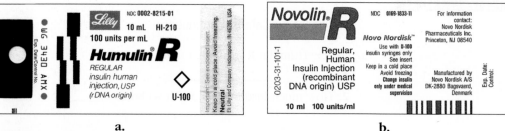

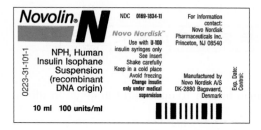

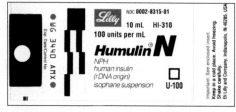

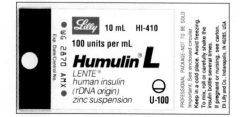

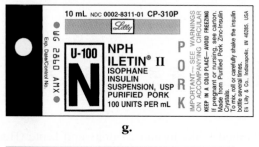

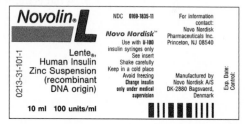

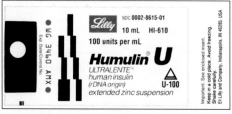

Figure 9-14a–j *Fast-acting, intermediate, and long-acting insulins (a, c, d, f, g, i, and j courtesy of Eli Lilly Pharmaceuticals, Indianapolis, IN) (b, e, and h courtesy of Novo Nordisk Pharmaceuticals, Inc., New York, NY)*

PRACTICE

Reading Insulin Labels (Continued)

a. *Order:* Humulin R Insulin 24 units subcut

    1. *Label:* _____

    2. How much insulin would you withdraw? _____ units

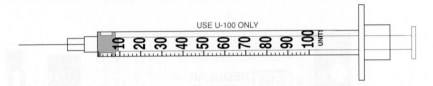

b. *Order:* Lente (Human) Insulin 46 units subcut

    1. *Label:* _____

    2. How much insulin would you withdraw? _____ units

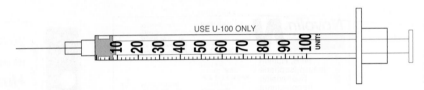

c. *Order:* Regular Human Insulin 10 units and Ultralente Insulin 42 units subcut

    1. *Labels:* _____

    2. Which insulin would be drawn up first? _____

    3. What is the total amount of insulin mixed in the syringe? _____ units

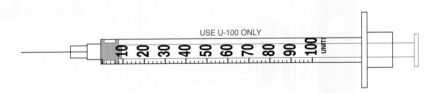

d. *Order:* Regular (Purified Pork) Insulin 24 units and Lente (Human) Insulin 42 units subcut

    1. *Labels:* _____

    2. Which insulin would be drawn up last? _____

    3. What is the total amount of insulin mixed in the syringe? _____ units

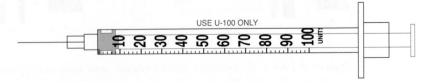

(**Note:** See Appendix G for answer key.)

INSULIN ADMINISTRA-TION

Insulin is ordered and measured in USP units. Almost universally used is the concentration of 100 units per milliliter, designated on the bottle as Unit 100 insulin. This means that 1 mL of the product contains 100 units of insulin. Insulin syringes for this strength are available in two sizes, a 1 mL size that measures up to 100 units and a 0.5 mL size that measures up to 50 units (Figure 9-15); these are referred to commonly as Unit-100 syringes. They usually are prepackaged with a 27 or 28 gauge, 1/2″ needle. Use of the unit-calibrated insulin syringe eliminates the need for calculation, because it is only necessary to draw up the ordered number of units. Neither a tuberculin syringe nor a 2–3 mL syringe gives precise enough measurement; these never should be used for Unit-100 insulin.

Insulin is also available in Unit-500 concentrations, 1 mL containing 500 units of insulin. Unit-500 insulin is a concentration of regular insulin that can be administered only subcutaneously. Because the amounts of Unit-500 insulin ordered are usually very small, a tuberculin-type syringe as well as the Unit-100 syringe can be used for measurement.

Insulin Injection

Because most persons who require insulin injections are eventually taught to self-administer this hormone, nurses must be alert to the learning needs of these clients and must teach and reinforce correct principles of insulin administration.

Because the insulin injection is repeated daily or more often, it is essential to rotate injection sites to prevent tissue damage or complications such as atrophy, thickening, or scarring, all of which can interfere with proper absorption. Clients should be taught to alternate sites using a site selection plan that will help ensure proper rotation.

The abdomen is the recommended site for subcutaneous administration of insulin (Figure 9-16). Any area of the abdomen may be used, including the lateral aspect above the iliac crest, making sure to stay at least 2 inches away from the umbilicus or any scar tissue. An alternative subcutaneous site is the upper outer thigh. Less desirable subcutaneous sites are also shown in Figure 9-16 if the preferred sites cannot be utilized.

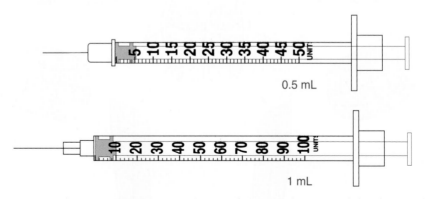

Figure 9-15 Insulin syringes

Preferred Sites

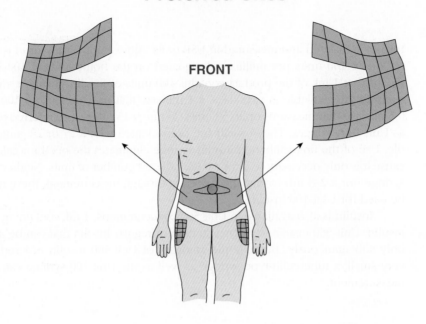

FRONT

Less Desirable Sites

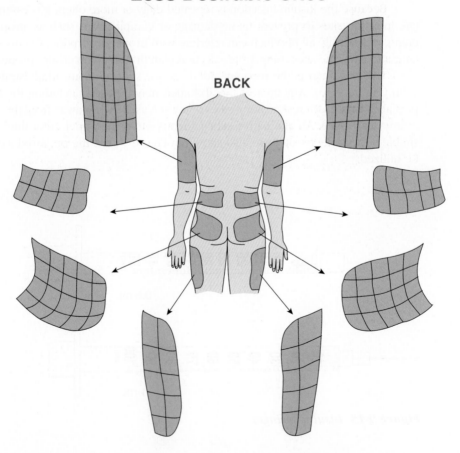

BACK

Figure 9-16 *Insulin injection sites and rotation patterns*

Clients may also need to learn how to mix combinations of insulin preparations in one syringe. It is important to stress that the short-acting (regular) insulin be withdrawn prior to withdrawal of long-acting (modified) insulin. It is essential that any air bubbles be eliminated from the syringe when obtaining the dose of insulin to have an accurate amount. The step for aspirating for blood prior to injection is omitted in teaching self-administration of insulin, because it is difficult for clients to do this one-handed.

In addition to the insulin syringe and needle, other insulin injection devices are currently available that offer accuracy, convenience, and versatility for persons who self-administer their insulin. These devices can be easily carried and facilitate daily single or multiple injections of premixed insulin, thereby greatly simplifying the procedure and routine of insulin self-administration.

One of the latest devices for administration of insulin is a "smart" insulin pump, which delivers a steady flow of insulin much like a healthy pancreas, thereby eliminating the need for injection. One example of an external pump is seen in Figure 9-17.

The learner is referred to Performance Criteria: Administration of Insulin checklist (Appendix H) for use as a guide in the administration of insulin.

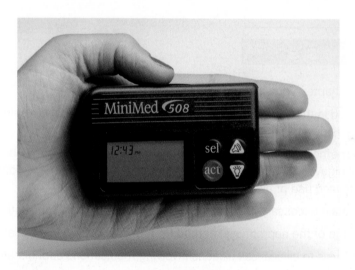

Figure 9-17 *External Insulin Pump (Courtesy of Medtronic MiniMed, Wilbraham, Pa.)*

CHAPTER 10

Calculations of Intravenous Medications and Solutions

Upon completion of this chapter, you should be able to:

- Identify equipment used in the administration of intravenous medications and solutions, including types of vascular access devices, infusion sets, and solution containers.

- Describe the various methods by which intravenous medications/solutions may be administered: continuous IV drip, IV piggyback, volume control set, peripheral lock, central venous catheters, IV bolus, implanted ports, and use of electronic infusion devices.

- Read drug labels to obtain necessary information for administration of IV medications and solutions.

- Demonstrate knowledge of the appropriate method for rounding off when calculating IV flow rates.

- Apply dimensional analysis to clinical calculations involving medications administered intravenously.

- Identify nursing responsibilities in relation to assessing and adjusting intravenous infusions.

Section I: Intravenous Equipment

INTRAVENOUS INJECTIONS AND INFUSIONS

Intravenous administration refers to the injection or infusion of medications and fluids into a vein. It is another example of parenteral administration. Because the medication enters the circulation directly, the effect of drugs given intravenously is immediate. The abbreviation IV is used for these medication orders.

This chapter deals with equipment and solutions used in administering IVs, reading labels and adding medications, and calculating IV drug dosages.

NEEDLELESS INFUSION SYSTEMS

Generally, a needleless system is used to administer intravenous fluids. This system consists of an administration set with tubing to which is connected some type of vascular access device (cannula, stylet, shielded or retracted needle) with attached intravenous catheter. Following venipuncture using the vascular access device, the catheter is advanced into the vein. The IV solution is then infused through the intravenous catheter.

Intravenous catheters vary in length from $1\frac{1}{4}''$–36" and gauge from 12 G (large diameter) to 22 G (small diameter). The size and length selected vary depending on site of insertion, size or age of client, and viscosity of solution.

Needleless IV systems greatly reduce the risk of IV contamination via air, blood, or touch and also reduce the risk of accidental needle-stick injuries. (See Figure 10-1.)

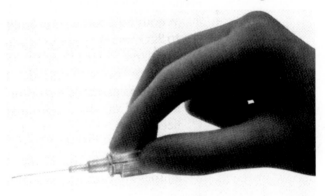

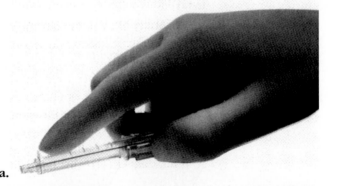

Figure 10-1 *The PROTECTIV™ IV Catheter Safety System has built-in needlestick protection. As the user slides the catheter off the introducer needle, a protective guard glides over the contaminated needle before it is removed from the catheter hub. A reassuring "click" tells the user when the needle is locked safely inside the guard (Courtesy Critikon, Inc.)*

a.

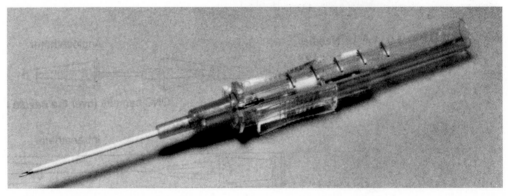

b.

EQUIPMENT

Infusion Sets

A variety of IV administration sets is available for use as primary setups for continuous infusion and secondary setups for intermittent infusion. All sets consist of intravenous tubing, some type of drip chamber, a roller clamp, and protective caps to maintain sterility.

The size of the opening into the drip chamber determines the size of the drop delivered by the infusion set. Macrodrip sets are calibrated to deliver 10, 15, or 20 drops per milliliter. Microdrip (minidrip) sets, calibrated to administer very precise amounts of fluid, deliver 60 drops per milliliter, Figure 10-2. The drop size, called the *drop factor,* is identified on the package. The drop factor refers to the number of drops needed to deliver 1 mL of fluid, and always should be determined prior to calculating or adjusting the flow rate, Figure 10-3.

The earlier IV infusion sets worked by gravity flow, and flow rate was calculated in number of drops per minute using a macrodrip infusion set; these drops were called macrodrops. While gravity flow systems are sometimes still used, for example, in emergency situations, they have been largely replaced by electronic pumps and controllers. These devices can be set to automatically provide both micro and macro rate programming.

Infusion sets may be used individually (primary line) or attached to each other (piggyback or secondary lines).

Intravenous Solution Containers

Intravenous solution containers are made of glass or plastic and come in a variety of sizes and shapes. Glass containers are vacuum sealed and have rubber stoppers with openings for the tubing, for venting, and for the addition of medications. Plastic containers have special ports for insertion of tubing and addition of medications. All containers are calibrated according to the amount of fluid contained and are labeled as to type of solution, instructions for use, and other pertinent information.

IV Drops

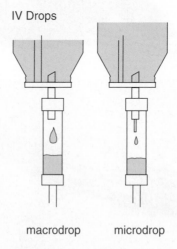

macrodrop   microdrop

Figure 10-2 IV drops

Interlink® System

2C6425s

Solution Set

101" (2.6 m)

2 Injection Sites, Male Luer Lock Adapter

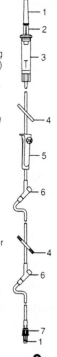

10 drops/mL
Approx.

Fluid path is sterile, nonpyrogenic.
Cautions: Do not use if tip protectors (1) are not in place. Do not place on sterile field.

Directions: Use aseptic technique
Close regulating clamp (5). Insert spike (2) into solution container. Fill drip chamber (3) to fill line. Open regulating clamp (5). Prime set, purge air. Close regulating clamp (5) until roller meets bottom of frame. Attach male Luer adapter (7) to Interlink® cannula or vascular access device using a firm push and twist motion and then engage the Luer lock collar to prevent accidental disconnection.

To properly set flow, always close regulating clamp (5) until roller meets bottom of frame, then reopen to establish flow rate. Repeat procedure if adjusting clamp from fully open position.

Cautions:
Do not allow air to be trapped in set. Puncturing set components may cause air embolism. If needle must be used, insert small gauge needle into perimeter of septum (6). Do not disconnect administration set, syringe or other component from cannula while cannula is still connected to Interlink® injection site.
Federal (USA) law restricts this device to sale by or on order of a physician.
Single use only. Do not resterilize.

Notes:
To stop flow without disturbing regulating device (5), close lowest slide clamp (4). Swab septum of injection site (6) with antiseptic prior to access. Access Interlink® injection site (6) (identified by a colored ring) with Interlink® cannula. See cannula directions. Replace per CDC guidelines.

For Product Information 1-800-933-0303

LDPE

Baxter

*Address Position Only

HIBC BAR CODE POSITION ONLY

* +H16Ø2C6425S1$ *

Figure 10-3 *(Courtesy of Baxter Healthcare Corporation, Deerfield, IL)*

Intravenous Solutions

Commonly used IV solutions and their abbreviations are:

Solution	*Abbreviation*
Water	W
Saline	S
Normal saline	NS
Dextrose	D
Ringer's	R
Lactated Ringer's	LR

READING LABELS: DROP FACTOR

From Figure 10-4, answer the following questions:

1. What is the calibration in drops per milliliter (drop factor) for each of the infusion sets?

   a. _____

   b. _____

   c. _____

2. Which is/are macrodrip set(s)? _____

3. Which is/are microdrip (minidrip) set(s)? _____

(**Note:** See Appendix G for answer key.)

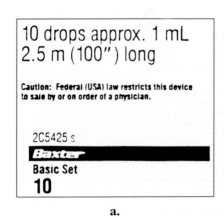

a.

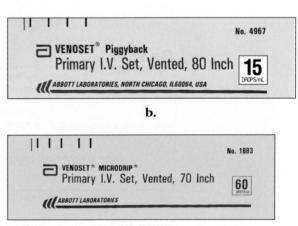

b.

c.

Figure 10-4 *(Part a courtesy of Baxter Healthcare Corporation, Deerfield, IL. **Note:** This product labeling is a sample and is subject to change at any time. Be sure to read the directions for use accompanying the product. Parts b and c photography courtesy of Abbott Laboratories)*

**READING IV
LABELS**

Refer to Figure 10-5.

1. What is the total amount of solution in the container? _____

2. What percentage of the solution is dextrose? _____ (this IV solution would be abbreviated D5W)

3. What is the name of the manufacturer? _____

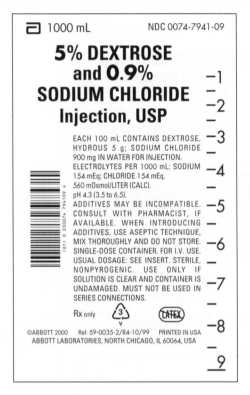

Figure 10-5 *(Photography courtesy of Abbott Laboratories)*

Refer to Figure 10-6.

1. What is the total amount of solution in the container? _____

2. What percentage of the solution is sodium chloride?* _____

    *This percentage solution is also called normal saline and orders may be written using the abbreviation NS.

> 250 ml
> 0.9% Sodium Chloride
> Inj., USP

Figure 10-6

Refer to Figure 10-7.

1. What is the total amount of solution in the container? _____

2. What percentage of the solution is dextrose? _____ (this IV solution would be abbreviated D5LR)

3. What other chemical ingredients does the solution contain? _____

(**Note:** See Appendix G for answer key.)

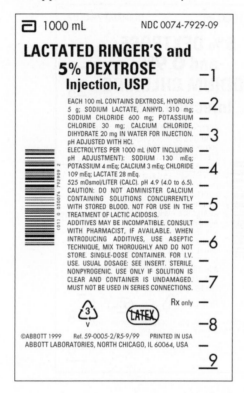

Figure 10-7 *(Photography courtesy of Abbott Laboratories)*

INTERMITTENT IV DRUG ADMINISTRATION

Various methods may be utilized to administer medications by the intravenous route. These include addition of a medication to the solution container of an existing (primary) IV line or to the mini bag container of an attached secondary line (called a piggyback infusion); or by bolus injection (IV push) through a peripheral (saline) lock or a central venous catheter.

IV Piggyback (IVPB)

Medications may be given intravenously by adding a secondary infusion line to an existing IV line. This is called the piggyback method and may be used to administer medications that are ordered at regularly scheduled times (i.e., intermittent drug administration) (e.g., q 6 hr).

Medications administered via piggyback usually are diluted in 50–100 mL of solution. They may be infused simultaneously or alternately with a primary infusion. The piggyback set includes a small IV bottle or bag (mini bag), a drip chamber, and short tubing with a spike that is inserted into the primary line through a special port, Figure 10-8.

Volume Control Set

This is a special infusion set designed to administer small amounts of fluid over a specified time period or to eliminate the possibility of accidentally infusing a greater volume of fluid or medication than is safe for the client. It consists of a small fluid chamber, drip chamber, and tubing and can be used as either a primary or secondary infusion line, Figure 10-9. The fluid chamber (burette) holds 100 mL or more, to which medications can be added through a medication port. The drip chamber is calibrated at 60 gtt per mL (micro- or minidrip) and the IV flow rate is regulated by adjusting the clamp below this chamber. These sets often are referred to by their brand names such as Buretrol, Volutrol, and Metriset.

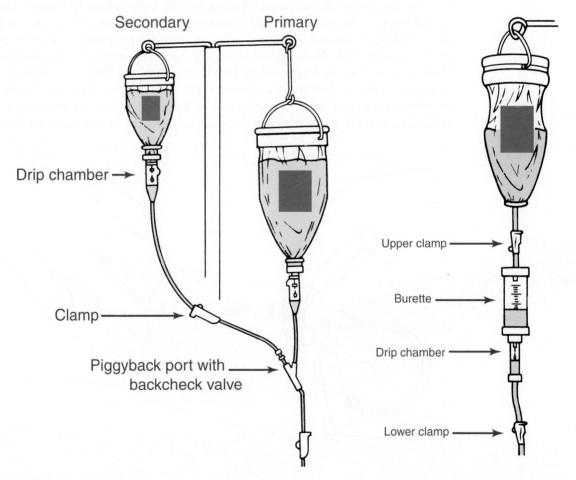

Figure 10-8 *IV piggyback*

Figure 10-9 *IV volume control set*

Peripheral Lock

The peripheral lock, also called P-lock, is a device that serves as an intermittent IV line. It may be used for administration of regularly scheduled IV medications for clients who do not also require parenteral fluids, thus eliminating the need for a continuous IV. In addition, a P-lock may be inserted for the purpose of administering IV medications that are incompatible with solutions or drugs concurrently being given IV through a primary line.

The lock consists of an IV catheter that terminates in a connecting device to which a cannula and syringe can be attached for the administration of medication at designated times, Figure 10-10. Alternatively, a mini bag and tubing can be attached for an IVPB. Because the catheter remains in the vein, it must be flushed periodically with saline to prevent clot formation and to maintain patency. In some instances, depending on hospital policy or provider's order, diluted heparin is injected following the saline flush. (The peripheral lock sometimes is referred to as the saline lock.)

Implanted Ports

Intravascular devices that can serve as infusion ports for long-term IV therapy (lasting several weeks to several years) can be surgically implanted into a large vein, such as the subclavian or femoral, or into an artery. As with the peripheral lock, medication can be injected or IV fluids infused through a latex diaphragm at designated times. These infusion ports are often used for long-term treatment such as chemotherapy, total parenteral nutrition (TPN), or long-term antibiotics. They are particularly useful for the infusion of irritant medications. Because of the length of time the needle remains in the vein, periodic flushing is essential, especially prior to and following medication

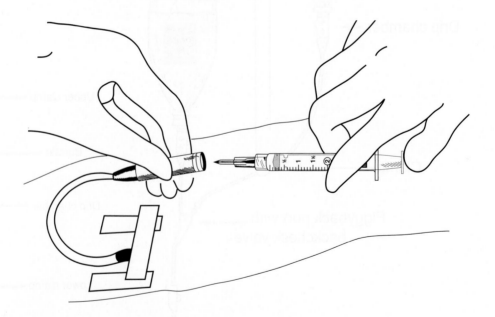

Figure 10-10 Peripheral lock

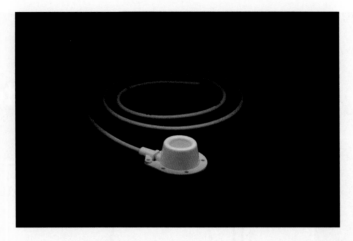

Figure 10-11 *Vortex LP chest port (Image courtesy of RITA Medical Systems)*

injection. As a rule, both saline and heparin are used for flushing. A specialized (90° angle) needle, called the Huber needle, is used for injection and flushing. The Vortex LP, pictured in Figure 10-11 is one type of chest port.

Central Venous Catheter

Medications can be infused through a catheter that is inserted into a major vein and usually advanced from this vein into the superior vena cava. If the catheter also is to be used for measuring central venous pressure, it is directed through the vena cava into or just proximal to the right atrium. Because the catheter is left in place, it can be used for a continuous or intermittent infusion line. Veins most commonly used for central venous lines are the subclavian and the external jugular, although the brachial and femoral veins are alternative routes.

A very useful modification of the central venous catheter is a multilumen catheter that permits a variety of treatment and monitoring procedures to be performed via a single venipuncture site.

One such device is pictured in Figure 10-12. This catheter, which contains three lumens, can be used in place of multiple central and peripheral lines for clients who require a multiplicity of intravenous therapy and monitoring, often several procedures simultaneously. This versatile central venous catheter provides routes for fluid administration, TPN, blood sampling, central venous pressure monitoring, and medication administration, including simultaneous infusion of incompatible drugs.

The multilumen catheter must be flushed periodically with saline to maintain patency of lumens that are used intermittently. The procedure is similar to that used with the peripheral lock. A lumen that is being used for a continuous IV infusion does not need to be flushed.

Another type of central venous catheter is called a peripherally inserted central catheter (PICC). This catheter, which comes in a variety of lengths and is available as a single-lumen or multiple-lumen device is designed for either long- or short-term use.

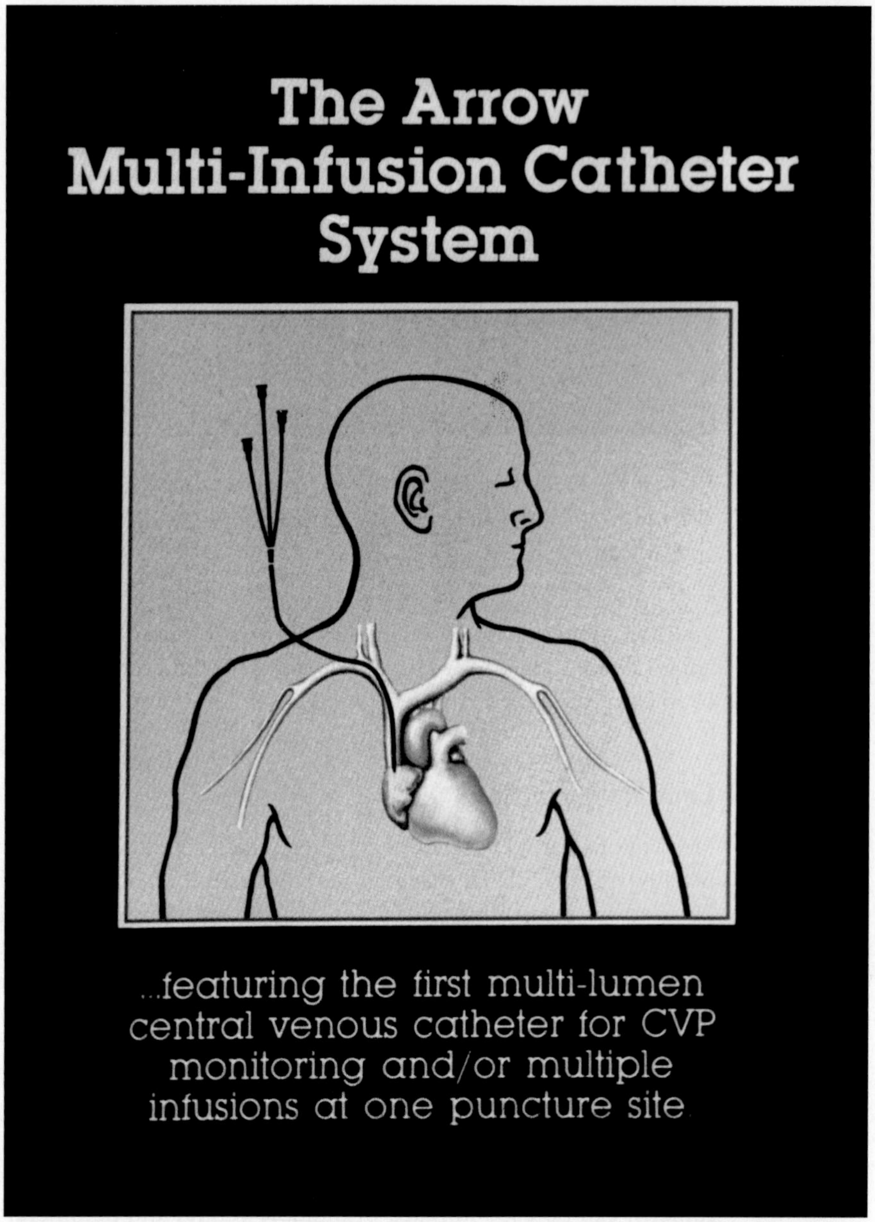

The Arrow Multi-Infusion Catheter System

...featuring the first multi-lumen central venous catheter for CVP monitoring and/or multiple infusions at one puncture site

Figure 10-12 *Multilumen central venous catheter for CVP monitoring or multiple infusions at one puncture site (Courtesy of Arrow International, Inc., Reading, PA)*

Because of its small diameter, it can be inserted into a peripheral vein, typically the basilic or cephalic vein, and threaded up toward the heart, usually as far as the subclavian vein or superior vena cava.

One advantage of the PICC line is that it does not require surgical insertion. Because it is easy to insert and maintain, the PICC line is being increasingly utilized over more invasive and expensive devices.

Flushing protocol is determined by agency policy and is similar to that used for other central venous catheter devices.

ELECTRONIC INFUSION DEVICES

Electronic infusion devices, sometimes referred to as EIDs, help provide accuracy and safety in administration of IV therapy. Rate controllers automatically regulate the drop rate of infusions wherein the force of gravity provides the needed pressure to maintain fluid flow, Figure 10-13. IV regulator pumps use positive pressure, which can be varied or adjusted as needed, to automatically deliver infusions at the ordered rate and volume, Figure 10-14.

A syringe pump, also called a mini infuser, is sometimes used when a small amount of medication (e.g., up to 60 mL) is administered. The medication is infused from a syringe that is inserted into the apparatus, Figure 10-15.

Pumps and controllers have a variety of mechanisms for automatically regulating drop rate and fluid volume and for providing warning alarms when there is a problem with the infusion or equipment. For example, the EID pictured in Figure 10-14 has alert/alarms indicating dose out of range, air in IV line, downstream occlusion, completion of IV, and other malfunctions.

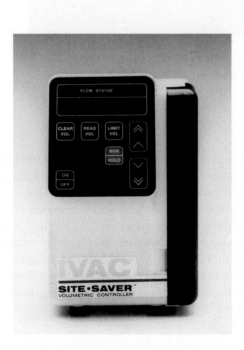

Figure 10-13 *Volumetric controller (Courtesy IVAC Corporation, San Diego, CA)*

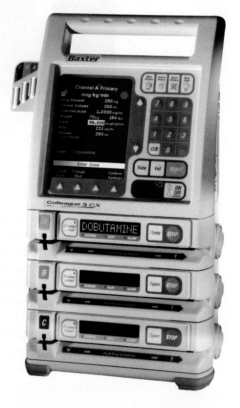

Figure 10-14 *Colleague CX electronic infusion device (Courtesy of Baxter Healthcare Corporation, Deerfield, IL)*

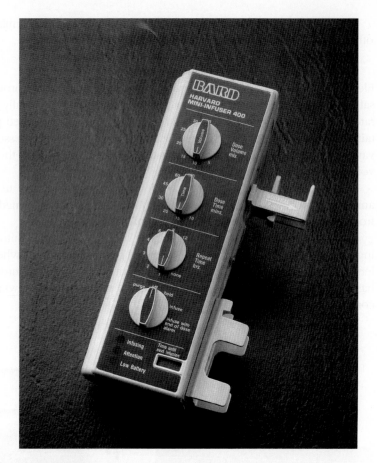

Figure 10-15 *Harvard mini infuser (Courtesy Bard® Med Systems Division, North Reading, MA)*

Pumps are available in a variety of sizes, some small enough to be used as ambulatory infusion devices that are powered by batteries and are particularly suitable for ambulatory clients and patient-controlled analgesia (PCA).

Infusions are ordered as to volume and rate, and nurses are responsible for setting and adjusting the infusion device and monitoring the infusion. The infusion rate, site, and client response should be monitored hourly, more often if problems arise.

If electronic (automatic) devices are not in use and the gravity flow system is utilized, the nurse manually sets and adjusts the flow rate to the desired drops per minute by use of a roller-clamp on the IV tubing. In this case, it is necessary to convert the ordered volume and rate to drops per minute.

Section II: Calculation of IV Flow Rate and Infusion Times

CALCULATION OF INTRAVENOUS FLOW RATES, INFUSION TIMES, INFUSION RATE, AND BOLUS USING DIMENSIONAL ANALYSIS

In calculating the flow rate for *drops per minute*, one minute becomes the labeled value that must be converted to an equivalent value: number of drops. *One minute*, therefore, is the starting factor and *drops* is the answer unit and these, as in all dimensional analysis conversions, form an equivalent relationship.

It is essential in calculating flow rate to know the drop factor. This refers to the size of the drop delivered by the particular infusion set being used: the number of drops required to make 1 mL. The drop factor always will be stated in practice problems requiring calculation of drops per minute.

Rounding Off

The rate of flow should be rounded to the nearest whole number.

1. 31.6 gtt per min; adjust to 32 gtt per min
2. 42.3 gtt per min; adjust to 42 gtt per min
3. 56.8 mL per hr; adjust to 57 mL per hr
4. 120.4 mL per hr; adjust to 120 mL per hr

CALCULATION OF IV FLOW RATE IN GTT PER MIN

EXAMPLE   **Order:** 1000 mL of D5W (5% Dextrose in water) IV to infuse over a period of 5 hr

Drop Factor: 10 gtt per mL

Starting Factor   Answer Unit
   1 min   gtt

Equivalents: 1000 mL = 5 hr, 10 gtt = 1 mL, 60 min = 1 hr

Conversion Equation:

$$1 \text{ min} \times \frac{1 \text{ hr}}{60 \text{ min}} \times \frac{1000 \text{ mL}}{5 \text{ hr}} \times \frac{10 \text{ gtt}}{1 \text{ mL}} = 33.3 = 33 \text{ gtt}$$

Flow Rate: 33 gtt per min

EXAMPLE   **Order:** 1500 mL of Sodium Chloride 0.9% (0.9% Sodium Chloride Solution) to infuse at a rate of 90 mL per hr

Drop Factor: 20 gtt per mL

Starting Factor   Answer Unit
   1 min   gtt

Equivalents: 90 mL = 1 hr, 20 gtt = 1 mL, 60 min = 1 hr

Conversion Equation:

$$1 \text{ min} \times \frac{1 \text{ hr}}{60 \text{ min}} \times \frac{90 \text{ mL}}{1 \text{ hr}} \times \frac{20 \text{ gtt}}{1 \text{ mL}} = 30 \text{ gtt}$$

Flow Rate: 30 gtt per min

EXAMPLE   **Order:** 1000 mL of 5% D $\frac{1}{2}$ NSS (5% Dextrose in $\frac{1}{2}$ Normal Saline Solution) to infuse at a rate of 100 mL per hr

Drop Factor: 60 gtt per mL

Starting Factor	Answer Unit
1 min	gtt

Equivalents: 100 mL = 1 hr, 60 gtt = 1 mL, 60 min = 1 hr

Conversion Equation:

$$1 \text{ min} \times \frac{1 \text{ hr}}{60 \text{ min}} \times \frac{100 \text{ mL}}{1 \text{ hr}} \times \frac{60 \text{ gtt}}{1 \text{ mL}} = 100 \text{ gtt}$$

*Flow rate: 100 gtt per min

***Note:** When using any infusion set having a drop factor of 60 gtt per mL (sometimes written as: drop factor microdrip), the flow rate per minute *always* will be the same as the number of mL per hour. For example:
Order: 50 mL per hr; flow rate: 50 gtt per min
Order: 70 mL per hr; flow rate: 70 gtt per min
Therefore, the flow rate calculation can be omitted for mL per hr.

Keep in mind that when a microdrip infusion set (60 gtt per mL) is used, the total number of drops per min will be much larger than when a macrodrip set is used (10–20 gtt per mL).

The abbreviation KVO stands for keep vein open (or TKO = to keep open). This means that the IV is to run at a very slow rate simply to have an infusion route available for emergency use or intermittent administration of drugs. A microdrip infusion set usually is used. A typical flow rate, which may vary according to hospital policy, is 10–20 mL per hr.

It can be seen from the box above that no calculation is necessary for a KVO order, because the flow rate will be the same as the stated mL per hr; in this case, 10–20 gtt per min.

EXAMPLE   **Order:** 500 mL D5W IV KVO at 10 mL per hr

Drop Factor: 60 gtt per mL (microdrip)

Starting Factor	Answer Unit
1 min	gtt

Equivalents: 60 min = 1 hr, 60 gtt = 1 mL, 10 mL = 1 hr

Conversion Equation:

$$1 \text{ min} \times \frac{1 \text{ hr}}{60 \text{ min}} \times \frac{10 \text{ mL}}{1 \text{ hr}} \times \frac{60 \text{ gtt}}{1 \text{ mL}} = 10 \text{ gtt}$$

Flow rate: 10 gtt per min

Note that the calculated flow rate of 10 gtt per minute is identical to the ordered flow rate of 10 mL per hour due to the cancellation of drop and minute values thus illustrating why the computation can be omitted for this type of order.

PRACTICE

Calculation of IV Flow Rate in gtt per min

1. *Order:* 1500 mL of D5W IV to infuse in 8 hr
   Drop Factor: 10 gtt per mL

2. *Order:* 1000 mL NS to infuse in 10 hr
   Drop Factor: 15 gtt per mL

3. *Order:* 800 mL 5% glucose in water in 4 hr
   Drop Factor: 15 gtt per mL

4. *Order:* 700 mL D5W IV in 5 hr
   Drop Factor: 10 gtt per mL

5. *Order:* 2500 mL 5% Dextrose in 0.45 NS IV in 24 hr
   Drop Factor: 20 gtt per mL

6. *Order:* 1250 mL D 2.5 W IV in 6 hr
   Drop Factor: 15 gtt per mL

PRACTICE

Calculation of IV Flow Rate in gtt per min (Continued)

7. *Order:* 500 mL Sodium Chloride 0.9% IV in 3 hr
   Drop Factor: 10 gtt per mL

8. *Order:* 100 mL Ringer's IV in 4 hr
   Drop Factor: 15 gtt per mL

9. *Order:* 300 mL D5W IV in 3 hr
   Drop Factor: 60 gtt per mL

10. *Order:* 50 mL Serum Albumin IV to infuse in 1 hr
    Drop Factor: 15 gtt per mL

11. *Order:* 1000 mL Ringer's IV to infuse at a rate of 125 mL per hr
    Drop Factor: 15 gtt per mL
    What should the flow rate be per minute?

12. *Order:* 1000 mL D5W IV to infuse at a rate of 100 mL per hr
    Drop Factor: 10 gtt per mL
    What should the flow rate be per minute?

PRACTICE

Calculation of IV Flow Rate in gtt per min (Continued)

13. ***Order:*** 1500 mL Sodium Chloride 0.9% IV to infuse at a rate of 150 mL per hr

Drop Factor: 15 gtt per mL

What should the flow rate be per minute?

14. ***Order:*** 2000 mL of D2.5W IV to infuse at a rate of 125 mL per hr

Drop Factor: 10 gtt per mL

What should the flow rate be per minute?

15. ***Order:*** 500 mL Isolyte M IV to infuse at a rate of 125 mL per hr

Drop Factor: 60 gtt per mL

What should the flow rate be per minute?

16. ***Order:*** Hyperalimentation (TPN) 1000 mL D20W IV to infuse at a rate of 80 mL per hr

Drop Factor: 15 gtt per mL

What should the flow rate be per minute?

17. ***Order:*** Hyperalimentation (TPN) 1000 mL Aminosyn 3.5% IV to infuse at a rate of 40 mL per hr

Drop Factor: 20 gtt per mL

What should the flow rate be per minute?

(***Note:*** See Appendix G for answer key.)

CALCULATION OF IV FLOW RATE IN ML PER HR

Electronic infusion pumps are useful because they maintain a more accurate flow rate than is possible with the standard IV (gravity) administration set. They are especially suitable for administering low hourly infusions, for example, 5 mL or less, 20 mL or less, for clients at risk for fluid overload. In addition, high-volume infusions, for example, over 150 mL per hr, that require specific hourly rates can be administered accurately and on time. Flow rates that are ordered in mL per hour are calculated as follows:

EXAMPLE   **Order:** 500 mL D5$\frac{1}{2}$NS IV to infuse at a 10 hr rate (i.e., over a period of 10 hr). Use an infusion pump.

How many mL per hr should be administered?

Starting Factor	Answer Unit
1 hr	mL

Equivalents: 500 mL = 10 hr

Conversion Equation:

$$1 \, \cancel{hr} \times \frac{500 \, mL}{10 \, \cancel{hr}} = 50 \, mL$$

PRACTICE

Calculation of the Number of mL per hr That Will Infuse

1. *Order:* 1000 mL 5% D/NS IV to infuse at an 8 hr rate

2. *Order:* 500 mL Lactated Ringer's IV to infuse at a 6 hr rate

3. *Order:* 1500 mL 2.5% D 0.45 NaCl IV to infuse at a 12 hr rate

4. *Order:* 250 mL D 2.5W IV to infuse at a 2 hr rate

PRACTICE

Calculation of the Number of mL per hr That Will Infuse (Continued)

5. *Order:* 2500 mL NS IV to infuse at a 24 hr rate

6. *Order:* Hyperalimentation (TPN) 2000 mL Liposyn II 20% IV to infuse in 24 hr

7. *Order:* Hyperalimentation (TPN) 3000 mL Aminosyn 8.5% IV to infuse in 24 hr

(***Note:*** See Appendix G for answer key.)

CALCULATION OF INFUSION TIME

Dimensional analysis can be used to calculate the anticipated length of time required for an infusion to be completed. (**Note:** When doing these problems, carry answers to hundredths and round to tenths. Convert to hr or min.)

EXAMPLE   **Order:** 1500 mL D2.5W IV
Drop Factor: 15 gtt per mL
Flow Rate: 40 gtt per min
How many hours will it take for the IV to infuse?
In this problem, the value sought is the length of time required to infuse a certain amount. The unit of time, therefore, becomes the answer unit. The quantity that will be converted to a unit of time (1500 mL) becomes the starting factor. The conversion equation is set up and solved in the usual manner.

Starting Factor   Answer Unit
1500 mL   hours

Equivalents: 15 gtt = 1 mL, 40 gtt = 1 min, 60 min = 1 hr
Conversion Equation:

$$1500 \text{ mL} \times \frac{15 \text{ gtt}}{1 \text{ mL}} \times \frac{1 \text{ min}}{40 \text{ gtt}} \times \frac{1 \text{ hr}}{60 \text{ min}} = 9.4 \text{ hr}$$

Convert 0.4 hr to min

Starting Factor   Answer Unit
0.4 hr   min

Equivalents: 60 min = 1 hr

Conversion Equation:

$$0.4 \text{ hr} \times \frac{60 \text{ min}}{1 \text{ hr}} = 24 \text{ min}$$

Therefore: 9.4 hr = 9 hr 24 min

PRACTICE

Calculation of Infusion Time

1. *Order:* 1500 mL Lactated Ringer's IV

Drop Factor: 10 gtt per mL

Flow Rate: 20 gtt per min

How long should it take the IV to infuse?

2. *Order:* 750 mL D10W IV

Drop Factor: 15 gtt per mL

Flow Rate: 21 gtt per min

How long should it take the IV to infuse?

3. *Order:* 500 mL of Sodium Chloride 0.9% IV

Drop Factor: 60 gtt per mL

Flow Rate: 125 gtt per min

How long should it take the IV to infuse?

PRACTICE

Calculation of Infusion Time (Continued)

4. *Order:* 2000 mL D5W

   Drop Factor: 15 gtt per mL

   Flow Rate: 34 gtt per min

   How long should it take the IV to infuse?

5. *Order:* 1000 mL D2.5NS IV

   Drop Factor: 10 gtt per mL

   Flow Rate: 23 gtt per min

   How long should it take the IV to infuse?

(***Note:*** See Appendix G for answer key.)

Section III: Adding Medications to IV Fluids and Calculating Flow Rates

CALCULATION OF FLOW RATE (GTT/MIN) WHEN IV CONTAINS MEDICATION

The IV flow rate is calculated the same whether or not medication has been added to the IV container. If medication is to be added, however, the additional numbers in the order may cause confusion in determining the conversion factors. It is, therefore, essential to carefully inspect the information given and select the correct equivalents for the conversion equation.

EXAMPLE   **Order:** Ampicillin 500 mg in 50 mL of Sodium Chloride 0.9% to infuse in 1 hr

Drop Factor: 60 gtt per mL

Starting Factor   Answer Unit
1 min   gtt

Equivalents: 50 mL = 1 hr, 60 gtt = 1 mL, 60 min = 1 hr

Conversion Equation:

$$1 \text{ min} \times \frac{1 \text{ hr}}{60 \text{ min}} \times \frac{50 \text{ mL}}{1 \text{ hr}} \times \frac{60 \text{ gtt}}{1 \text{ mL}} = 50 \text{ gtt}$$

Flow Rate: 50 gtt/min

(*Note:* The medication (Ampicillin 500 mg) that is added to the total amount of IV solution (50 mL) and the 0.9% NaCl are not pertinent to the computation of the flow rate and are not included in the conversion equation.)

PRACTICE

Calculation of Flow Rate When IV Contains Medication

1. *Order:* 1000 mL D5NS with KCl 40 mEq IV to infuse in 4 hr
   Drop Factor: 15 gtt per mL

2. *Order:* 250 mL D5W with Aminophylline 0.5 g IV to infuse in 2 hr
   Drop Factor: 60 gtt per mL

3. *Order:* Geopen (carbenicillin disodium) 2 g in 50 mL Sodium Chloride 0.9% to infuse in 30 min
   Drop Factor: 15 gtt per mL

4. *Order:* Erythromycin 500 mg in 100 mL D5W to infuse in 20 min
   Drop Factor: 10 gtt per mL

5. *Order:* Cleocin (clindamycin) 600 mg in 100 mL D5W to infuse in 60 min
   Drop Factor: 20 gtt per mL

(*Note:* See Appendix G for answer key.)

ADDING MEDICATIONS TO INTRAVENOUS FLUIDS

Intravenous medications can be administered in several ways. They may be added directly to a traditional IV setup, called a primary line, for continuous drip. For intermittent doses (e.g., every 8 or 12 hours), medications may be added to a second line that is then connected to the primary line, or they may be infused through a central venous line. Medications also can be injected directly into a vein (IV bolus) using a syringe and needle; through a primary line via the flashball or a Y-port; or through a peripheral lock. The medication order should state clearly the desired IV route of administration.

If two or more medications are added to the same IV, it is essential that the substances be compatible. The person mixing and adding substances to an IV has responsibility for ascertaining compatibility. Information about drug compatibility is obtained from the pharmacist, a drug reference book, the manufacturer's product insert, or a drug incompatibility chart.

Whenever a substance is added to an IV, the container must be labeled with the corresponding name, dosage, date, and time. A safety rule to observe when adding medications to an IV is to prepare the medication **before** the IV container is labeled. Add the medication, check once more to be sure the correct drug and amount has been added, then affix the label to the IV container.

Medications that are dispensed in liquid form may be added to the IV container through a medication port for infusion or through the tubing or peripheral lock for injection. Medications that are dispensed as dry powders or crystals must be reconstituted just prior to infusion or injection. Instructions for reconstitution are printed in the package insert or on the medication label. Reconstitution and mixing of intravenous medications usually is done by a registered pharmacist in a controlled area (for example, under laminar air flow hood) in the pharmacy. In some instances, nurses may reconstitute medication, add medication to existing infusions, or both.

Remember that only solvents designated in the directions should be used for reconstitution, because these have been determined to be compatible with this particular drug. In addition, when reconstituted drugs are added to IV solutions, it is likewise essential that drug and solution are compatible.

Adding Drugs to IVs and Calculating Flow Rate in gtt/min

EXAMPLE **Order:** Vibramycin 75 mg in 1000 mL Normosol-M in D5W IV to run in 24 hr

Label: Vibramycin (doxycycline hyclate) 100 mg

Directions for reconstitution: Add 10 mL sterile water for injection to yield a concentration of 10 mg per mL.

1. How much of the reconstituted solution must be added to the IV bottle to provide the ordered dose of Vibramycin 75 mg?

Equivalent: 10 mg = 1 mL

Conversion Equation: $75 \text{ mg} \times \dfrac{1 \text{ mL}}{10 \text{ mg}} = 7.5 \text{ mL}$

Add Vibramycin 7.5 mL to 1000 mL Normosol-M in D5W.

2. What should the flow rate be for this IV order?

Drop Factor: 15 gtt per mL

Equivalents: 1000 mL = 24 hr, 60 min = 1 hr, 15 gtt = 1 mL

Conversion Equation:

$$1 \text{ min} \times \frac{1 \text{ hr}}{60 \text{ min}} \times \frac{1000 \text{ mL}}{24 \text{ hr}} \times \frac{15 \text{ gtt}}{1 \text{ mL}} = 10.4 = 10 \text{ gtt}$$

EXAMPLE   **Order:** Ticar 3 g in 100 mL Lactated Ringer's IV to run in 2 hr

Label: Ticar (ticarcillin disodium) 3 g

Directions for reconstituting: Add 12 mL sterile water for injection to yield a concentration of 200 mg per mL.

1. How much of the reconstituted solution must be added to the IV bottle to provide the ordered dose of Ticar 3 g?

Equivalents: 1 g = 1000 mg   200 mg = 1 mL

Conversion Equation:

$$3 \text{ g} \times \frac{1000 \text{ mg}}{1 \text{ g}} \times \frac{1 \text{ mL}}{200 \text{ mg}} = 15 \text{ mL}$$

Add Ticar 15 mL to 100 mL Lactated Ringer's solution.

2. What should the flow rate be for this IV order?

Drop Factor: 60 gtt per mL

Equivalents: 1 hr = 60 min   100 mL = 2 hr   60 gtt = 1 mL

Conversion Equation:

$$1 \text{ min} \times \frac{1 \text{ hr}}{60 \text{ min}} \times \frac{100 \text{ mL}}{2 \text{ hr}} \times \frac{60 \text{ gtt}}{1 \text{ mL}} = 50 \text{ gtt}$$

PRACTICE

Adding Drugs to IVs and Calculating Flow Rate in gtt per min

1. *Order:* Kefzol 350 mg in 100 mL 5% D/LR IV to run in 60 min.

Label: Figure 10-16. What is the generic name? _____

Drop Factor: 15 gtt/mL

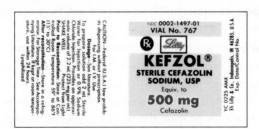

Figure 10-16 *(Courtesy of Eli Lilly Pharmaceuticals, Indianapolis, IN)*

Adding Drugs to IVs and Calculating Flow Rate in gtt per min (Continued)

a. How much diluent must be added to the vial to reconstitute the drug for intravenous use?

b. How much of the resulting solution must be added to the IV bottle to provide the ordered dose of Kefzol 350 mg?

c. What should the flow rate be for this IV order?

2. *Order:* Folic Acid 12 mg in 500 mL D5W in 4 hours

   Label: Figure 10-17

   Drop Factor: 60 gtt per mL

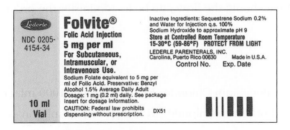

Figure 10-17 *(Courtesy of Lederle Laboratories, Pearl River, NY)*

a. How many mL of Folvite must be added to the IV bottle to provide the ordered dose?

b. What should the flow rate be for this IV order?

PRACTICE

Adding Drugs to IVs and Calculating Flow Rate in gtt per min (Continued)

3. **Order:** Ampicillin Sodium 150 mg in 1000 mL M/6 Sodium Lactate IV to infuse at a rate of 150 mL per hr

   Label: Figure 10-18. What is the trade name? _____

   Drop Factor: 15 gtt per mL

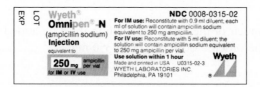

Figure 10-18 *(Courtesy of Wyeth Laboratories, Philadelphia, PA)*

   a. How many mL of Ampicillin Sodium must be added to the IV bottle to provide the total ordered dose?

   b. What should the flow rate be to administer the ordered number of mL per hr?

4. **Order:** Potassium Chloride (KCl) 30 mEq in 1000 mL D5NS IV in 6 hr

   Label: Potassium Chloride (KCl) injection 40 mEq in 20 mL vial, Figure 10-19

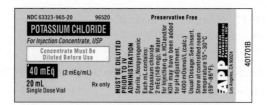

Figure 10-19 *(Courtesy of American Pharmaceutical Partners, Schaumberg, IL)*

(**Note:** This medication is already in solution; therefore, reconstitution is not necessary.)

   Drop Factor: 10 gtt per mL

Adding Drugs to IVs and Calculating Flow Rate in gtt per min (Continued)

a. How many mL of this medication must be added to the IV bottle to provide the ordered dose?

b. What should the flow rate be for this IV order?

5. *Order:* Tetracycline 150 mg in 100 mL Sodium Chloride 0.9% to infuse in 40 min via Volutrol

Label: Tetracycline 250 mg

Directions: Dilute with 5 mL sterile water for injection and add to ordered IV solution.

Drop Factor: 60 gtt per mL

a. How many mL of the reconstituted solution should be added to the IV solution?

b. What should the flow rate be for this IV order?

6. *Order:* Cefoxitin Sodium 2 g IV in 100 mL Lactated Ringer's Solution to infuse in 60 min

Label: Cefoxitin Sodium 2 g

Directions: Reconstitute with 20 mL sterile water for injection to yield 2 g per 21 mL.

Drop factor: 60 gtt per mL

What should the flow rate be?

7. *Order:* Ampicillin Sodium 250 mg IVPB in 100 mL D5W to infuse in 60 min

Label: Ampicillin Sodium 1 g

Directions: Reconstitute with 3.5 mL sterile water for injection to yield 1 g per 4 mL.

Drop Factor: 10 gtt per mL

Adding Drugs to IVs and Calculating Flow Rate in gtt per min (Continued)

    a. How many mL of the reconstituted solution should be added to the IV solution?

    b. What should the flow rate be?

8. *Order:* Coly-Mycin M 100 mg in 500 mL D5W to infuse at 5 mg per hr

    Label: Coly-Mycin M (colistimethate sodium) 150 mg

    Directions: Reconstitute with 2 mL sterile water for injection to yield 75 mg per mL and add to IV solution.

    Drop factor: 60 gtt per mL

    a. How many mL of reconstituted solution should be added to the IV solution?

    b. What should the flow rate be?

9. *Order:* Mithracin 1534 mcg in 1000 mL D5W to infuse in 6 hr

    Label: Mithracin (plicamycin) 2.5 mg

    Directions: Reconstitute with 4.9 mL of sterile water for injection to yield 0.5 mg per mL and add to IV solution.

    Drop Factor: 60 gtt per mL

    a. How many mL of reconstituted Mithracin should be added to the ordered IV solution?

    b. What should the flow rate be?

PRACTICE

Adding Drugs to IVs and Calculating Flow Rate in gtt per min (Continued)

10. **Order:** Penicillin G Potassium 5 million units in 100 mL D5W IV to infuse over 1 hr

    Label: Penicillin G Potassium 20,000,000 units dry powder

    Directions: Reconstitute with 31.6 mL sterile water for injection to yield concentration of 500,000 units per mL.

    Drop Factor: 15 gtt per mL

    a. How many mL of the reconstituted Penicillin G should be added to the 100 mL D5W?

    b. What should the flow rate be?

(**Note:** See Appendix G for answer key.)

Section IV: Special Applications of IV Therapy

CRITICAL CARE IV CALCULATIONS

Adding Drugs to IVs and Calculating the Drug Infusion Rate

The provider may order the IV medication to be infused at the rate of a specified concentration (amount) of drug per unit of time. We call this the *drug infusion rate*.

The drug infusion rate can be calculated in terms of either:

    a. *volume of solution* per unit of time (e.g., mL per hr or mL per min)

        OR

    b. *concentration of drug* per unit of time (e.g., mg, mcg, units per hr or min).

EXAMPLE   A drug infusion rate of 2.5 units per hr means that:

    1. the IV flow rate (volume per unit of time) that will infuse 2.5 units of the drug per hour must be determined.

           OR

    2. the concentration of drug contained in a specified amount of solution per hour must be determined.

Because these are usually potent drugs that require the most accurate method of infusion, they are administered using an electronic infusion device, such as a volumetric pump or controller, or a syringe pump. These devices automatically infuse the correct amount per hour or per minute.

EXAMPLE **Order:** Heparin 20,000 units in 500 mL Sodium Chloride 0.9% IV to infuse at 1200 units per hr. Use an infusion pump.

How many mL per hr should be administered?

Starting Factor	Answer Unit
1 hr	mL

Equivalents: 1200 units = 1 hr   20,000 units = 500 mL

Conversion Equation:

$$1 \text{ hr} \times \frac{1200 \text{ units}}{1 \text{ hr}} \times \frac{500 \text{ mL}}{20,000 \text{ units}} = 30 \text{ mL}$$

Flow Rate: 30 mL per hr

Set the infusion pump at the gtt per min setting that corresponds to 30 mL per hr.

EXAMPLE **Order:** Heparin 20,000 units in 500 mL Sodium Chloride 0.9% IV to infuse at 30 mL per hr

How many units will be infused per hour?

Starting Factor	Answer Unit
1 hr	units

Equivalents: 30 mL = 1 hr   20,000 units = 500 mL

Conversion Equation:

$$1 \text{ hr} \times \frac{30 \text{ mL}}{1 \text{ hr}} \times \frac{20,000 \text{ units}}{500 \text{ mL}} = 1200 \text{ units}$$

EXAMPLE **Order:** Aminophylline 280 mg in 350 mL D5W into central venous catheter. Infuse 250 mL in 75 min and the remainder at 20 mL per hr. Use an infusion pump.

Label: See Figure 10-20.

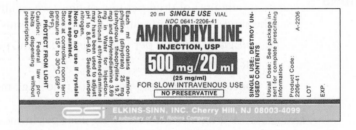

Figure 10-20 *(Courtesy of Elkins-Sinn Pharmaceuticals, Cherry Hill, NJ)*

1. How many mL of medication should be added to the IV bottle?

Equivalents: 500 mg = 20 mL

Conversion Equation:

$$280 \text{ mg} \times \frac{20 \text{ mL}}{500 \text{ mg}} = 11.2 \text{ mL}$$

Answer: Add Aminophylline 11.2 mL to 350 mL D5W.

2. How many mg would the client receive per minute at the infusion rate of 250 mL per 75 min?
Equivalents: 250 mL = 75 min   350 mL = 280 mg
Conversion Equation:

$$1 \text{ min} \times \frac{250 \text{ mL}}{75 \text{ min}} \times \frac{280 \text{ mg}}{350 \text{ mL}} = 2.7 \text{ mg}$$

3. Determine the mL per hr to which the infusion pump should be set to infuse the first 250 mL of IV solution at the ordered rate.
Equivalents: 60 min = 1 hr   250 mL = 75 min
Conversion Equation:

$$1 \text{ hr} \times \frac{60 \text{ min}}{1 \text{ hr}} \times \frac{250 \text{ mL}}{75 \text{ min}} = 200 \text{ mL}$$

Answer: Regulate the infusion pump to deliver 200 mL per hr.

4. How long will it take to infuse the remaining solution at the ordered rate?
Equivalent: 20 mL = 1 hr
Conversion Equation:

$$100 \text{ mL} \times \frac{1 \text{ hr}}{20 \text{ mL}} = 5 \text{ hr}$$

EXAMPLE   **Order:** Heparin 1000 units per hr via IV pump from Heparin 30,000 units in 500 mL D5W. How many mL per hr should be administered?
Equivalents: 1 hr = 1000 units, 30,000 units = 500 mL
Conversion Equation:

$$1 \text{ hr} \times \frac{1000 \text{ units}}{1 \text{ hr}} \times \frac{500 \text{ mL}}{30,000 \text{ units}} = 16.6 = 17 \text{ mL}$$

PRACTICE

Calculation of the Volume of Solution or Concentration of Drug

1. *Order:* Pitocin 25 units in 1000 mL Sodium Chloride 0.9% IV to infuse at a drug infusion rate of 2.5 units per hr

Label: Pitocin (oxytocin) 10 units per mL

a. How many mL of Pitocin must be added to the IV bottle?

b. How many mL per hr should be administered?

PRACTICE

Calculation of the Volume of Solution or Concentration of Drug (Continued)

2. *Order:* Humulin R Insulin 100 units in 500 mL Sodium Chloride 0.9% to infuse at 5 units per hr via IV pump

   How many mL per hr should be administered?

3. *Order:* Morphine Sulfate 100 mg in 250 mL D5W to infuse at 3.2 mg per hr via IV pump

   How many mL per hr should be administered?

4. *Order:* Heparin 20,000 units in 1000 mL Sodium Chloride 0.9% to infuse at 1000 units per hr via IV pump

   How many mL per hr should be administered?

5. *Order:* Minocin (minocycline) 100 mg in 500 mL D5W to infuse at 20 mg per hr via IV pump

   How many mL per hr should be administered?

6. *Order:* Coly-Mycin-M 150 mg in 100 mL D5W to infuse in 60 minutes (via IV mini-bottle/saline lock)

   Label: Coly-Mycin-M (colestimethate sodium) 150 mg

   Directions: Reconstitute with 2 mL sterile water for injection to yield 75 mg per mL and add to ordered amount of IV solution.

   How many mL per hr should be administered?

PRACTICE

Calculation of the Volume of Solution or Concentration of Drug (Continued)

7. *Order:* Cefizox 1 g in 50 mL Ringer's Solution IV to infuse in 30 min via IV pump

   Label: Cefizox (ceftizoxime sodium) 1 g

   Directions: Reconstitute with 10 mL sterile water for injection to yield 1 g per 10.7 mL.

   How many mL per hr should be administered via the IV pump?

8. *Order:* Pipracil 2 g in 100 mL D5W IV to infuse in 30 min

   Label: Pipracil (piperacillin sodium) 2 g

   How many mL per hr should be administered via the IV pump?

9. *Order:* Cleocin 300 mg IV (Buretrol) in 50 mL D5W to infuse at dose rate of 30 mg per min (use an infusion pump)

   Label: Cleocin (clindamycin) 300 mg per 2 mL

   Directions: Dilute in 50 mL of D5W and administer via volume control set.

   a. Determine the mL per hr to which the infusion pump should be set.

   b. At this rate, how many minutes will it take to infuse the ordered 50 mL?

10. *Order:* Heparin 2500 units per hr via IV pump from Heparin 50,000 units in 1000 mL D5W

    How many mL per hr should be administered?

Calculation of the Volume of Solution or Concentration of Drug (Continued)

11. *Order:* Lidocaine 2 g in 500 mL D5W to infuse at 60 mL per hr via IV pump

How many mg will infuse in 1 min?

12. *Order:* Isuprel (isoproterenol hydrochloride) 2 mg in 500 mL D5W to infuse at 45 mL per hr via IV pump

How many mcg will infuse in 1 min?

13. *Order:* Cordarone Intravenous 360 mg in 500 mL D5W to infuse at 85 mL per hr via IV pump

How many mg will infuse in 1 hr?

14. *Order:* Dopamine 400 mg in 250 mL D5W to infuse at 60 mL per hr via IV pump

How many mg will infuse in 1 hr?

15. *Order:* Aminophylline 250 mg in 250 mL D5W into central venous catheter. Infuse 200 mL in 45 minutes and the remainder at 17 mL per hr. Use an IV pump.

Label: Aminophylline 250 mg per 10 mL

a. How many mL of medication should be added to the IV bottle?

b. Determine the mL per hr to which the IV pump should be set to infuse the first 200 mL of solution at the ordered rate.

PRACTICE

Calculation of the Volume of Solution or Concentration of Drug (Continued)

    c. How long will it take to infuse the remaining solution at the ordered rate?

16. **Order:** Magnesium Sulfate 20 g in 1000 mL D5W IV via pump. Infuse 600 mL in 90 min and the remainder (400 mL) at 50 mL per hr.

    Label: Magnesium Sulfate 5 g per 10 mL

    a. How many mL should be added to the IV?

    b. How many g would the client receive per minute at the infusion rate of 600 mL per 90 min?

    c. Determine the mL per hr to which the IV pump should be set to infuse the first 600 mL of solution at the ordered rate.

    d. How long will it take to infuse the remaining solution at the ordered rate?

17. **Order:** Ritadrine Hydrochloride 150 mg in 500 mL Ringer's IV (via IV pump) to infuse at 0.1 mg per min and increase by 0.05 mg per min every 10 min until uterine contractions cease

    Label: Ritadrine Hydrochloride 50 mg per 5 mL

    a. How many mL of the medication should be added to the IV bottle?

PRACTICE

Calculation of the Volume of Solution or Concentration of Drug (Continued)

b. What is the concentration of the resulting solution per mL (i.e., mg of Ritadrine per mL)?

c. How many mL per hr should be administered to infuse the initial dose of 0.1 mg per min?

d. Ten minutes later, the flow rate should be increased to how many mL per hr to infuse the ordered dose (0.1 mg + 0.05 mg = 0.15 mg)?

e. Ten minutes later, the flow rate should be increased to how many mL per hr to infuse the ordered dose (0.15 mg + 0.05 mg = 0.2 mg)?

(*Note:* See Appendix G for answer key.)

Calculating IV Dosage and Flow Rate Based on Body Weight

IV medications may be ordered according to a *specified amount* (e.g., mcg per kg of body weight) to be administered within a *specified unit* of time (e.g., per minute). The medication is added to a *specified volume* and type of IV solution. The total desired dose per minute must first be determined and then the infusion rate calculated that will administer the correct mL per hr or gtt per min.

EXAMPLE **Order:** Infuse Nipride (nitroprusside sodium) 50 mg in 250 mL D5W at 3 mcg/kg/min.
Weight: 215 lb
Drop Factor: 60 gtt per mL

1. How many mcg per min must be administered?

$$215 \text{ lb} \times \frac{1 \text{ kg}}{2.2 \text{ lb}} \times \frac{3 \text{ mcg per min}}{1 \text{ kg}} = 293.2 \text{ mcg per min}$$

2. How many mL per hr will provide the required dose?

$$1 \text{ hr} \times \frac{60 \text{ min}}{1 \text{ hr}} \times \frac{293.2 \text{ mcg}}{1 \text{ min}} \times \frac{1 \text{ mg}}{1000 \text{ mcg}} \times \frac{250 \text{ mL}}{50 \text{ mg}} = 87.9 = 88 \text{ mL per hr}$$

3. How many gtt per min will provide the required dose?

$$1 \text{ min} \times \frac{293.2 \text{ mcg}}{1 \text{ min}} \times \frac{1 \text{ mg}}{1000 \text{ mcg}} \times \frac{250 \text{ mL}}{50 \text{ mg}} \times \frac{60 \text{ gtt}}{1 \text{ mL}} = 87.9 = 88 \text{ gtt per min}$$

*OR

$$215 \text{ lb} \times \frac{1 \text{ kg}}{2.2 \text{ lb}} \times \frac{3 \text{ mcg}}{1 \text{ kg}} \times \frac{1 \text{ mg}}{1000 \text{ mcg}} \times \frac{250 \text{ mL}}{50 \text{ mg}} \times \frac{60 \text{ gtt}}{1 \text{ mL}} = 87.9 = 88 \text{ gtt per min}$$

4. How many mcg per gtt will be administered?

$$1 \text{ gtt} \times \frac{1 \text{ min}}{88 \text{ gtt}} \times \frac{293.2 \text{ mcg}}{1 \text{ min}} = 3.3 \text{ mcg per gtt}$$

*_Note:_ When calculating gtt per min, the step of calculating mcg per min can be omitted.

EXAMPLE **Order:** Infuse Heparin 10,000 units in 250 mL D5W at 0.4 units/kg/min.
Weight: 59 kg
Drop Factor: 60 gtt per mL

1. How many units per min must be administered?

$$59 \text{ kg} \times \frac{0.4 \text{ units per min}}{1 \text{ kg}} = 23.6 \text{ units per min}$$

2. How many mL per hr will provide the required dose?

$$1 \text{ hr} \times \frac{60 \text{ min}}{1 \text{ hr}} \times \frac{23.6 \text{ units}}{1 \text{ min}} \times \frac{250 \text{ mL}}{10,000 \text{ units}} = 35 \text{ mL per hr}$$

3. How many gtt per min will provide the required dose?

$$1 \text{ min} \times \frac{23.6 \text{ units}}{1 \text{ min}} \times \frac{250 \text{ mL}}{10,000 \text{ units}} \times \frac{60 \text{ gtt}}{1 \text{ mL}} = 35 \text{ gtt per min}$$

OR

$$59 \text{ kg} \times \frac{0.4 \text{ units}}{1 \text{ kg}} \times \frac{250 \text{ mL}}{10,000 \text{ units}} \times \frac{60 \text{ gtt}}{1 \text{ mL}} = 35 \text{ gtt per min}$$

4. How many units per gtt will be administered?

$$1 \text{ gtt} \times \frac{1 \text{ min}}{35 \text{ gtt}} \times \frac{23.6 \text{ units}}{1 \text{ min}} = 0.7 \text{ units per gtt}$$

IV Flow Rate and Dosages Based on Body Weight

1. *Order:* Infuse Amrinone 250 mg in 500 mL D5W at 5 mcg/kg/min.

Weight: 202 lb

Drop Factor: 60 gtt per mL

   a. How many mcg per min must be administered?

   b. How many mL per hr will provide the required dose?

   c. How many gtt per min will provide the required dose?

   d. How many mcg per gtt will be administered?

2. *Order:* Infuse Dobutamine 250 mg in 250 mL D5W at 7 mcg/kg/min.

Weight: 73.6 kg

Drop Factor: 60 gtt per mL

   a. How many mcg per min must be administered?

   b. How many mL per hr will provide the required dose?

IV Flow Rate and Dosages Based on Body Weight (Continued)

    c. How many gtt per min will provide the required dose?

    d. How many mcg per gtt will be administered?

3. ***Order:*** Infuse Nitroprusside 50 mg in 250 mL D5W at 1.5 mcg/kg/min.
Weight: 198 lb
Drop Factor: 60 gtt per mL
    a. How many mcg per min must be administered?

    b. How many mL per hr will provide the required dose?

    c. How many gtt per min will provide the required dose?

    d. How many mcg per gtt will be administered?

4. ***Order:*** Intropin (dopamine hydrochloride) 800 mg in 250 mL D5W at 8 mcg/kg/min
Weight: 72.8 kg

IV Flow Rate and Dosages Based on Body Weight (Continued)

Drop Factor: 60 gtt per mL

   a. How many mcg per min must be administered?

   b. How many mL per hr will provide the required dose?

   c. How many gtt per min will provide the required dose?

   d. How many mcg per gtt will be administered?

5. *Order:* Infuse Dobutamine 250 mg in 150 mL D5W at 5 mcg/kg/min.

Weight: 83.2 kg

Drop Factor: 60 gtt per mL

   a. How many mcg per min must be administered?

   b. How many mL per hr will provide the required dose?

   c. How many gtt per min will provide the required dose?

PRACTICE

IV Flow Rate and Dosages Based on Body Weight (Continued)

d. How many mcg per gtt will be administered?

(*Note:* See Appendix G for answer key.)

Titrated Infusions

Some very potent drugs are administered according to the client's physiologic responses to the medication. That is, the dose is increased or decreased until the desired effect has been achieved. This effect may be raising or lowering the blood pressure, controlling arrhythmias or seizures, relieving chest pain, or treating other often life-threatening situations.

The technique of adjusting dose/flow rate to obtain a precise desired effect is called *titration*. Examples of drugs administered by titration include dopamine, nitroprusside, nitroglycerin, lidocaine, oxytocin, and magnesium sulfate.

Titrated drugs are given IV, either continuous or intermittent, depending on the volume or frequency of administration, or both, and equipment available. Small volume infusions may be administered via syringe or peripheral lock, and large volume infusions via an IV line, usually with a controlled volume infusion set and always using an electronic infusion device, such as a controller or a volumetric or syringe pump.

Titrated drug orders are written as a range of dosage between which the therapeutic dosage for the client should fall (e.g., 5–10 mcg/kg/min). It is necessary, therefore, to determine the IV flow rates that will administer the upper and lower limits of the ordered range of dosage. The gtt per min or mL per hr may be increased or decreased depending on the client's response to the current flow rate, not exceeding the upper limit. Administration is initiated at the lowest dosage and adjusted upward as needed.

In addition, titration calculations can be used to determine the amount of drug infusing at a given time (e.g., any time a flow rate adjustment is made). Because titrated infusions require frequent dosage adjustments, it follows that the electronic infusion device settings must be readjusted simultaneously. Titration is continued until the desired effect is achieved.

Several steps are necessary for calculating titrated infusions. Each step can be performed by using dimensional analysis, thus eliminating the need to memorize a confusing array of formulas. Each of the following steps has been presented in the preceding section; they are now arranged in the correct sequence for titration.

Steps in calculating titrated infusions:

1. Determine the amount of drug that will administer the upper and lower limits of the ordered titration range.

2. Determine the flow rate (mL per hr or gtt per min) that will administer the upper and lower limits of the ordered titration range. (Remember that when the drop factor is 60, the mL per hr and gtt per min are identical.)

3. Determine needed increases or decreases of flow rate as indicated by the client's physiologic response.

4. Determine the amount of drug infusing after adjustments in flow rate.

EXAMPLE **Order:** Infuse Nipride (nitroprusside) 50 mg in 250 mL D5W. Titrate 3–6 mcg/kg/min to maintain the systolic blood pressure at 150 mm Hg. Weight: 135 lb

  1. How many mcg per min will administer the ordered range of titration?
    Lower (3 mcg/kg/min):
    Equivalents: 1 kg = 2.2 lb   1 kg = 3 mcg per min
    Conversion Equation:

$$135 \text{ lb} \times \frac{1 \text{ kg}}{2.2 \text{ lb}} \times \frac{3 \text{ mcg per min}}{1 \text{ kg}} = 184 \text{ mcg per min}$$

    Upper (6 mcg/kg/min):
    Equivalents: 1 kg = 2.2 lb   1 kg = 6 mcg per min
    Conversion Equation:

$$135 \text{ lb} \times \frac{1 \text{ kg}}{2.2 \text{ lb}} \times \frac{6 \text{ mcg per min}}{1 \text{ kg}} = 368 \text{ mcg per min}$$

    The range of dosage for this client is 184–368 mcg per min.

  2. How many mL per hr or gtt per min will administer the ordered range of titration?
    Lower:
    Equivalents: 1 hr = 60 min   1 min = 184 mcg
    50 mg = 250 mL   1mg = 1000 mcg
    Conversion Equation:

$$1 \text{ hr} \times \frac{60 \text{ min}}{1 \text{ hr}} \times \frac{184 \text{ mcg}}{1 \text{ min}} \times \frac{1 \text{ mg}}{1000 \text{ mcg}} \times \frac{250 \text{ mL}}{50 \text{ mg}}$$
$$= 55 \text{ mL per hr or } 55 \text{ gtt per min}$$

    Upper:
    Equivalents: 1 hr = 60 min   1 min = 368 mcg per min   50 mg = 25 mL   1 mg = 1000 mcg
    Conversion Equation:

$$1 \text{ hr} \times \frac{60 \text{ min}}{1 \text{ hr}} \times \frac{368 \text{ mcg}}{1 \text{ min}} \times \frac{1 \text{ mg}}{1000 \text{ mcg}} \times \frac{250 \text{ mL}}{50 \text{ mg}}$$
$$= 110 \text{ mL per hr or } 110 \text{ gtt per min}$$

    The range of mL per hr and gtt per min for this IV is 55–110 mL per hr or 55–110 gtt per min.

3. The present systolic blood pressure reading is 170 mm Hg, indicating the dosage needs to be increased. Increase the lower limit (mL per hr) by 5 mL. How many mcg per min will the client now be receiving?

Equivalents: 1 hr = 60 min   1 hr = 60 mL

50 mg = 250 mL   1 mg = 1000 mcg

Conversion Equation:

$$1 \text{ min} \times \frac{1 \text{ hr}}{60 \text{ min}} \times \frac{60 \text{ mL}}{1 \text{ hr}} \times \frac{50 \text{ mg}}{250 \text{ mL}} \times \frac{1000 \text{ mcg}}{1 \text{ mg}} = 200 \text{ mcg per min}$$

4. After 1 hr, the systolic blood pressure reading is 120 mm Hg, indicating the dosage needs to be decreased. Decrease the lower limit (mL per hr) by 6 mL. How many mcg per min will the client be receiving?

Equivalents: 1 hr = 54 mL   1 hr = 60 min

50 mg = 250 mL   1 mg = 1000 mcg

Conversion Equation:

$$1 \text{ min} \times \frac{1 \text{ hr}}{60 \text{ min}} \times \frac{54 \text{ mL}}{1 \text{ hr}} \times \frac{50 \text{ mg}}{250 \text{ mL}} \times \frac{1000 \text{ mg}}{1 \text{ mg}} = 180 \text{ mcg per min}$$

PRACTICE

Titration Infusions

1. **Order:** Infuse Esmolol Hydrochloride 500 mL D5W. Titrate 50–100 mcg/kg/min to maintain the systolic blood pressure at 120 mm Hg.

   Weight: 140 lb

   a. How many mcg per min will administer the ordered range of titration?
   Lower (50 mcg/kg/min):

   Upper (100 mcg/kg/min):

   b. How many mL per hr or gtt per min will administer the ordered range of titration?
   Lower:

   Upper:

Titration Infusions (Continued)

    c. The present systolic blood pressure reading is 160 mm Hg. Increase the lower limit (mL per hr) by 5 mL. How many mcg per min will the client now be receiving?

2. *Order:* Infuse Dopamine 400 mg in 500 mL D5W. Titrate 5–10 mcg/kg/min to maintain the systolic blood pressure greater than 100 mm Hg.

    Weight: 175 lb

    a. How many mcg per min will administer the ordered range of titration?
    Lower (5 mcg/kg/min):

    Upper (10 mcg/kg/min):

    b. How many mL per hr or gtt per min will administer the ordered range of titration?
    Lower:

    Upper:

    c. The present systolic blood pressure reading is 68 mm Hg. Increase the lower limit (mL per hr) by 10 mL. How many mcg per min will the client now be receiving?

3. *Order:* Infuse Amrinone Lactate 250 mg in 50 mL NS. Titrate 5–10 mcg/kg/min to maintain the diastolic blood pressure below 90 mm Hg.

    Weight: 70 kg

    a. How many mcg per min will administer the ordered range of titration?
    Lower (5 mcg/kg/min):

    Upper (10 mcg/kg/min):

PRACTICE

Titration Infusions (Continued)

b. How many mL per hr or gtt per min will administer the ordered range of titration?
Lower:

Upper:

c. The present diastolic blood pressure reading is 100 mm Hg. Increase the lower limit (mL per hr) by 2 mL. How many mcg per min will the client now be receiving?

4. *Order:* Infuse Nitropress (nitroprusside sodium) 50 mg in 500 mL D5W. Titrate 1.5–3 mcg/kg/min to maintain the systolic blood pressure at 100 mm Hg.

Weight: 200 lb

a. How many mcg per min will administer the ordered range of titration?
Lower (1.5 mcg/kg/min):

Upper (3 mcg/kg/min):

b. How many mL per hr or gtt per min will administer the ordered range to titration?
Lower:

Upper:

c. The present systolic blood pressure reading is 90 mm Hg. Decrease the lower limit (mL per hr) by 5 mL. How many mcg per min will the client now be receiving?

5. *Order:* Infuse Dopamine Hydrochloride 200 mg in 500 mL D5W. Titrate 2–5 mcg/kg/min to maintain the systolic blood pressure at a minimum of 100 mm Hg.

Weight: 165 lb

PRACTICE

Titration Infusions (Continued)

a. How many mcg per min will administer the ordered range of titration?
Lower (2 mcg/kg/min):
Upper (5 mcg/kg/min):

b. How many mL per hr or gtt per min will administer the ordered range of titration?
Lower:

Upper:

c. The present systolic blood pressure reading is 80 mm Hg. Increase the lower limit (mL per hr) by 5 mL. How many mcg per min will the client now be receiving?

(*Note:* See Appendix G for answer key.)

Drugs Administered by IV Bolus

When a small amount of medication is injected directly into a vein, it is called an IV bolus or IV push. A venipuncture can be performed in any accessible vein and the medication injected by means of a syringe. If an IV is already in place, the medication can be injected through a Y-port or the flashball at the end of the infusion tubing. An IV bolus also can be given through the peripheral lock. Some infusion pumps are designed to deliver an IV bolus at a controlled rate.

Because drugs given by IV bolus will have an immediate effect, the rate of injection becomes extremely important. **Administering IV injections too quickly can result in adverse side effects or speed shock, or both.** Many drugs are ordered to be injected over a period of 1–30 minutes. On the other hand, some drugs must be given rapidly, even within a period of seconds, because an immediate effect is desired or necessary. It is, therefore, essential to determine the correct IV injection rate and to time this accurately using a clock or wristwatch with a second hand. The need for precision in this regard cannot be overemphasized.

EXAMPLE   **Order:** Chloromycetin 300 mg IV bolus via peripheral lock
Label: Chloromycetin (chloramphenicol) 1 g
Directions: Reconstitute with 10 mL sterile water for injection to yield 100 mg per mL. Safe injection rate is 1 g per min.
   1. How many mL of Chloromycetin should be administered?
      Equivalents: 1 g = 10 mL   1000 mg = 1 g

Conversion Equation:

$$300 \text{ mg} \times \frac{1 \text{ g}}{1000 \text{ mg}} \times \frac{10 \text{ mL}}{1 \text{ g}} = 3 \text{ mL}$$

2. How many seconds should it take to administer this IV bolus?

Equivalents: 1 g = 10 mL   1000 mg = 1 g   60 sec = 1 min

Conversion Equation:

$$3 \text{ mL} \times \frac{1 \text{ g}}{10 \text{ mL}} \times \frac{1 \text{ min}}{1 \text{ g}} \times \frac{60 \text{ sec}}{1 \text{ min}} = 18 \text{ sec}$$

OR

$$300 \text{ mg} \times \frac{1 \text{ g}}{1000 \text{ mg}} \times \frac{1 \text{ min}}{1 \text{ g}} \times \frac{60 \text{ sec}}{1 \text{ min}} = 18 \text{ sec}$$

PRACTICE

IV Bolus

1. **Order:** Metoprolol tartrate injectable 5 mg IV bolus via P-lock

   Label: Metoprolol tartrate injectable 1 mg per 1 mL

   Directions: Safe injection rate is 3 mg per 60 sec.

   a. How many mL should be injected?

   b. How long should it take to administer this IV bolus?

2. **Order:** Naloxone 0.6 mg IV bolus via primary infusion line

   Label: Figure 10-21

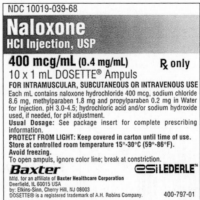

Figure 10-21 (*Courtesy of Baxter Healthcare Corporation, Deerfield, IL*)

IV Bolus (Continued)

Directions: Do not exceed rate of 0.5 mg per min for IV bolus.

  a. How many mL of Naloxone should be administered?

  b. How long should it take to administer this IV bolus of Naloxone?

3. *Order:* Demerol 30 mg IV bolus via Y-tube/primary line

  Label: Figure 10-22

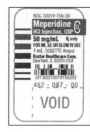

Figure 10-22 *(Courtesy of Baxter Healthcare Corporation, Deerfield, IL)*

Directions: Do not exceed rate of 25 mg per min for IV bolus.

  a. What is the total amount of solution to be injected?

  b. How long should it take to administer this IV bolus?

4. *Order:* Furosemide 35 mg IV bolus via peripheral lock

  Label: Figure 10-23

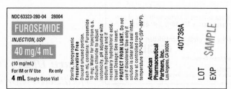

Figure 10-23 *(Courtesy of American Pharmaceutical Partners, Los Angeles, CA)*

PRACTICE

IV Bolus (Continued)

Directions: Administer undiluted. Maximum injection rate = 20 mg per min.

a. What is the total amount of solution to be injected?

b. How long should it take to administer this IV bolus?

5. **Order:** Aminophylline 240 mg IV bolus via peripheral lock

   Label: Aminophylline 25 mg per mL

   Directions: Do not exceed rate of 25 mg per min for IV bolus.

   a. How many mL of aminophylline should be administered?

   b. How long should it take to administer this IV bolus of aminophylline into the peripheral lock?

6. **Order:** Bretylium 5 mg per kg IV bolus

   Label: Bretylium 500 mg per mL

   Directions: Do not exceed injection rate of 25 mg per min.

   a. How many mg should be administered via bolus? (client weighs 135 lb)

   b. How many mL would the bolus contain?

PRACTICE

IV Bolus (Continued)

    c. How long should it take to administer this bolus?

7. **Order:** Lidocaine 1 mg per kg IV bolus. Follow by Lidocaine drip 1000 mg per 250 mL of D5W and run at 2 mg per min.

Label: Bolus-Lidocaine (1%) 10 mg per mL

Label: IV-Lidocaine (20%) 200 mg per mL

Directions: Do not exceed injection rate of 35 mg per min.

    a. How many mg of Lidocaine (1%) would be administered via bolus? (client weighs 170 lb)

    b. How many mL would the bolus contain?

    c. How long should it take to administer this bolus?

    d. How many mL of Lidocaine (20%) should be added to the IV?

    e. How many mL per hr should be administered IV?

(**Note:** See Appendix G for answer key.)

PARENTERAL NUTRITION

When nutritional needs cannot be met by enteral intake, supplementary or total nutrition can be provided via parenteral routes. Basic nutrients, electrolytes, and vitamins, as well as fluid requirements, can be administered intravenously through a peripheral or central vein. Choice of route depends on tonicity or concentration of the solution, as well as anticipated duration of parenteral nutrition administration.

Terms associated with parenteral nutrition include:

TPN: total parenteral nutrition—all nutrients essential for tissue maintenance are provided intravenously.

CPN: refers to IV nutrition via a central vein, usually the superior vena cava. The terms *TPN* and *CPN* often are used interchangeably.

PTPN: peripheral total parenteral nutrition (or PPN—peripheral parenteral nutrition) refers to IV nutrition via a peripheral vein, usually the radial, basilic, or cephalic vein of the arm.

Hyperalimentation: refers to the provision of nutrients in excess of maintenance needs.

Regardless of the route used for administration, it is important to remember that parenteral nutrition solutions are natural culture mediums for bacterial growth and should not hang in excess of 12 hr.

Nutrition calculations can be used to determine the amounts of nutrients and energy contained in a parenteral nutrition formula (IV solution). Generally, they are concerned with the caloric value, expressed as kilocalories (kcal) of the glucose, amino acid, or fat emulsion content of the IV solution.

Equivalents necessary for setting up the conversion equations include:

*1 g glucose = 3.4 kcal

1 g amino acid (protein) = 4 kcal

1 g of 10% fat emulsion = 1.1 kcal

1 g of 20% fat emulsion = 2 kcal

In a percentage solution, the symbol % refers to *parts of substance (solid) per 100 parts of solution* (liquid) (i.e., a 1% solution would contain 1 g of solid in 100 mL of liquid). See Appendix F, Percentage Solutions: Equivalent Units for Solids and Liquids.

Thus:

a 5% solution indicates 5 g per 100 mL

a 2.5% solution indicates 2.5 g per 100 mL

***Note:** kcal values for intravenous CHO and fat are different from the kcal values for the same orally ingested nutrients. Protein values are unchanged.

4 kcal per g of CHO (carbohydrate)

4 kcal per g of protein

9 kcal per g of fat

EXAMPLE   **Order:** TPN 1000 mL D5W (carbohydrate), 500 mL Liposyn II 10% (fat), 500 mL Aminosyn 3.5% (protein) IV

How many kcal of carbohydrates, fats, and proteins are provided by this IV?

Carbohydrates:

Equivalents: 5 g = 100 mL   1 g = 3.4 kcal

Conversion Equation:

$$1000 \text{ mL} \times \frac{5 \text{ g}}{100 \text{ mL}} \times \frac{3.4 \text{ kcal}}{1 \text{ g}} = 170 \text{ kcal}$$

Fats:

Equivalents: 10 g = 100 mL   1 g = 1.1 kcal

Conversion Equation:

$$500 \text{ mL} \times \frac{10 \text{ g}}{100 \text{ mL}} \times \frac{1.1 \text{ kcal}}{1 \text{ g}} = 55 \text{ kcal}$$

Protein:

Equivalents: 3.5 g = 100 mL   1 g = 4 kcal

Conversion Equation:

$$500 \text{ mL} \times \frac{3.5 \text{ g}}{100 \text{ mL}} \times \frac{4 \text{ kcal}}{1 \text{ g}} = 70 \text{ kcal}$$

PRACTICE

Nutrition Calculations

1. *Order:* TPN 1500 mL D5W IV

   How many kcal of carbohydrate are provided?

2. *Order:* TPN 1000 mL Aminosyn 3.5% IV

   How many kcal of protein are provided?

3. *Order:* CPN 1000 mL Liposyn II 10% IV

   How many kcal of fat are provided?

Nutrition Calculations (Continued)

4. *Order:* TPN 500 mL 2.5% Dextrose in Water IV

How many kcal of carbohydrate are provided?

5. *Order:* PTPN 1500 mL Aminosyn PF 7% IV

How many kcal of protein are provided?

6. *Order:* TPN 2500 mL D10W IV

How many kcal of carbohydrate are provided?

7. *Order:* CPN 1500 mL Intralipid 20% IV

How many kcal of fat are provided?

8. *Order:* TPN 3000 mL 20% Dextrose in Water IV

How many kcal of carbohydrate are provided?

9. *Order:* TPN 1000 mL Aminosyn II 5% and 500 mL 25% Dextrose in Water IV

   a. How many kcal of protein are provided?

PRACTICE

Nutrition Calculations (Continued)

b. How many kcal of carbohydrates are provided?

10. *Order:* TPN 1000 mL Aminosyn II 4.25% and 1000 mL D10W IV

  a. How many kcal of protein are provided?

  b. How many kcal of carbohydrate are provided?

(***Note:*** See Appendix G for answer key.)

Section V: Assessment and Adjustment of IVs

One of the major responsibilities of the nurse who is caring for clients with intravenous infusions is observation and assessment. The flow rate is assessed by counting the drops per minute (gtt per min) and determining what adjustments need to be made in the event the rate has changed. A checklist, such as the example in Figure 10-24, may be useful in performing the IV assessment.

A variety of factors can affect the flow rate, including positional changes that may alter the angle of the needle or catheter, a clot that partially obstructs the infusion flow, improper height of the container, tubing dangling below insertion site, dislodgement of needle or clamp, and infiltration or irritation at the insertion site.

Regardless of the infusion system used (e.g., gravity [infusion], controller, or pump), nursing assessment is of prime importance, because early observation and correction of undesirable factors are essential to maintain the infusion at the designated rate and to prevent adverse occurrences. Even if the IV is attached to an automatic infusion pump or controller, frequent observation is necessary to be sure the system is working properly and the desired flow rate is being maintained.

Although the previous section dealt with the use of dimensional analysis to calculate the initial flow rate, most nurses will be much more frequently involved with maintaining IV infusions than starting them. This involves periodic observation of the amount of fluid remaining to be infused and recalculation of the flow rate to determine if adjustments need to be made to complete the IV within the ordered time pe-

---

IV Assessment

Client Initials _____ Room # _____

Name of IV fluid being infused _____

_____

#mL left in bag/bottle _____

Flow rate: _____   mL per hr or _____ gtt per min

Without disturbing dressing, what is condition of IV site?_____

_____

What time do you anticipate the IV bag will need to be changed? _____

What IV solution will be hung next? _____

Figure 10-24 IV assessment

riod. Dimensional analysis lends itself equally well to determining the need for adjustment of the flow rate when any of the previously mentioned factors have caused it to speed up or slow down.

EXAMPLE • **Starting IV**

Order: 1000 mL of Sodium Chloride 0.9% to infuse over a period of 8 hr.

Drop Factor: 15 gtt per mL

Question: What should the flow rate be when the IV is started?

Answer:

$$1 \text{ min} \times \frac{1 \text{ hr}}{60 \text{ min}} \times \frac{1000 \text{ mL}}{8 \text{ hr}} \times \frac{15 \text{ gtt}}{1 \text{ mL}} = 31 \text{ gtt}$$

• **Assessing the IV**

After the IV has been running 5 hr, there are still 450 mL left to infuse. Does the IV flow rate need to be adjusted to complete the infusion in the ordered time period?

Two factors must be noted in this problem. First, the total amount of solution is now 450 mL; second, the total number of hours remaining is 3. The conversion equation is written exactly as before, substituting the new values in the conversion factor mL per hr.

$$1 \text{ min} \times \frac{1 \text{ hr}}{60 \text{ min}} \times \frac{450 \text{ mL}}{3 \text{ hr}} \times \frac{15 \text{ gtt}}{1 \text{ mL}} = 37.5 = 38 \text{ gtt}$$

• **Adjusting the IV**

The IV flow rate must be adjusted to 38 gtt per min.

REMEMBER

Although minor adjustments in flow rate are permissible (usually less than 25% increase over the initial flow rate), larger increases require a provider's order. One exception is in the administration of parenteral nutrition when any flow rate increase could be hazardous. Whenever there is a question, consult the provider.

PRACTICE

Adjusting IVs (Calculate in gtt/min)

1. **Order:** 2500 mL of D5W IV to infuse over a period of 12 hr

   Drop Factor: 10 gtt per mL

   a. What should the flow rate be when the IV is started?

   b. After the IV has been running 8 hours, there are still 800 mL left to infuse. To what should the flow rate be adjusted to have the IV completed on schedule?

2. **Order:** 1000 mL Lactated Ringer's IV in 6 hr

   Drop Factor: 15 gtt per mL

   a. What should the initial flow rate be?

   b. After 4 hr, 350 mL remain. To what should the flow rate be adjusted to have the IV completed on schedule?

PRACTICE

Adjusting IVs (Calculate in gtt/min) (Continued)

3. *Order:* 3000 mL D5W IV in 24 hr

Drop Factor: 20 gtt per mL

   a. What should the initial flow rate be?

   b. After 18 hr, 600 mL remain. What should the adjusted flow rate be?

4. *Order:* 1500 mL D2.5W IV in 12 hr

Drop Factor: 10 gtt per mL

   a. What should the initial flow rate be?

   b. After 7 hr, 800 mL remain. What should the adjusted flow rate be?

5. *Order:* 500 mL Sodium Chloride 0.9% IV in 8 hr

Drop Factor: 60 gtt per mL

   a. What should the initial flow rate be?

   b. After 5 hr, 150 mL remain. What should the adjusted flow rate be?

PRACTICE

Adjusting IVs (Calculate in gtt/min) (Continued)

6. **Order:** 750 mL Ringer's IV in 4 hr

   Drop Factor: 10 gtt per mL

   a. What should the initial flow rate be?

   b. After $2\frac{1}{2}$ hr, 300 mL remain. What should the adjusted flow rate be?

7. **Order:** 2000 mL D5W IV in 18 hr

   Drop Factor: 15 gtt per mL

   a. What should the initial flow rate be?

   b. After 11 hr, 900 mL remain. What should the adjusted flow rate be?

8. **Order:** 250 mL Isolyte M IV in 5 hr

   Drop Factor: 60 gtt per mL

   a. What should the initial flow rate be?

   b. After 2 hr, 120 mL remain. What should the adjusted flow rate be?

PRACTICE

Adjusting IVs (Calculate in gtt/min) (Continued)

9. **Order:** 1250 mL D2.5NS IV in 9 hr

   Drop Factor: 15 gtt per mL

   a. What should the initial flow rate be?

   b. After 3 hr, 750 mL remain. What should the adjusted flow rate be?

10. **Order:** 125 mL Sodium Chloride 0.9% in 2 hr IV

    Drop Factor: 60 gtt per mL

    a. What should the initial flow rate be?

    b. After $1\frac{1}{2}$ hr, 30 mL remain. What should the adjusted flow rate be?

(**Note:** See Appendix G for answer key.)

CHAPTER 11

Administration of Intravenous Medications and Solutions

OBJECTIVES

Upon completion of this chapter, you should be able to:

- Identify safe and suitable sites for intravenous injections and infusions.
- Identify nursing responsibilities in relation to administering, assessing, and monitoring intravenous injections and infusions.
- Follow infection-control guidelines with respect to safe handling or manipulation of IV equipment.
- Identify performance criteria related to IV medications and solutions.

INTRAVENOUS ADMINISTRATION

A variety of methods can be used when medications or fluids are given intravenously. The traditional method was a gravity-flow infusion system regulated by a simple controller clamp. This method is still used, to some extent, in an emergency situation, or when a mechanical regulator is not available. Currently, infusions are regulated by a variety of electronic pumps or controllers. Infusions are employed for the purpose of administering fluids and medications directly into the blood rather than via the gastrointestinal route. Infusions, referred to as IVs, can be continuous or intermittent. Intermittent infusions may be administered via IV piggyback, a volume control set, or some type of vascular access device, for example, a peripheral lock or port or a central venous catheter.

Implantation or insertion of most intravascular devices requires specialized knowledge and ability and these are inserted by specially trained physicians, nurses, or technicians. Some such devices are implanted surgically.

As a rule, nurses are responsible for starting IVs and administering infusion therapy. These activities are regulated by nurse practice acts, by agency policy, by the

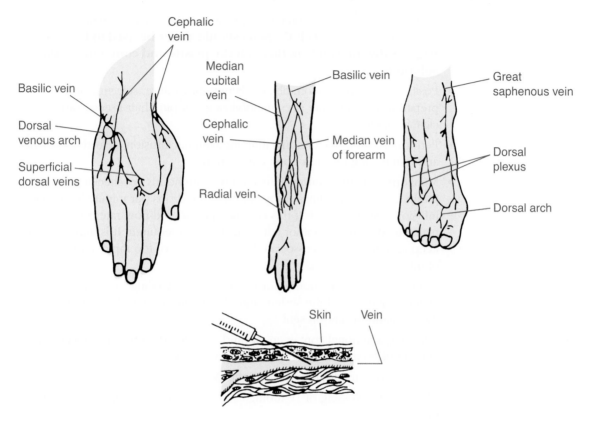

Figure 11-1 Intravenous infusion sites

Infusion Nurses Society (INS), by the Occupational Safety and Health Administration (OSHA), and by the Centers for Disease Control and Prevention (CDC). Nurses should be aware of their professional and legal responsibilities with respect to intravenous administration.

INFUSION SITES

Any easily accessible vein may be chosen for venipuncture. Most commonly used are the hand and lower arm, the antecubital fossa, and the upper arm (Figure 11-1). Less desirable are veins in the legs and feet because of the greater risk of thrombophlebitis and embolism. In infants, a scalp vein or the dorsum of the foot is often used. An intravascular device may be used for infusion directly through a major vein such as the subclavian or the femoral.

NURSING RESPONSIBIL-ITIES RELATIVE TO INTRAVEN-OUS ADMINIS-TRATION

In addition to the principles for administration of medications listed in Chapters 7 and 9, specific nursing responsibilities in relation to intravenous injections and infusions include the following:

- Setting up for an intravenous infusion: obtaining correct solution, infusion set, and needle; attaching and priming tubing; adding medication if ordered; and labeling container appropriately (e.g., client's name, solution, rate, date, and time). **Felt tip pens should never be used to label IV bags, as the ink can leak through the plastic and contaminate the solution.**

- Positioning client comfortably, explaining procedure, selecting and preparing venipuncture site: immobilizing, clipping hair if necessary, cleansing, etc.

- Performing venipuncture, initiating intravenous infusion, adjusting flow rate, and terminating infusion upon completion.

- Monitoring the intravenous infusion flow rate hourly by checking the pump/controller readings or by counting the drops per minute if a gravity infusion system is used. If this is done, the ordered flow rate can be maintained with very minor adjustments being required. It is important to keep in mind the risks associated with too slow or too rapid administration of intravenous solutions.

- Inspecting the IV site hourly for redness, heat, swelling, or pain and checking patency of the system and placement of the catheter if any of these conditions are present.

- Attaching additional containers of fluid as ordered; noting and recording amount of fluid administered per agency policy.

- Administering medication through the IV.

- Changing IV dressing or IV tubing as necessary or according to hospital policy.

- Providing physical care for the client, including assistance with meals, ambulation, comfort, and hygiene.

- Observing for complications associated with intravenous administration:
  1. Fluid overload (overhydration) resulting from too rapid administration of intravenous solutions.
     Signs: rapid breathing
               shortness of breath
               dilation of neck veins
               increase in blood pressure
               decreased fluid output in relation to fluid intake
  2. Adverse effects resulting from too rapid administration of intravenous medication, especially bolus injection.
     Signs: headache
               flushed face
               irregular pulse
               decrease in blood pressure (shock)

(**Note:** The nurse should use caution in increasing the IV flow rate even if it is running behind schedule. Speeding up the IV in an attempt to catch up and complete in the specified time could cause fluid overload or adverse medication reaction. If major adjustments in flow rate are deemed necessary, a provider's order should be obtained.)

3. Infiltration (leakage) of IV solution into subcutaneous tissue surrounding venipuncture site due to displacement of needle or intracatheter.

   Signs: sluggish flow rate
   absence of blood backflow
   localized swelling, pallor, pain
   area cool to touch

4. Thrombophlebitis (injury or irritation to a vein) resulting in clot formation at end of intracatheter.

   Signs: sluggish flow rate
   redness, pain or tenderness, heat at IV site or along affected vein

5. Allergic reaction to IV fluid or additive.

   Signs: rash
   itching
   shortness of breath

6. Infection at venipuncture site related to improper care of IV site (e.g., dressing changes, etc.).

   Signs: discharge
   inflammation

7. Systemic infection related to contamination of equipment or solutions.

   Signs: elevated TPR
   chills, malaise

8. Air embolism resulting from air in tubing due to loose connections or containers running dry.

   Signs: cyanosis
   hypotension
   weak, rapid pulse
   loss of consciousness

9. Catheter embolism resulting from improper insertion, accidental breakage, or dislodgment.

   Signs: same as air embolism, plus discomfort in involved vein

Any adverse effects observed resulting from administration of IV therapy should be reported immediately, and appropriate treatment or intervention instituted.

PRECAUTIONS IN HANDLING IV EQUIPMENT

Because the administration of IV fluids and medications involves the risk of coming into contact with blood or body fluids, it is essential that:

- sterile technique be maintained in performing venipuncture, changing site dressings, and manipulating any equipment that subjects the client to the risk of infection.

- personnel observe blood and body fluid precautions as recommended by the Centers for Disease Control and Prevention. This includes wearing gloves when flushing lumens, starting and terminating IVs, or performing any procedure that subjects personnel to a risk of infection through contact with blood or body fluids.

* all vascular access devices used in administration of intravenous therapy be discarded into puncture-resistant containers.

RECORDING

Intravenous medications and solutions are recorded in a variety of locations depending on policies of the agency. These may include the MAR, a special intravenous form, nurses notes, or the intake/output record. The initial notation should include information relative to time, type, site, and flow rate. Subsequent notations document ongoing assessment, observations, flow rate, additives, client's response, adverse effects, and time of termination.

The learner is referred to a nursing text or skills manual for detailed instruction on performance of venipuncture and administration of continuous intravenous infusion.

The learner is referred to Performance Criteria checklists in Appendix H for use as a guide when performing the following procedures: Setting Up an IV; Starting IV (with an Over-the-Needle Type Catheter); Assessment and Termination of IV; Preparation and Administration of IV Piggyback (IVPB) through infusing IV.

CHAPTER 12

Pediatric Dosage

OBJECTIVES

Upon completion of this chapter, you should be able to:

- Identify special considerations related to safety and comfort when administering medications to infants and children.

- Identify adaptations and special considerations related to administration of oral and parenteral medications to infants and children and when giving intramuscular injections and intravenous infusions.

- Apply dimensional analysis to clinical calculations of pediatric dosage based on body weight and body surface area.

There are several methods for calculating pediatric medication dosage based on various combinations of age, height, weight, body surface area, and adult dose. Because children of the same age can vary widely in size and weight, most of the usual methods are not applicable in all cases. Furthermore, rules or formulas do not take into consideration the physical condition of the child and the variety of responses or susceptibilities to the effects of drugs possible in individual children. **Because of the serious consequences that may result from overdosage or underdosage, accuracy of calculating and precision of administering medications to infants and children is of prime importance.**

GENERAL CONSIDERATIONS IN ADMINISTERING ORAL AND PARENTERAL MEDICATIONS TO CHILDREN

- Be sure positive identification has been made by comparison of name tag with medication administration guide or other means. Do not rely on child's response to spoken name.

- Corroborate calculated dosages by double-checking with another nurse or referring to a drug information source, or both. This is particularly important when administering insulin, heparin, or digoxin.

- Exercise particular caution in maintaining security of drugs, medication cart, needles, syringes, etc., making sure they are not accessible to children.

- Be sure child is awake and alert before administering oral medications. Never administer oral medications to a crying or resisting child or an injection to a sleeping child.

- Make explanations according to child's developmental level of understanding regarding reasons for medication, route of administration, expected sensations, taste, etc. Allow child to express feelings; be accepting of negative reactions.

- Maintain a firm but friendly manner. Give praise and comfort following administration.

- Restrain child gently but firmly. Obtain assistance as necessary, particularly for injections.

- Children up to 3 years of age are unable to swallow pills, and even older children may have much difficulty. Crush and dissolve pills and tablets (exclusive of enteric coated) as necessary. Administer liquids via cup, spoon, dropper, or syringe. For infants, liquid or dissolved medications can be placed in an empty nipple, from which the infant can suck while the nurse holds the nipple in an upright position.

ADMINISTRATION OF PARENTERAL MEDICATIONS TO INFANTS AND CHILDREN

Intramuscular Injections

The site of choice for intramuscular injections in neonates, infants, and children under the age of 3 is the anterolateral aspect of the upper thigh, the vastus lateralis muscle. The reason for this is that in children under the age of 3 years, the gluteal muscle is very small and poorly developed, and injection in this area is dangerously close to the sciatic nerve. The vastus lateralis site is located by measuring two to three finger breadths above the knee and below the trochanter depending on the size of the child.

The ventrogluteal site is acceptable in children over 3 years who have been walking for 1 year or more, and is a good site because it is free of major nerves and blood vessels. Figure 12-1 illustrates the method for locating this site. The thumb is placed on the anterior superior iliac spine and the index finger is abducted posteriorly. The injection site is located between the thumb and index finger. The dorsogluteal site should be avoided until the child is over age 4.

In older children, over age 5, the deltoid muscle is an acceptable site as long as the number and volume of injections is limited.

For any of the IM sites, volume of injections should be limited to a maximum of:

0.5 mL—neonate

1 mL—infant to 5 years

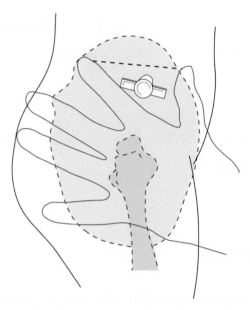

Figure 12-1 *Ventrogluteal site in child*

2 mL—6 to 12 years

3 mL—adolescent

Special consideration must be given to safety aspects of administering injections. Needles with a smaller diameter and shorter length should be used. For most infants and small children, a 25 gauge, 1″ needle is preferable unless solution is too viscous. Children must be restrained to avoid injury. A mummy restraint is suitable for infants; older children can be gently but firmly restrained by the person giving the injection or by another individual, if necessary. Make explanations brief, give injections quickly but safely, and allow the child to cry or express feelings. It is especially important for the nurse or parent to pick up, soothe, and comfort infants and young children following an injection.

Intravenous Infusions

Because infants have such small arm and hand veins, the four scalp veins (temporal area) and the dorsum of the foot are used as intravenous sites. For venipunctures on infants and children, a wing tip (butterfly) needle of suitable length may be used. On infants, a scalp vein butterfly needle may be preferable, Figure 12-2. In young children, the external jugular veins, the veins on the dorsal surface of the hand or flexor surface of the wrist, and the leg and foot veins are acceptable intravenous sites. The antecubital site is used least often because of the difficulty of preventing dislodgement.

These procedures are performed by specially trained personnel. It is important to have extra help when starting an IV on a child. Infants and young children must be restrained adequately during insertion of the IV catheter and the duration of the infusion. Mummy or elbow restraints and sandbags are effective methods. Armboards or

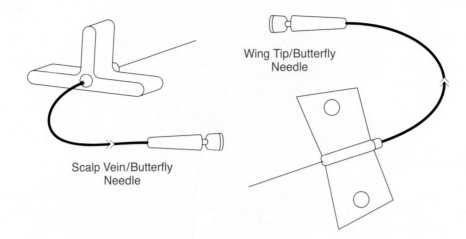

Figure 12-2 *Butterfly needles*

other immobilizing devices may be used for older children. Commercial protective devices are available to cover the area and help prevent dislodgement.

Intravenous infusions must be checked as often as every 15–30 minutes. Because of the greater risk of fluid overload, an automatic rate-flow infusion pump always should be used to regulate and maintain the rate of flow. A pediatric infusion set featuring volume control is an additional safety measure to prevent IV fluid overload. The minidrip feature of the volume control infusion set allows for easier regulation of the flow rate and more precise intravenous administration. A syringe-pump (mini-infuser) is useful in administering small amounts of intravenous fluids at a controlled rate. It is essential to maintain an accurate record of fluid intake and output on children receiving IV infusions.

PEDIATRIC DOSAGE BASED ON BODY WEIGHT— ORAL MEDICATIONS

EXAMPLE **Order:** Digoxin Elixir Pediatric 15 mcg per kg of body weight per dose PO

Label: Digoxin 0.05 mg per mL

Weight: 60 lb

How many mL should the child receive per dose?

Starting Factor	Answer Unit
60 lb	mL

Equivalents: 1 kg = 2.2 lb 15 mcg = 1 kg
1000 mcg = 1 mg   0.05 mg = 1 mL

Conversion Equation:

$$60 \text{ lb} \times \frac{1 \text{ kg}}{2.2 \text{ lb}} \times \frac{15 \text{ mcg}}{1 \text{ kg}} \times \frac{1 \text{ mg}}{1000 \text{ mcg}} \times \frac{1 \text{ mL}}{0.05 \text{ mg}} = 8.2 \text{ mL}$$

EXAMPLE **Order:** Ziagen Oral Solution 8 mg per kg of body weight per day PO to be given in two divided doses

Label: Ziagen Oral Solution (abacavir sulfate) 20 mg per mL

Weight: 4.5 kg

How many drops should be administered per dose?

Equivalents: 20 mg = 1 mL, 8 mg = 1 kg, 15 gtt = 1 mL   2 doses = 4.5 kg

Conversion Equation:

$$4.5 \text{ kg} \times \frac{8 \text{ mg}}{1 \text{ kg}} \times \frac{1 \text{ mL}}{20 \text{ mg}} \times \frac{15 \text{ gtt}}{1 \text{ mL}} = \frac{27 \text{ gtt}}{2 \text{ doses}} = 13.5 = 14 \text{ gtt}$$

Because it is important to administer the exact amount ordered, the computation should be carried out to two decimal places and rounded to the nearest tenth. To obtain a more precise measurement than is possible with a medicine cup, the medication should be measured using a syringe. It then may be administered directly from the syringe.

PRACTICE

Calculating Pediatric Dosage Based on Body Weight—Oral Medications

1. **Order:** Cefpodoxime proxetil Oral Suspension 5 mg per kg per dose PO

   Label: Figure 12-3. What is the trade name? _____

   Weight: 40 lb

   How many mL should the child receive?

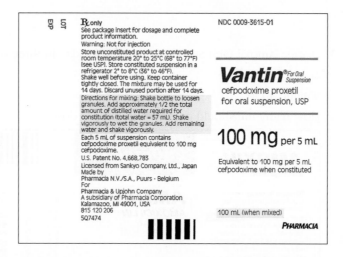

Figure 12-3 *(Courtesy of Pharmacia Corporation, Peapack, NJ)*

Calculating Pediatric Dosage Based on Body Weight—Oral Medications (Continued)

2. Order: Augmentin Oral Suspension 30 mg per kg in two divided doses per day PO

Label: Figure 12-4

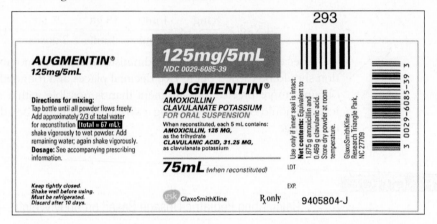

Figure 12-4 *(Reproduced with permission of Glaxo Smith Kline Group of Companies, all rights reserved)*

Weight: 22 lb

How many mL should be administered per dose?

3. Order: Amoxil Oral Suspension 40 mg/kg/day in three divided doses PO

Label: Figure 12-5

Weight: 40 lb

How many mL should be administered per dose?

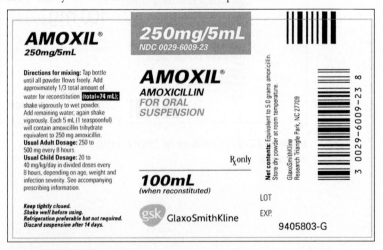

Figure 12-5 *(Reproduced with permission of GlaxoSmithKline Group of Companies, all rights reserved)*

Calculating Pediatric Dosage Based on Body Weight—Oral Medications (Continued)

4. *Order:* Gantrisin Pediatric Suspension 150 mg per kg PO in four divided doses per day

Label: Gantrisin Pediatric Suspension (sulfisoxazole) 0.5 g per tsp

Weight: 40 lb

How many mL should be administered per dose?

5. *Order:* Aminophylline Oral Liquid 2.5 mg per lb per dose PO

Label: Aminophylline Oral Liquid 105 mg per tsp

Weight: 18 kg

How many mL should the child receive per dose?

6. *Order:* Omnipen Oral Suspension 50 mg per kg per day in four divided doses PO

Label: Omnipen (ampicillin) Oral Suspension 125 mg per 5 mL

Weight: 33 lb

How many mL should be administered per dose?

7. *Order:* Velosef Oral Suspension 25 mg per kg in two divided doses PO

Label: Velosef (cephradine) Oral Suspension 250 mg per 5 mL

Weight: 44 lb

How many mL should be administered per dose?

Calculating Pediatric Dosage Based on Body Weight—Oral Medications
(Continued)

8. *Order:* Tetracycline Hydrochloride 25 mg per kg per day in four divided doses PO

   Label: Tetracycline Hydrochloride 125 mg per 5 mL

   Weight: 37 kg

   How many mL should be administered per dose?

9. *Order:* Ampicillin Oral Suspension 50 mg per kg per day in four divided doses PO

   Label: Ampicillin Oral Suspension 125 mg per 5 mL

   Weight: 42 lb

   How many mL should be administered per dose?

10. *Order:* Antiminth Oral Suspension 5 mg per lb single dose PO

    Label: Antiminth (pyrantil pamoate) Oral Suspension 50 mg per mL

    Weight: 45 lb

    How many mL should be administered per dose?

11. *Order:* Cleocin Pediatric 8 mg per kg per day in four divided doses PO

    Label: Cleocin (clindamycin) Pediatric 75 mg per 5 mL

    Weight: 84 lb

    How many mL should be administered per dose?

PRACTICE

Calculating Pediatric Dosage Based on Body Weight—Oral Medications (Continued)

12. *Order:* Theophylline Oral Solution 0.3 mL/lb/dose PO

    Label: Theophylline Oral Solution 80 mg per 15 mL

    Weight: 44 lb

    How many mL should be administered per dose?

13. *Order:* Furadantin Oral Suspension 5 mg per kg in four divided doses PO

    Label: Furadantin (nitrofurantoin) Oral Suspension 25 mg per 5 mL

    Weight: 15 lb

    How many mL should be administered per dose?

14. *Order:* Biaxin Oral Suspension 15 mg/kg/day in two divided doses PO

    Label: Biaxin Oral Suspension (clarithromycin) 125 mg per 5 mL

    Weight: 38 lb

    How many mL should be administered per dose? Administer via a syringe.

15. *Order:* Penbritin Oral Suspension 5 mg/lb/dose PO

    Label: Penbritin (ampicillin trihydrate) Oral Suspension 125 mg per 5 mL

    Weight: 12 lb

    How many mL should be administered per dose?

(*Note:* See Appendix G for answer key.)

CALCULATING PEDIATRIC DOSAGE— INJECTIONS

EXAMPLE   **Order:** Bicillin LA 50,000 units/kg/day IM in four divided doses

Label: Bicillin LA (penicillin G benzathine) 300,000 units per mL

Weight: 50 lb

How many mL will be administered per dose?

Equivalents: 1 kg = 2.2 lb, 300,000 units = 1 mL,
                   50,000 units = 1 kg

Conversion Equation:

$$50 \text{ lb} \times \frac{1 \text{ kg}}{2.2 \text{ lb}} \times \frac{50,000 \text{ units}}{1 \text{ kg}} \times \frac{1 \text{ mL}}{300,000 \text{ units}} = \frac{3.78 \text{ mL}}{4 \text{ doses}} = 0.95 \text{ mL} = 1 \text{ mL}$$

(**Note:** When the resulting dosage is less than 1 mL, the answer may be carried to three decimal places and rounded to the nearest hundredth, and the medication may be measured and administered in a tuberculin syringe. If the dosage is 1 mL or more, carry the answer to two decimal places and round to the nearest tenth.)

PRACTICE

Calculating Pediatric Dosage—Injections (see note above)

1. *Order:* Cleocin Phosphate 15 mg per kg in four divided doses per day IM

   Label: Figure 12-6. What is the generic name? _____

LOT/EXP	
Single Dose Container. See package insert for complete product information. Store at controlled room temperature 20° to 25°C (68° to 77°F). Do not refrigerate. 812 823 707 Pharmacia & Upjohn Company Kalamazoo, MI 49001, USA	NDC 0009-0902-11 6 mL Vial **Cleocin Phosphate®** clindamycin injection, USP **900 mg** Equivalent to 900 mg clindamycin

   Figure 12-6 *(Courtesy of Pharmacia and Upjohn Company, Kalamazoo, MI)*

   Weight: 20 kg

   How many mL should the child receive per dose?

2. *Order:* Lasix 3 mg per kg IM

   Label: Figure 12-7. What is the generic name? _____

   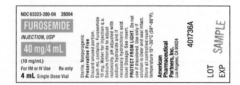

   Figure 12-7 *(Courtesy of American Pharmaceutical Partners, Los Angeles, CA)*

PRACTICE

Weight: 25 lb

How many mL should the child receive?

3. *Order:* Ancef 50 mg/kg/day in four divided doses IM

Label: Ancef (cefazolin sodium) 225 mg per mL

Weight: 15 lb

How many mL should the child receive per dose?

Use a tuberculin syringe.

4. *Order:* Streptomycin 30 mg/kg/day in two divided doses IM

Label: Streptomycin 1 g per 2.5 mL

Weight: 20 lb

How many mL should the child receive per dose?

Use a tuberculin syringe.

5. *Order:* Pipracil 100 mg/kg/day in four divided doses IM

Label: Pipracil (piperacillin sodium) 1 g per 2.5 mL

Weight: 55 lb

How many mL should the child receive per dose?

6. *Order:* Apresoline 1.7 mg/kg/day in four divided doses IM

Label: Apresoline (hydralazine hydrochloride) 20 mg per mL

Weight: 12 lb

How many mL should the child receive per dose?

PRACTICE

Calculating Pediatric Dosage—Injections (see note above) (Continued)

7. *Order:* Humatrope 0.06 mg/kg/day IM

Label: Humatrope (somatropin) 5 mg per 4 mL

Weight: 12.2 kg

How many mL should the children receive per dose?

8. *Order:* Penicillin G Potassium 35,000 units/kg/day in four divided doses IM

Label: Penicillin G Potassium 250,000 units per mL

Weight: 72 lb

How many mL should the child receive per dose?

9. *Order:* Rocephin 50 mg/kg/day in two divided doses IM

Label: Rocephin (cetriaxone) 250 mg per mL

Weight: 22.7 kg

How many mL should the child receive per dose?

10. *Order:* Digoxin 0.002 mg/kg/day in two divided doses IM

Label: Digoxin 0.5 mg per 2 mL

Weight: 25 lb

How many mL should the child receive per dose?

(***Note:*** See Appendix G for answer key.)

CALCULATING PEDIATRIC DOSAGE—IVS

EXAMPLE **Order:** Dopamine 5 mcg/kg/min IV. Dilute 100 mg dopamine in 100 mL D5$\frac{1}{2}$NS

Label: Figure 12-8

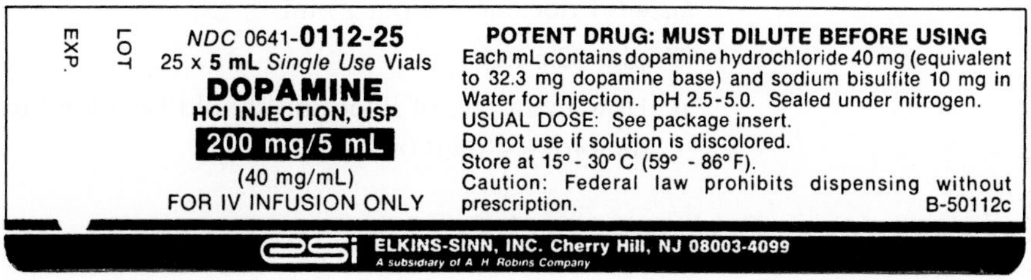

| EXP. | LOT | NDC 0641-**0112-25**
25 x **5 mL** *Single Use* Vials
DOPAMINE
HCI INJECTION, USP
200 mg/5 mL
(40 mg/mL)
FOR IV INFUSION ONLY | **POTENT DRUG: MUST DILUTE BEFORE USING**
Each mL contains dopamine hydrochloride 40 mg (equivalent to 32.3 mg dopamine base) and sodium bisulfite 10 mg in Water for Injection. pH 2.5-5.0. Sealed under nitrogen.
USUAL DOSE: See package insert.
Do not use if solution is discolored.
Store at 15° - 30° C (59° - 86° F).
Caution: Federal law prohibits dispensing without prescription. B-50112c |

ELKINS-SINN, INC. Cherry Hill, NJ 08003-4099
A subsidiary of A. H. Robins Company

Figure 12-8 (*Courtesy of Elkins-Sinn, Inc., Cherry Hill, NJ*)

Weight: 10 lb

1. How many mL of dopamine should be added to the 100 mL D5$\frac{1}{2}$NS to obtain the ordered dilution?

$$100 \text{ mg} \times \frac{5 \text{ mL}}{200 \text{ mg}} = 2.5 \text{ mL}$$

2. How many mcg of dopamine should the child receive per min?

$$10 \text{ lb} \times \frac{1 \text{ kg}}{2.2 \text{ lb}} \times \frac{5 \text{ mcg per min}}{1 \text{ kg}} = 22.7 \text{ mcg per min}$$

3. How many mcg of dopamine should the child receive per hr?

$$1 \text{ hr} \times \frac{60 \text{ min}}{1 \text{ hr}} \times \frac{22.7 \text{ mcg}}{1 \text{ min}} = 1362 \text{ mcg}$$

4. What should the flow rate be in mL per hr to infuse the calculated dose?

$$1 \text{ hr} \times \frac{1362 \text{ mcg}}{1 \text{ hr}} \times \frac{1 \text{ mg}}{1000 \text{ mcg}} \times \frac{100 \text{ mL}}{100 \text{ mg}} = 1 \text{ mL}$$

OR

$$1 \text{ hr} \times \frac{60 \text{ min}}{1 \text{ hr}} \times \frac{22.7 \text{ mcg}}{1 \text{ min}} \times \frac{1 \text{ mg}}{1000 \text{ mcg}} \times \frac{100 \text{ mL}}{100 \text{ mg}} = 1 \text{ mL}$$

Calculating Pediatric Dosage—IVs

1. **Order:** Lidocaine 30 mcg/kg/min IV. Dilute 300 mg lidocaine in 250 mL D5W

   Label: Lidocaine 1 g per 25 mL

   Weight: 32.6 kg

   a. How many mL of lidocaine should be added to the 250 mL D5W to obtain the ordered dilution?

   b. How many mcg of lidocaine should the child receive per min?

   c. How many mg of lidocaine should the child receive per hr?

   d. What should the flow rate be in mL per hr to infuse the calculated dose?

   e. At the calculated rate, how many hours should it take for the total IV to infuse?

2. **Order:** Nitropress 2 mcg/kg/min IV. Dilute 30 mg in 250 mL D5$\frac{1}{2}$NS

   Label: Nitropress (nitroprusside sodium) 50 mg per 2 mL

   Weight: 18.5 kg

   a. How many mL of Nitropress should be added to the 250 mL D5$\frac{1}{2}$NS to obtain the ordered dilution?

PRACTICE

Calculating Pediatric Dosage—IVs (Continued)

b. How many mcg of Nitropress should the child receive per min?

c. How many mg of Nitropress should the child receive per hr?

d. What should the flow rate be in mL per hr to infuse the calculated dose?

3. *Order:* Aminophylline 0.3 mg per kg in 30 mL D5W IV to infuse over 20 min

Label: Figure 12-9

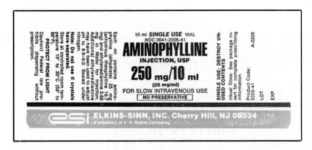

Figure 12-9 *(Courtesy of Elkins-Sinn, Inc., Cherry Hill, NJ)*

Weight: 45 lb

a. How many mg should the child receive as a total dose?

b. How many mL of aminophylline should be added to the 30 mL D5W?

PRACTICE

Calculating Pediatric Dosage—IVs (Continued)

4. *Order:* Verapamil Hydrochloride 0.2 mg per kg via IV bolus

Label: Verapamil Hydrochloride 2.5 mg per mL

Weight: 10 lb

Directions: Administer over a 2 min period.

How much solution should be administered per dose?

5. *Order:* Isoptin 0.3 mg per kg via IV bolus

Label: Isoptin (verapamil hydrochloride) 5 mg per 2 mL

Weight: 60 lb

Directions: Administer over a 2 min period.

How much solution should be administered per dose?

6. *Order:* Vancocin IV 20 mg per kg in 100 mL D5W. Infuse in 60 min.

Label/Product Insert: Figure 12-10

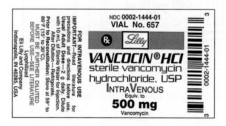

PREPARATION AND STABILITY

At the time of use, reconstitute by adding either 10 mL of Sterile water for Injection to the 500-mg vial or 20 mL of Sterile water for Injection to the 1-g vial, or dry sterile vancomycin powder. Vials reconstituted in this manner will give a solution of 50 mg/mL. FURTHER DILUTION IS REQUIRED.

After reconstitution, the vials may be stored in a refrigerator for 14 days without significant loss of potency. Reconstituted solutions containing 500 g of vancomycin must be diluted with at least 500 mL of diluent. Reconstituted solutions containing 1 g of vancomycin must be diluted with at least 200 mL of diluent. The desired dose, diluted in this manner, should be administered by intermittent intravenous infusion over a period of at least 60 minutes.

Figure 12-10 *(Courtesy of Eli Lilly Pharmaceuticals, Indianapolis, IN)*

PRACTICE

Calculating Pediatric Dosage—IVs (Continued)

Weight: 40 lb

Drop Factor: 60 gtt per mL

   a. How many mL of sterile diluent should be added to the vial?

   b. What is the concentration of the resulting solution?

   c. How many mL of reconstituted Vancocin IV will contain the ordered dose?

   d. What should the flow rate be?

   e. What is the maximum refrigeration period?

7. *Order:* Tagamet 5 mg per kg IV in 100 mL D5W. Infuse in 20 min.

   Label: Tagamet (cimetidine) 300 mg per 2 mL

   Weight: 50 lb

   Drop Factor: 60 gtt per mL

   a. How much Tagamet should be added to the 100 mL D5W?

   b. What should the flow rate be?

Calculating Pediatric Dosage—IVs (Continued)

8. **Order:** Cosmegen 0.015 mg per kg IV in 50 mL D5W. Administer in 15 min.

Label: Cosmegen (dactinomycin) 0.5 mg per mL

Weight: 64 lb

Drop Factor: 60 gtt per mL

a. How much Cosmegen should be added to the 50 mL D5W?

b. What should the flow rate be?

(**Note:** See Appendix G for answer key.)

CALCULATION OF PEDIATRIC DOSAGE BASED ON BODY SURFACE AREA

Pediatric dosage can be calculated on the basis of the body surface area of the child, which can be determined by the use of a nomogram, Figure 12-11. This method can be used for children up to 12 years of age. The child's weight and height are located on the chart; a straight line drawn between them intersects the body-surface column (SA) at the number indicating the child's body surface area (BSA). The surface area measurement is expressed in square meters (M^2). This figure is then plugged into a modified dimensional analysis equation, Figure 12-12, to calculate pediatric dosage using BSA estimates.

The child's body surface area in M^2 is located on the nomogram (Figure 12-11) in the following manner:

Child's height: 26 in

Child's weight: 22 lb

Place a ruler at the level of the child's weight (22 lb) in the right-hand column and line the edge up with the child's height (26 in) in the left-hand column. Read the surface area (SA) measurement at the point where the ruler intersects the SA column. The body surface area for this child is 0.45 M^2.

The enclosed (center) column on the nomogram can be used as an estimate of body surface of children of average height and build using weight alone.

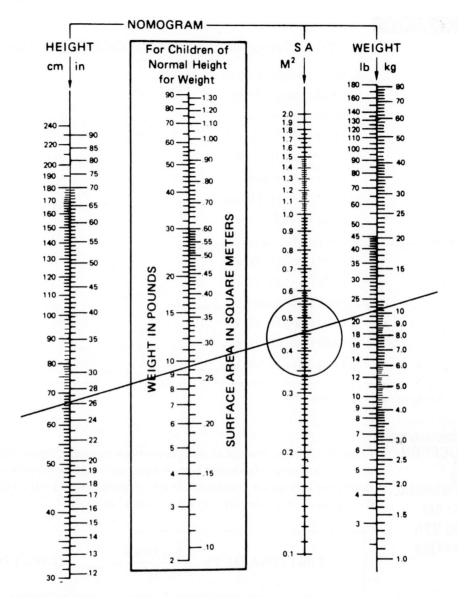

Figure 12-11 *West Nomogram (Modified and reprinted with permission from Behrman, R.E., Kliegman, R.M., and Arvin, A.M.* Nelson Textbook of Pediatrics, *15th ed., W.B. Saunders Company, Philadelphia, PA)*

PRACTICE

Use the Nomogram to Determine the Child's Body Surface Area

1. Child's height: 149 cm

   Child's weight: 36 kg

   Body surface area: _____

2. Child's height: 46 in

   Child's weight: 44 lb

   Body surface area: _____

3. Child's height: 138 cm

   Child's weight: 32 kg

   Body surface area: _____

4. Child's height: 29 in

   Child's weight: 22 lb

   Body surface area: _____

5. Child's height: 82 cm

   Child's weight: 12 kg

   Body surface area: _____

(**Note:** See Appendix G for answer key.)

APPLICATION OF DIMENSIONAL ANALYSIS USING BSA ESTIMATES

From the BSA dimensional analysis conversion equation, Figure 12-12, it can be seen that the equivalent relationship between *average adult body surface area* (1.7 M^2) and *adult dose* becomes a conversion factor or bridge whereby the *child's BSA* (M^2) and the *child's dose* also become an equivalent relationship.

$$\text{Child's BSA } (M^2) \times \frac{\text{Adult Dose}}{1.7 \, M^2} = \_\_\_\_\_ \text{ (Child's Dose)}$$

Figure 12-12 *BSA dimensional analysis conversion equation*

EXAMPLE Find the child's dose of amoxicillin.

Adult dose: Amoxicillin 250 mg

Child's height: 104 cm

Child's weight: 9.6 kg

From Nomogram: BSA = 0.51 M^2

Starting Factor	Answer Unit
Child's BSA (M^2)	Child's dose in mg
0.51 M^2	_____ mg

Equivalent: 1.7 M^2 = 250 mg

Conversation Equation:

$$0.51 \, \cancel{M^2} \times \frac{250 \text{ mg}}{1.7 \, \cancel{M^2}} = 75 \text{ mg}$$

PRACTICE

Use Nomogram (Figure 12-11) and Dimensional Analysis to Calculate Pediatric Dosages

(*Note:* Carry to two decimal places and round to nearest tenth.)

1. Child's height: 25 in
   Child's weight: 14 lb
   Adult dose: Meperidine 50 mg
   Find the child's dose.

2. Child's height: 108 cm
   Child's weight: 18 kg
   Adult dose: Mellaril (thioridazine) 10 mg
   Find the child's dose.

3. Child's height: 46 in
   Child's weight: 50 lb
   Adult dose: Xylocaine Hydrochloride 200 mg
   Find the child's dose.

4. Child's height: 54 in
   Child's weight: 70 lb
   Adult dose: Ceftin (cefuroxime) 250 mg
   Find the child's dose.

PRACTICE

Use Nomogram (Figure 12-11) and Dimensional Analysis to Calculate Pediatric Dosages

5. Child's height: 150 cm

Child's weight: 38 kg

Adult dose: Augmentin (amoxicillin and potassium clavulanete) 250 mg

Find the child's dose.

(*Note:* See Appendix G for answer key.)

CHAPTER 13

Clinical Calculations

Upon completion of this chapter, you should be able to:

- Apply dimensional analysis to solve, with 100% accuracy, any type of clinical calculation involved in the administration of medication.

The following clinical problems represent the type of calculations that commonly are encountered in the administration of medications. The prescription orders, the label information, and the conversions required are truly representative of clinical practice. Successful completion of these problems would indicate acceptable competence in performing clinical calculations. With the mastery of this systematic, unified method of problem solving, the learner also should have developed a measure of confidence in his or her ability to solve new problems as they may occur in the clinical setting.

Although most of the equivalent relationships should have been memorized by now, it may be helpful to detach the table of equivalents (printed on the back of title page) for use as a reference in completing the following calculations and for future use in the clinical area.

Before beginning this unit, you may wish to review the method (and modifications) for determining the starting factor and answer unit.

- In general, the starting factor is the known quantity and its unit which is to be converted to a desired unit (quantity of medication).

EXAMPLE   Starting Factor   Answer Unit
                gr, g   mg, cap, tsp

- In calculations based on body weight, the starting factor is the particular quantity of weight that is to be converted to a desired unit (quantity of medication).

EXAMPLE | Starting Factor | Answer Unit
lb, kg | mL, mg, tab ÷ number of doses

- In calculations based on body surface area, the starting factor is the particular amount of body surface area that is to be converted to a desired unit (child's dose).

EXAMPLE | Starting Factor | Answer Unit
BSA (M^2) | mg, mL, gtt

- In calculations for IV flow rate in gtt per min, the starting factor is the particular amount of time (1 min) that is to be converted to a desired unit (number of drops).

EXAMPLE | Starting Factor | Answer Unit
min | gtt

- In calculations for IV flow rate in mL per hr, the starting factor is the particular amount of time (1 hr) that is to be converted to a desired unit (number of mL).

EXAMPLE | Starting Factor | Answer Unit
hr | mL

- In calculations for IV infusion time, the starting factor is the particular amount of solution (mL) that is to be converted to a desired unit (amount of time).

EXAMPLE | Starting Factor | Answer Unit
mL | hr, min, sec

PRACTICE

Solve Using Dimensional Analysis

(**Note:** Round in the appropriate manner.)

1. **Order:** Restoril gr $\frac{1}{2}$ PO

   Label: Figure 13-1

Solve Using Dimensional Analysis (Continued)

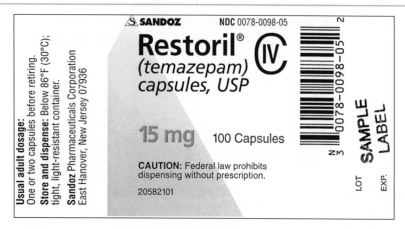

Figure 13-1 *(Used with permission of Novartis Pharmaceuticals Corporation)*

2. ***Order:*** Colchicine gr $\frac{1}{200}$ PO

Label: Colchicine 0.6 mg per tab (scored)

3. ***Order:*** Lanoxin 0.125 mg PO

Label: Lanoxin (digoxin) 0.25 mg per tab (scored)

4. ***Order:*** Dynapen Oral Suspension 125 mg PO

Label: Dynapen (dicloxacillin sodium) Oral Suspension 62.5 mg per 5 mL

5. ***Order:*** Glucophage 0.5 g PO

Label: Glucophage (metformin hydrochloride) 500 mg per tab

Solve Using Dimensional Analysis (Continued)

6. *Order:* Dramamine 100 mg PO

   Label: Dramamine (dimenhydrinate) 50 mg per tab

7. *Order:* Keflex 0.5 g PO

   Label: Figure 13-2

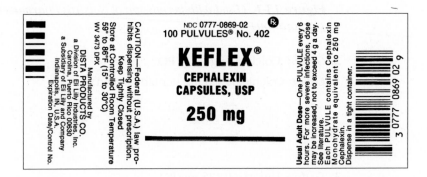

NDC 0777-0869-02
100 PULVULES® No. 402

KEFLEX®

CEPHALEXIN
CAPSULES, USP

250 mg

CAUTION—Federal (U.S.A.) law prohibits dispensing without prescription.
Keep Tightly Closed
Store at Controlled Room Temperature
59° to 86°F (15° to 30°C)
WV 3473 DPX

DISTA PRODUCTS CO.
a Division of Eli Lilly Industries, Inc.
Carolina, Puerto Rico 00630
a Subsidiary of Eli Lilly and Company
Indianapolis, IN, U.S.A.
Manufactured by

Expiration Date/Control No.

Usual Adult Dose—One PULVULE every 6 hours. For more severe infections, dose may be increased, not to exceed 4 g a day.
See literature.
Each PULVULE contains Cephalexin Monohydrate equivalent to 250 mg Cephalexin.
Dispense in a tight container.

3 0777 0869 02 9

Figure 13-2 *(Courtesy of Eli Lilly Pharmaceuticals, Indianapolis, IN)*

8. *Order:* Zyloprim 0.3 g PO

   Label: Zyloprim (allopurinol) 100 mg per tab

9. *Order:* Vibramycin Syrup 125 mg PO

   Label: Vibramycin (doxycycline calcium oral suspension) Syrup 50 mg per tsp

   Give _____ mL.

PRACTICE

Solve Using Dimensional Analysis (Continued)

10. *Order:* Codeine Sulfate gr 1 PO

Label: Figure 13-3

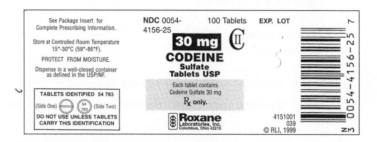

Figure 13-3 *(Courtesy of Roxane Laboratories, Inc., Columbus, OH)*

11. *Order:* Penicillin VK Oral Suspension 125 mg PO

Label: Penicillin VK (penicillin V potassium) Oral Suspension 250 mg per 5 mL

12. *Order:* Chloral Hydrate Syrup 1000 mg PO

Label: Chloral Hydrate Syrup 0.5 g per 5 mL

Give _____ mL.

13. *Order:* Furosemide 0.04 g PO

Label: Figure 13-4

PRACTICE

Solve Using Dimensional Analysis (Continued)

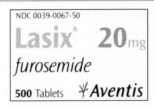

Figure 13-4   *(Courtesy of Aventis Pharmaceuticals, Kansas City, MO)*

14. Order: Mysoline Suspension 125 mg PO

Label: Mysoline (primidone) Suspension 0.25 g per 5 mL

15. Order: Vistaril Oral Suspension 50 mg PO

Label: Figure 13-5

Give _____ tsp.

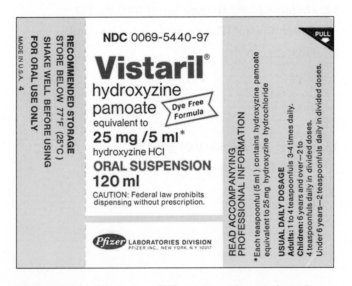

Figure 13-5   *(Courtesy of Pfizer, Inc., New York, NY)*

PRACTICE

Solve Using Dimensional Analysis (Continued)

16. *Order:* Lipitor 0.02 g PO

  Label: Lipitor (atorvastatin calcium) 10 mg per tab

17. *Order:* Diucardin 0.15 g PO

  Label: Diucardin (hydroflumethiazide) 50 mg per tab

18. *Order:* Klorvess 30 mEq PO

  Label: Klorvess (potassium chloride) 20 mEq per 15 mL

19. *Order:* Antivert 0.05 g PO

  Label: Figure 13-6

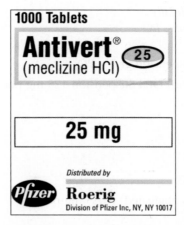

Figure 13-6 *(Courtesy of Pfizer, Inc., New York, NY)*

PRACTICE

Solve Using Dimensional Analysis (Continued)

20. **Order:** Claritin 0.01 g PO

    Label: Claritin (loratadine) 10 mg per tab

21. **Order:** Achromycin 0.5 g PO

    Label: Achromycin (tetracycline hydrochloride) 125 mg per 5 mL

22. **Order:** Phenobarbital gr $\frac{1}{2}$ PO

    Label: Figure 13-7

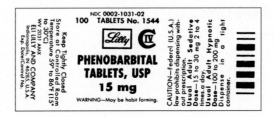

Figure 13-7   *(Courtesy of Eli Lilly*
Pharmaceuticals, Indianapolis, IN)

23. **Order:** Omnipen-N Oral Suspension gr $7\frac{1}{2}$ PO

    Label: Omnipen-N (ampicillin) Oral Suspension 125 mg per 5 mL

24. **Order:** Premarin 1.25 mg PO

    Label: Premarin (estrogens conjugated) 0.625 mg per tab

PRACTICE

Solve Using Dimensional Analysis (Continued)

25. *Order:* Declomycin 0.3 g PO

Label: Declomycin (demeclocycline hydrochloride) 150 mg per tab

26. *Order:* Mebaral 0.016 g PO

Label: Mebaral (mephobarbital) 32 mg per tab (scored)

27. *Order:* HydroDIURIL 0.1 g PO

Label: HydroDIURIL (hydrochlorothiazide) 50 mg per tab

28. *Order:* Eskalith cap 600 mg PO

Label: Figure 13-8

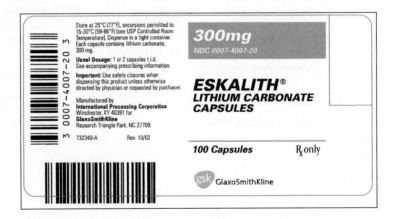

Store at 25°C (77°F), excursions permitted to 15-30°C (59-86°F) [see USP Controlled Room Temperature]. Dispense in a tight container. Each capsule contains lithium carbonate, 300 mg.

Usual Dosage: 1 or 2 capsules t.i.d. See accompanying prescribing information.

Important: Use safety closures when dispensing this product unless otherwise directed by physician or requested by purchaser.

Manufactured by
International Processing Corporation
Winchester, KY 40391 for
GlaxoSmithKline
Research Triangle Park, NC 27709

732340-A   Rev. 10/02

0007-4007-20 3

300mg
NDC 0007-4007-20

ESKALITH®
LITHIUM CARBONATE
CAPSULES

100 Capsules   R̠ only

gsk GlaxoSmithKline

Figure 13-8 *(Reproduced with permission of GlaxoSmithKline Group of Companies, all rights reserved)*

Solve Using Dimensional Analysis (Continued)

29. *Order:* Lanoxicaps 0.05 mg PO

    Label: Lanoxicaps (digoxin) 50 mcg per tab

30. *Order:* Quinora 0.6 g PO

    Label: Quinora (quinidine sulfate) 200 mg per tab

31. *Order:* Methadone Hydrochloride 0.01 g PO

    Label: Figure 13-9

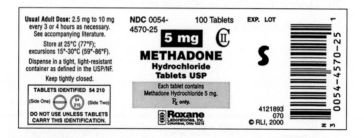

Figure 13-9 *(Used with permission of Roxane Laboratories, Inc.)*

32. *Order:* Procainamide hydrochloride Extended-Release Tab 1 g PO

    Label: Figure 13-10

PRACTICE

Solve Using Dimensional Analysis (Continued)

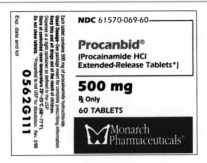

Figure 13-10 *(Used with permission of King Pharmaceuticals, Inc., Bristol, TN)*

33. *Order:* Tylenol gr 5 PO

Label: Tylenol (acetaminophen) 325 mg per tab

34. *Order:* Pen-Vee K 250 mg PO

Label: Pen-Vee K (penicillin V potassium) 125 mg per tsp

Give _____ mL.

35. *Order:* Mellaril 75 mg PO

Label: Mellaril (thioridazine) 25 mg per 5 mL

36. *Order:* Choledyl Elixir 0.2 g PO

Label: Choledyl (oxtriphylline) Elixir 100 mg per 5 mL

PRACTICE

| Solve Using Dimensional Analysis (Continued) |

37. *Order:* Caffeine gr 3 PO

    Label: Caffeine 0.2 g per tab

38. *Order:* Brethine 0.005 g PO

    Label: Figure 13-11

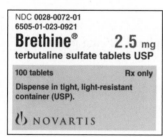

Figure 13-11 *(Courtesy of Novartis Pharmaceuticals, East Hanover, NJ)*

39. *Order:* Prazosin hydrochloride 0.004 g PO

    Label: Figure 13-12

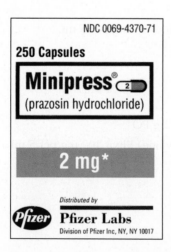

Figure 13-12 *(Courtesy of Pfizer, Inc., New York, NY)*

PRACTICE

Solve Using Dimensional Analysis (Continued)

40. *Order:* Aldomet 500 mg PO

 Label: Aldomet (methyldopa) 125 mg per tab

41. *Order:* Phenergan 25 mg PO

 Label: Phenergan (promethazine hydrochloride) 12.5 mg per tab

42. *Order:* Erythromycin 0.75 g PO

 Label: Erythromycin 250 mg per cap

43. *Order:* Hydroxyzine pamoate Oral Suspension 60 mg PO

 Label: Figure 13-13

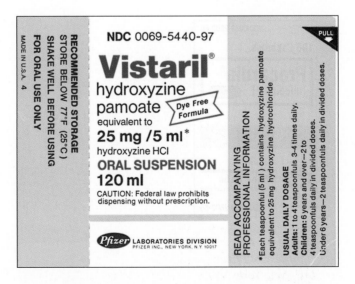

Figure 13-13 *(Courtesy of Pfizer, Inc., New York, NY)*

Solve Using Dimensional Analysis (Continued)

44. *Order:* Quinidine Sulfate Tablet gr 6 PO
   Label: Quinidine Sulfate Tablet 0.2 g per tab

45. *Order:* Novo-soxazole 2 g PO
   Label: Novo-soxazole (sulfisoxazole) 500 mg per tab

46. *Order:* Nitroglycerin gr $\frac{1}{600}$ sublingual
   Label: Nitroglycerin 0.1 mg per tab

47. *Order:* Nifedipine 0.03 g PO
   Label: Figure 13-14

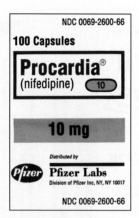

Figure 13-14
*(Courtesy of Pfizer,
Inc., New York, NY)*

PRACTICE

Solve Using Dimensional Analysis (Continued)

48. ***Order:*** Chloral Hydrate Syrup 0.25 g PO

   Label: Chloral Hydrate Syrup 250 mg per 5 mL

49. ***Order:*** Penicillin V Potassium Oral Solution 100,000 units PO

   Label: Figure 13-15

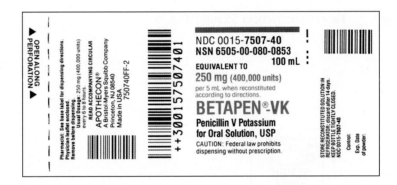

Figure 13-15 *(Courtesy of Apothecon Bristol-Myers Squibb, Princeton, NJ)*

50. ***Order:*** Narcan 400 mcg IM

   Label: Narcan (naloxone hydrochloride) 0.4 mg per mL

51. ***Order:*** Pfizerpen 200,000 units IM

   Label: Pfizerpen (penicillin G potassium procaine) 1,000,000 units per 10 mL

Solve Using Dimensional Analysis (Continued)

52. *Order:* Librium 25 mg IM

Label: Librium (chlordiazepoxide) 100 mg per 2 mL

53. *Order:* Terramycin 100 mg IM

Label: Terramycin (oxytetracycline) 250 mg per 2 mL

54. *Order:* Nebcin 55 mg IM

Label: Figure 13-16

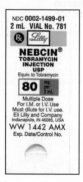

Figure 13-16 *(Courtesy of Eli Lilly Pharmaceuticals, Indianapolis, IN)*

55. *Order:* Meperidine 60 mg IM

Label: Meperidine 75 mg per 1.5 mL

PRACTICE

Solve Using Dimensional Analysis (Continued)

56. *Order:* Methergine 0.15 mg IM

  Label: Methergine (methylergonovine maleate) 0.2 mg per mL

57. *Order:* Vitamin B$_{12}$ 600 mcg IM

  Label: Vitamin B$_{12}$ (cyanocobalamin) 1000 mcg per mL

58. *Order:* Diazepam 2 mg IM

  Label: Figure 13-17

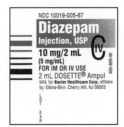

Figure 13-17 *(Courtesy of Baxter Healthcare Corporation, New Providence, NJ)*

59. *Order:* Maxipime 250 mg IM

  Label: Maxipime (cefepime hydrochloride) 280 mg per mL

PRACTICE

Solve Using Dimensional Analysis (Continued)

60. *Order:* Kefzol 500 mg IM

  Label: Kefzol (cefazolin sodium) 330 mg per mL

61. *Order:* Vistaril 25 mg IM

  Label: Vistaril (hydroxyzine hydrochloride) 100 mg per 2 mL

62. *Order:* Digoxin 0.25 mg IM

  Label: Digoxin 500 mcg per 2 mL

63. *Order:* Promethazine gr $\frac{1}{6}$ IM

  Label: Promethazine 25 mg per mL

64. *Order:* Hydroxyzine hydrochloride 0.075 g IM

  Label: Figure 13-18

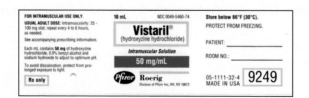

Figure 13-18 *(Courtesy of Pfizer, Inc., New York, NY)*

Solve Using Dimensional Analysis (Continued)

65. *Order:* Lasix 40 mg IM

   Label: Lasix (furosemide) 10 mg per mL

66. *Order:* Thorazine 15 mg IM

   Label: Thorazine (chlorpromazine) 25 mg per mL

67. *Order:* Atropine sulfate gr $\frac{1}{150}$ (0.4 mg) subcut

   Label: Atropine sulfate 400 mcg per mL

68. *Order:* Ancef 250 mg IM

   Label: Figure 13-19

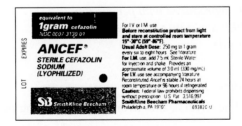

Figure 13-19 *(Courtesy of SmithKline Beecham Pharmaceuticals, Philadelphia, PA)*

69. *Order:* Terramycin100 mg IM

   Label: Terramycin (oxytetracycline) 250 mg per 2 mL

Solve Using Dimensional Analysis (Continued)

70. *Order:* Meperidine 15 mg IM

    Label: Meperidine 25 mg per mL

71. *Order:* Nydrazid 0.15 g IM

    Label: Nydrazid (isoniazid) 100 mg per mL

72. *Order:* Thorazine 12.5 mg IM

    Label: Figure 13-20

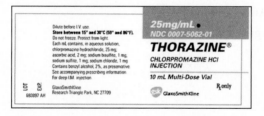

Figure 13-20 *Reproduced with permission of GlaxoSmithKline Group of Companies, all rights reserved)*

73. *Order:* Apresoline 25 mg IM

    Label: Apresoline (hydralazine hydrochloride) 20 mg per mL

74. *Order:* Phenergan 35 mg IM

    Label: Phenergan 50 mg per mL

Solve Using Dimensional Analysis (Continued)

75. *Order:* Ancef 250 mg IM

    Label: Ancef (cefazolin sodium) 225 mg per mL

76. *Order:* Unasyn 1 g IM

    Label: Unasyn (ampicillin sodium) 1.5 g per 4 mL

77. *Order:* Demerol 30 mg IM

    Label: Figure 13-21

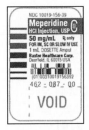

Figure 13-21
*(Courtesy Baxter
Healthcare
Corporation)*

78. *Order:* Morphine sulfate gr $\frac{1}{12}$ subcut

    Label: Morphine sulfate 10 mg per mL

PRACTICE

Solve Using Dimensional Analysis (Continued)

79. *Order:* Atropine sulfate gr $\frac{1}{150}$ IM

   Label: Figure 13-22

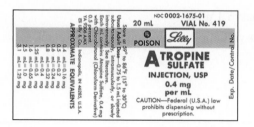

Figure 13-22 *(Courtesy of Eli Lilly Pharmaceuticals, Indianapolis, IN)*

80. *Order:* Morphine sulfate 10 mg IM

   Label: Figure 13-23
   Use a tuberculin syringe.

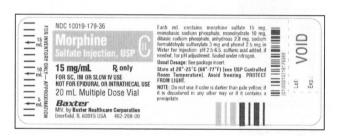

Figure 13-23 *(Courtesy of Baxter Healthcare Corporation)*

81. *Order:* Tagamet 200 mg IM

   Label: Tagamet (cimetidine) 300 mg per 2 mL in prefilled syringe

   Give _____ mL.

   Discard _____ mL.

PRACTICE

Solve Using Dimensional Analysis (Continued)

82. Order: Terramycin 150 mg IM

   Label: Terramycin (oxytetracycline) 50 mg per mL

83. Order: Depo-Provera 600 mg IM

   Label: Figure 13-24

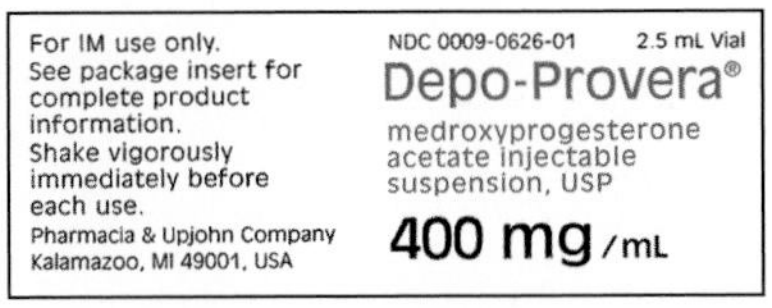

For IM use only.
See package insert for complete product information.
Shake vigorously immediately before each use.
Pharmacia & Upjohn Company
Kalamazoo, MI 49001, USA

NDC 0009-0626-01   2.5 mL Vial
Depo-Provera®
medroxyprogesterone acetate injectable suspension, USP
400 mg /mL

Figure 13-24 *(Courtesy of Pharmacia Corporation, Peapack, NJ)*

84. Order: Nembutal 60 mg IM

   Label: Nembutal (pentobarbital) 100 mg per 2 mL

85. Order: Kefzol 750 mg IM

   Label: Kefzol (cefazolin) 1 g per 3 mL

86. Order: Heparin sodium 7000 unit subcut

   Label: Figure 13-25

PRACTICE

Solve Using Dimensional Analysis (Continued)

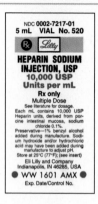

Figure 13-25
(Courtesy of Eli Lilly Pharmaceuticals, Indianapolis, IN)

87. ***Order:*** Valium 8 mg IM

    Label: Valium (diazepam) 5 mg per mL

88. ***Order:*** Atropine sulfate 0.3 mg IM

    Label: Atropine sulfate 0.4 mg per mL
    Use a tuberculin syringe.

89. ***Order:*** Vitamin B_{12} 750 mcg IM

    Label: Vitamin B_{12} 1000 mcg per mL
    Use a tuberculin syringe.

90. ***Order:*** Ceftazidime 0.25 g IM

    Label: Figure 13-26

PRACTICE

Solve Using Dimensional Analysis (Continued)

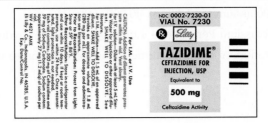

Figure 13-26   *(Courtesy of Eli Lilly Pharmaceuticals, Indianapolis, IN)*

91. *Order:* Aqua Mephyton 0.5 mg IM

   Label: Aqua Mephyton (phytonadione) 2 mg per mL

92. *Order:* Unasyn 0.5 g IM

   Label: Unasyn (ampicillin sodium/sulbactam sodium) 1.5 g dry powder
   Reconstitution: Add 3.2 mL sterile water for injection to yield 1.5 g per 4 mL.

93. *Order:* Streptomycin 400 mg IM

   Label: Streptomycin 1 g dry powder
   Reconstitution: Add 3.2 mL sterile water for injection to yield 250 mg per mL.

94. *Order:* Penbritin 350 mg IM

   Label: Penbritin (ampicillin sodium) 2 g dry powder
   Reconstitution: Add 6.8 mL sterile water for injection to yield 250 mg per mL.

PRACTICE

Solve Using Dimensional Analysis (Continued)

95. *Order:* Potassium Penicillin G 40,000 units IM

    Label: Potassium Penicillin G 1,000,000 units dry powder

    Reconstitution: Add 10 mL sterile saline for injection to yield 100,000 units per /mL.

96. *Order:* Ampicillin 500 mg IM

    Label: Ampicillin 1 g dry powder

    Reconstitution: Add 2.4 mL sterile water for injection to yield 1 g per 2.5 mL.

97. *Order:* Ticar 650 mg IM

    Label: Figure 13-27

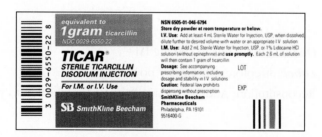

Figure 13-27 *(Courtesy of SmithKline Beecham Pharmaceuticals, Philadelphia, PA)*

98. *Order:* Pfizerpen 600,000 units IM

    Label: Buffered Pfizerpen (penicillin G potassium) 5,000,000 units dry powder

    Reconstitution: Add 4.8 mL sterile water for injection to yield 750,000 units per mL.

PRACTICE

Solve Using Dimensional Analysis (Continued)

99. ***Order:*** Megacillin 60,000 units IM

 Label: Megacillin (penicillin G potassium) 1,000,000 units dry powder

 Reconstitution: Add 20 mL sterile diluent to yield 50,000 units per mL.

100. ***Order:*** Cefizox 400 mg IM

 Label: Cefizox (ceftizoxime) 500 mg dry powder

 Reconstitution: Add 1.5 mL sterile diluent to yield 280 mg per mL.

101. ***Order:*** Kefzol 250 mg IM

 Label: Figure 13-28

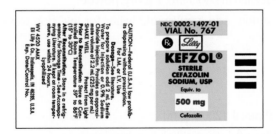

Figure 13-28 *(Courtesy of Eli Lilly Pharmaceuticals, Indianapolis, IN)*

102. ***Order:*** Tazicef (ceftazidime) 250 mg IM

 Label: Figure 13-29

 Directions: Calculate dosages based on each amount of diluent stated on the label.

 a.

 b.

Solve Using Dimensional Analysis (Continued)

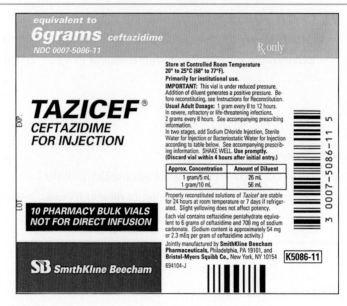

Figure 13-29 *(Reprinted with permission from GlaxoSmithKline)*

103. *Order:* Mezlin 0.6 g IM

   Label: Mezlin (mezlocillin) 1 g dry powder

   Reconstitution: Add 4 mL sterile water for injection to yield 250 mg per mL.

104. *Order:* Pipracil 1200 mg IM

   Label: Pipracil (piperacillin) 2 g dry powder

   Reconstitution: For each gram, add 2 mL of sterile diluent to yield 1 g per 2.5 mL.

105. *Order:* Ampicillin 150 mg IM

   Label: Ampicillin 1 g dry powder

   Reconstitution: Add 3.4 mL sterile water for injection to yield 1 g per 4 mL.

PRACTICE

Solve Using Dimensional Analysis (Continued)

106. *Order:* Ancef 500 mg IM

    Label: Ancef (cefazolin for injection) 1 g dry powder

    Reconstitution: Add 2.5 mL sterile water for injection to yield 330 mg per mL.

107. *Order:* Thorazine 35 mg IM

    Label: Figure 13-30

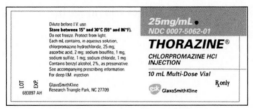

Figure 13-30 *(Reproduced with permission of GlaxoSmithKline Group of Companies, all rights reserved)*

108. *Order:* BCG vaccine 400,000 units ID

    Label: BCG vaccine 8,000,000 units per mL

109. *Order:* Vitamin A 17,500 units IM

    Label: Vitamin A 50,000 units per mL

110. *Order:* Vitamin A 35,000 units IM

    Label: Vitamin A 50,000 units per mL

PRACTICE

Solve Using Dimensional Analysis (Continued)

For 111–160, calculate flow rate in gtt/min unless directed otherwise.

111. *Order:* 3000 mL D5W IV in 24 hr

Drop Factor: 15 gtt per mL

112. *Order:* 750 mL 5% D5NS IV in 6 hr

Drop Factor: 15 gtt per mL

113. *Order:* 2500 mL Lactated Ringer's IV in 24 hr

Drop Factor: 15 gtt per mL

114. *Order:* 1000 mL D5W IV in 4 hr

Drop Factor: 10 gtt per mL

115. *Order:* 1.5 L NS IV in 8 hr

Drop Factor: 20 gtt per mL

116. *Order:* 1000 mL Ringer's Solution IV in 8 hr

Drop Factor: 15 gtt per mL

PRACTICE

Solve Using Dimensional Analysis (Continued)

117. *Order:* 250 mL packed blood cells IV in 4 hr

Drop Factor: 10 gtt per mL

118. *Order:* 650 mL D5W in 3 hr, IV

Drop Factor: 10 gtt per mL

119. *Order:* 1000 mL Ringer's Solution IV in 8 hr

Drop Factor: 10 gtt per mL

120. *Order:* 300 mL 10% Glucose in 8 hr, IV

Drop Factor: 10 gtt per mL

121. *Order:* 100 mL 10% Glucose in 3 hr, IV

Drop Factor: 15 gtt per mL

122. *Order:* 2000 mL D5W in 12 hr, IV

Drop Factor: 10 gtt per mL

PRACTICE

Solve Using Dimensional Analysis (Continued)

123. *Order:* 500 mL D5W in 4 hr, IV
Drop Factor: 10 gtt per mL

124. *Order:* 1200 mL D5W in 8 hr, IV
Drop Factor: 15 gtt per mL

125. *Order:* 900 mL NS in 6 hr, IV
Drop Factor: 10 gtt per mL

126. *Order:* 500 mL D5W in 3.5 hr, IV
Drop Factor: 15 gtt per mL

127. *Order:* 2000 mL of D5W in 24 hr, IV
Drop Factor: 10 gtt per mL

128. *Order:* 500 mL Normal Saline in 12 hr, IV
Drop Factor: 60 gtt per mL

PRACTICE

Solve Using Dimensional Analysis (Continued)

129. *Order:* 3000 mL D5W in 24 hr, IV

Drop Factor: 15 gtt per mL

130. *Order:* 1000 mL Lactated Ringer's in 12 hr, IV

Drop Factor: 60 gtt per mL

131. *Order:* 750 mL Ringer's Solution in 5 hr, IV

Drop Factor: 10 gtt per mL

132. *Order:* Vistide 200 mg in 250 mL sterile water IV in $1\frac{1}{2}$ hr

Drop Factor: 15 gtt per mL

133. *Order:* Floxin IV 400 mg in 1000 mL Isotonic Saline IV in 24 hr

Drop Factor: 10 gtt per mL

134. *Order:* Cosyntropin 0.25 mg in 500 mL D5W IV in 8 hr

Drop Factor: 15 gtt per mL

Solve Using Dimensional Analysis (Continued)

135. *Order:* Cardizem 100 mg in 200 mL NS IV to infuse at 15 mg per hr

Drop Factor: 60 gtt per mL

136. *Order:* Penicillin G Potassium 15,000,000 units IV in 1000 mL D5W to infuse over 24 hr

Label: Penicillin G Potassium 20,000,000 units

Reconstitution: Dilute with 31.6 mL of D5W to yield 500,000 units per mL.

Drop Factor: 15 gtt per mL

a. How much should be added to the 1000 mL of D5W?

b. What should the flow rate be?

137. *Order:* 2500 mL D5W IV

Drop Factor: 10 gtt per mL

Flow Rate: 40 gtt per min

How long should it take the IV to infuse?

138. *Order:* Zovirax 5 mg per kg IVPB in 100 mL D5W in 60 min

Weight: 70 kg

Label: Zovirax (acyclovir) 500 mg dry powder

Drop Factor: 60 gtt per mL

Directions: Reconstitute by adding 10 mL sterile diluent to yield 50 mg per mL.

a. How many mL of reconstituted Zovirax should be added to the 100 mL D5W?

Solve Using Dimensional Analysis (Continued)

b. What should the flow rate be?

139. *Order:* Aminophylline 1 g in 1000 mL D5 $\frac{1}{2}$ NS IV to infuse at 35 mg per hr

Drop Factor: 60 gtt per mL

What should the flow rate be?

140. *Order:* Mefoxin 2 g IVPB in 100 mL Sodium Chloride 0.9% IV in 60 min

Label: Mefoxin (cefoxitan sodium) 1 g dry powder

Reconstitution: Dilute with 10 mL sterile water for injection to yield 1 g per 10.5 mL.

Drop Factor: 15 gtt per mL

a. How many mL Mefoxin should be added to the IV solution?

b. What should the flow rate be?

141. *Order:* Cefazolin Sodium 1 g in 100 mL 10% DW IV to infuse in 60 min via Volutrol

Label: Cefazolin Sodium 1 g dry powder

Reconstitution: Dilute with 2.5 mL sterile water for injection to yield 1 g per 3 mL.

Drop Factor: 60 gtt per mL

What should the flow rate be?

PRACTICE

Solve Using Dimensional Analysis (Continued)

142. *Order:* Heparin sodium 30,000 units in 250 mL D5W IV to infuse at 10 mL/hr (via IV pump)

Label: Heparin sodium 20,000 units per mL

Drop Factor: 60 gtt per mL

  a. How many mL of heparin should be added to the IV solution?

  b. What should the flow rate be?

143. *Order:* Heparin sodium 10,000 units in 100 mL D5W IV to infuse at 1200 units per hr

Label: Heparin sodium 10,000 units per mL

Drop Factor: 60 gtt per mL

  a. What should the flow rate be?

  b. How many hours will it take to complete the IV?

144. *Order:* Regular Insulin 10 units per hr IV in 500 mL NS to infuse in 6 hr

Label: Regular Insulin 100 units per mL

How many units of insulin should be added to the IV solution in order to administer the insulin over a period of 6 hr?

Solve Using Dimensional Analysis (Continued)

145. *Order:* Lidocaine hydrochloride 1 g in 250 mL D5W (IV minibottle/peripheral lock) to infuse at a rate of 2 mg per min

Label: Lidocaine hydrochloride 1g per 5 mL

Drop Factor: 60 gtt per mL

What should the flow rate be?

146. *Order:* Dopamine hydrochloride 400 mg in 500 mL D5W to infuse at 5 mcg/kg/min IV

Weight: 75 kg

Drop Factor: 60 gtt per mL

    a. How many mcg per min should be administered?

    b. How many mL per hr will provide the required dose?

    c. How many gtt per min will provide the required dose?

    d. How many mcg per gtt will be administered?

147. *Order:* Heparin sodium 7000 units in 250 mL D5W at 0.4 units/kg/min IV

Weight: 129 lb

Drop Factor: 60 gtt per mL

    a. How many units per min should be administered?

PRACTICE

Solve Using Dimensional Analysis (Continued)

    b. How many mL per hr will provide the required dose?

    c. How many gtt per min will provide the required dose?

148. *Order:* Nipride (nitroprusside sodium) 50 mg in 250 mL D5W at 4 mcg/kg/min IV

Weight: 77.6 kg

Drop Factor: 60 gtt per mL

    a. How many mcg per min should be administered?

    b. How many mL per hr will provide the required dose?

    c. How many gtt per min will provide the required dose?

    d. How many mcg per gtt will be administered?

149. *Order:* Dobutamine hydrochloride 250 mg in 500 mL 5% Dextrose in Lactated Ringer's at 10 mcg/kg/min IV

Weight: 181 lb

Drop Factor: 60 gtt per mL

PRACTICE

Solve Using Dimensional Analysis (Continued)

a. How many mcg per min should be administered?

b. How many mL per hr will provide the required dose?

c. How many gtt per min will provide the required dose?

d. How many mcg per gtt will be administered?

150. ***Order:*** Intropin (dopamine hydrochloride) 400 mg in 500 mL D5W at 10 mcg/kg/min IV

Weight: 88.6 kg

Drop Factor: 60 gtt per mL

a. How many mcg per min should be administered?

b. How many mL per hr will provide the required dose?

c. How many gtt per min will provide the required dose?

PRACTICE

Solve Using Dimensional Analysis (Continued)

d. How many mcg per gtt will be administered?

151. *Order:* Nitroprusside sodium 50 mg in 250 mL D5W at 4 mcg/kg/min IV

Weight: 109 lb

Drop Factor: 60 gtt per mL

a. How many mcg per min should be administered?

b. How many mL per hr will provide the required dose?

c. How many gtt per min will provide the required dose?

d. How many mcg per gtt will be administered?

152. *Order:* Infuse Nitroprusside sodium 50 mg in 250 mL D5W. Titrate 0.5–1.5 mcg/kg/min to maintain the systolic blood pressure below 140 mm Hg.

Weight: 198 lb

a. What is the concentration of the solution in mcg per mL?

b. How many mcg per min will administer the ordered range of titration?

Solve Using Dimensional Analysis (Continued)

Lower (0.5 mcg/kg/min):

Upper (1.5 mcg/kg/min):

c. How many mL per hr or gtt per min will administer the ordered range of titration?

Lower:

Upper:

d. What is the titration (concentration) factor in mcg per gtt?

e. The present systolic blood pressure reading is 155 mm Hg. Increase the gtt per min by 5 gtt. How many mcg per min will the client now be receiving?

153. *Order:* Heparin Sodium 25,000 units in 500 mL D5W IV to infuse over 24 hr via IV pump

To how many mL per hr should the IV pump be set?

154. *Order:* Penicillin G Potassium 8 million units IVPB in 100 mL D5W to infuse over 1 hr

Label: Penicillin G Potassium 20,000,000 units dry powder

Solve Using Dimensional Analysis (Continued)

Reconstitution: Add 11.5 mL sterile water for injection to yield 1,000,000 units per mL.

Drop Factor: 15 gtt per mL

a. How many mL of reconstituted solution should be added to 100 mL D5W?

b. What should the flow rate be?

155. *Order:* KCl 40 mEq in 1000 mL D5W IV

   Drop Factor: 15 gtt per mL

   Flow Rate: 35 gtt per min

   How long should it take the IV to infuse?

156. *Order:* Aminophylline 150 mg IVPB in 100 mL D5W to infuse in 60 min

   Label: Aminophylline 250 mg per 10 mL

   Drop Factor: 60 gtt per mL

   a. How many mL should be added to the 100 mL D5W?

   b. What should the flow rate be?

157. *Order:* Zovirax (acyclovir) 5 mg per kg IVPB in 100 mL D5W to infuse in 60 min

   Label: Zovirax 500 mg dry powder

   Weight: 130 lb

Solve Using Dimensional Analysis (Continued)

Reconstitution: Add 10 mL sterile water for injection to yield 500 mg per 10 mL.

Drop Factor: 60 gtt per mL

a. How many mL should be added to the 100 mL D5W?

b. What should the flow rate be?

158. **Order:** Cefizox (ceftizoxime for injection) 2 g IVPB in 100 mL D5W to infuse in 1 hour

Label: Cefizox 2 g dry powder

Reconstitution: Add 20 mL sterile diluent to yield 95 mg per mL.

Drop Factor: 15 gtt per mL

a. How many mL of reconstituted solution should be added to 100 mL D5W?

b. What should the flow rate be?

159. **Order:** Kefurox 750 mg in 100 mL NS IV via Metriset

Drop Factor: 60 gtt per mL

Flow Rate: 100 gtt per min

How long should it take the IV to infuse?

160. **Order:** 1000 mL D5$\frac{1}{2}$ NS IV via central venous catheter to infuse at 150 mL per hr for first 500 mL. Add MVI 10 mL to remaining 500 mL and continue infusion at 75 mL per hr. Use an IV pump.

Solve Using Dimensional Analysis (Continued)

Label: MVI 10 mL per ampule

Drop Factor: 60 gtt per mL

a. What should the flow rate be for the first 500 mL?

b. To what should the rate be adjusted for the remaining 500 mL?

161. *Order:* Heparin sodium 10,000 units in 100 mL D5W IV to infuse at 10 gtt per min

Drop Factor: 60 gtt per mL

How many units of heparin is the client receiving in 24 hours?

162. *Order:* Digoxin 0.375 mg IV push at a rate of 0.5 mL per min

Label: Digoxin 0.25 mg per mL

a. How many mL of digoxin should be administered?

b. How long should it take to administer the IV digoxin?

163. *Order:* Lidocaine hydrochloride 1 mg per kg via IV push

Weight: 154 lb

How many mg should be administered per dose?

164. *Order:* Adriamycin 30 mg per M^2 via IV bolus at a rate of 3 mg per min. BSA = 0.5 M^2

Label: Adriamycin (doxorubicin hydrochloride) 10 mg. Dilute in 5 mL sodium chloride for injection.

Solve Using Dimensional Analysis (Continued)

    a. How many mL should be administered per dose?

    b. How long should it take to inject the Adriamycin?

165. *Order:* Valium 0.3 mg per kg via IV bolus at a rate of 5 mg per min

    Label: Valium (diazepam) 5 mg per mL

    Weight: 40 lb

    a. How many mL of Valium should the child receive per dose?

    b. How long should it take to inject the Valium?

166. *Order:* Mivacron 0.15 mg per kg of body weight via IV push over a period of 10 sec

    Label: Mivacron (mivacurium chloride) 2 mg per mL

    Weight: 35 lb

    How many mL of Mivacron should the child receive per dose?

167. *Order:* TPN 1000 mL Liposyn II 20% IV

    How many kcal of fat are provided?

PRACTICE

Solve Using Dimensional Analysis (Continued)

168. *Order:* CPN 1000 mL 5% dextrose in 0.9% Sodium Chloride IV
How many kcal of carbohydrate are provided?

169. *Order:* PTPN 500 mL Aminosyn II 3.5% IV
How many kcal of protein are provided?

170. *Order:* Hyperalimentation 1500 mL Liposyn 10% IV
How many kcal of fat are provided?

171. *Order:* Methimazole 0.4 mg per kg PO in three divided doses
Label: Methimazole 5 mg per tab (scored)
Weight: 79 lb

172. *Order:* Valproic Acid per 5 mg per kg PO in three divided doses
Label: Valproic Acid 250 mg per 5 mL
Weight: 165 lb

173. *Order:* Isoniazid 5 mg per kg PO
Label: Isoniazid 100 mg per tab
Weight: 60 kg

Solve Using Dimensional Analysis (Continued)

174. *Order:* Sus-Phrine 0.02 mg per kg subcut

   Label: Sus-Phrine (epinephrine) 1:1000 1 mg per mL

   Weight: 44 lb

175. *Order:* Velosef Expectorant 25 mg/kg/day PO in two divided doses

   Label: Velosef (cephradine expectorant) 125 mg per 5 mL

   Weight: 32 lb

   How many mL should be administered per dose?

176. *Order:* Symmetrel Syrup 8.8 mg/kg PO in two divided doses

   Label: Symmetrel (amantadine) Syrup 50 mg per 5 mL

   Weight: 35 lb

177. *Order:* Terramycin 3 mg/lb/day in two divided doses IM

   Label: Terramycin (oxytetracycline) 100 mg per 2 mL

   Weight: 20 lb

178. *Order:* Kefzol 40 mg/kg/day in three divided doses IM

   Label: Kefzol (cefazolin sodium) 330 mg per mL

   Weight: 55 lb

Solve Using Dimensional Analysis (Continued)

179. *Order:* Naloxone 0.01 mg per kg IM stat

   Label: Figure 13-31

   Weight: 6 lb

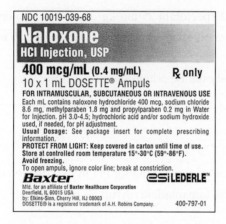

NDC 10019-039-68

Naloxone
HCl Injection, USP

400 mcg/mL (0.4 mg/mL)   R only
10 x 1 mL DOSETTE® Ampuls
FOR INTRAMUSCULAR, SUBCUTANEOUS OR INTRAVENOUS USE
Each mL contains naloxone hydrochloride 400 mcg, sodium chloride
8.6 mg, methylparaben 1.8 mg and propylparaben 0.2 mg in Water
for Injection. pH 3.0-4.5; hydrochloric acid and/or sodium hydroxide
used, if needed, for pH adjustment.
Usual Dosage: See package insert for complete prescribing
information.
PROTECT FROM LIGHT: Keep covered in carton until time of use.
Store at controlled room temperature 15°-30°C (59°-86°F).
Avoid freezing.
To open ampuls, ignore color line; break at constriction.
Baxter   **eSiLEDERLE**™
Mfd. for an affiliate of Baxter Healthcare Corporation
Deerfield, IL 60015 USA
by: Elkins-Sinn, Cherry Hill, NJ 08003
DOSETTE® is a registered trademark of A.H. Robins Company.   400-797-01

Figure 13-31 *(Courtesy of Baxter Healthcare Corporation, Deerfield, IL)*

180. *Order:* Vibramycin Syrup 4.4 mg/kg/day in two divided doses PO

   Label: Vibramycin Syrup (dorycycline calcium) 50 mg per tsp

   Weight: 60 lb

   Give _____ mL/dose.

181. *Order:* Nebcin 7.5 mg/kg/day in four divided doses IM

   Label: Figure 13-32

   Weight: 15 kg

PRACTICE

Solve Using Dimensional Analysis (Continued)

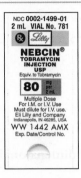

Figure 13-32   *(Courtesy of Eli Lilly Pharmaceuticals, Indianapolis, IN)*

182. **Order:** Dobutrex 250 mg in 500 mL 5% Dextrose IV at 5 mcg per kg per min

   Label: Dobutrex (dobutamine hydrochloride) 250 mg per 20 mL

   Weight: 143 lb

183. **Order:** Dilantin 5 mg/kg/day in two divided doses PO

   Label: Dilantin (phenytoin) 125 mg per 5 mL

   Weight: 62 lb

184. **Order:** Kefzol 25 mg/kg/day in four divided doses IM

   Label: Kefzol (cefazolin sodium) 250 mg dry powder

   Weight: 30 lb

   Reconstitution: Dilute in 2 mL sterile water for injection to yield 125 mg per mL.

PRACTICE

Solve Using Dimensional Analysis (Continued)

185. *Order:* Acetaminophen Elixir 10 mg/kg/dose PO

    Label: Acetaminophen Elixir 160 mg per 5 mL

    Weight: 54 lb

For 186–190, use the West nomogram and dimensional analysis.

186. Child's height: 33 in

    Child's weight: 28 lb

    Adult dose: Dilantin (phenytoin sodium) 100 mg

    Find the child's dose.

187. Child's height: 95 cm

    Child's weight: 15 kg

    Adult dose: Lomotil (diphenoxylate hydrochloride and atropine sulfate) 5 mL

    Find the child's dose.

188. Child's height: 104 cm

    Child's weight: 17 kg

    Adult dose: Atropine sulfate 0.4 mg

    Find the child's dose.

189. Child's height: 52 in

    Child's weight: 50 lb

PRACTICE

Solve Using Dimensional Analysis (Continued)

Adult dose: Digoxin 0.125 mg
Find the child's dose.

190. Child's height: 58.5 cm
Child's weight: 5.9 kg
Adult dose: Valium (diazepam) 2 mg
Find the child's dose.

For 191–200, use the drug labels in Figure 13-33 and calculate the correct dosage.

191. *Order:* Ticar (ticarcillin) 250 mg IM

192. *Order:* Cefpodoxime proxetil for Oral Suspension 10 mg/kg/PO
Weight: 31 lb

193. *Order:* Depo-Provera 1000 mg IM

194. *Order:* Heparin sodium 3000 units subcut

PRACTICE

Solve Using Dimensional Analysis (Continued)

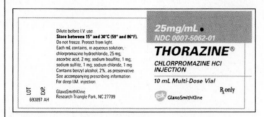

a.

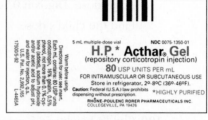

b.

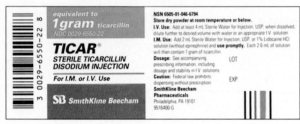

c.

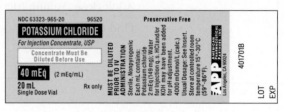

d.

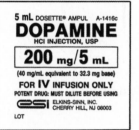

e.

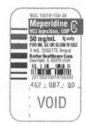

f.

g.

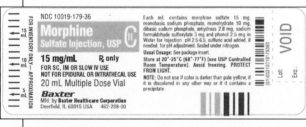

h.

i.

PRACTICE

Solve Using Dimensional Analysis (Continued)

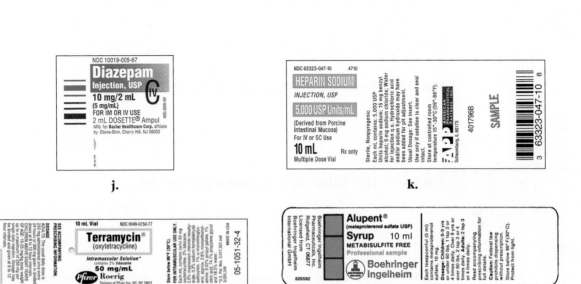

j.

k.

l.

m.

Figure 13-33 *(a and c courtesy of GlaxoSmithKline Group of Companies, all rights reserved; b, courtesy of Rhône-Poulenc Rorer Pharmaceuticals, Inc., Collegeville, PA; d, i, and k courtesy of American Pharmaceutical Partners, e courtesy of Elkins-Sinn, Inc., Cherry Hill, NJ; g and h, courtesy of Pharmacia Corporation, Peapack, NJ; j, courtesy of Baxter Healthcare Corporation, Deerfield, IL; l, Courtesy of Pfizer, Inc., New York, NY; m, courtesy of Boehringer Ingelheims Pharmaceuticals, Inc., Ridgefield, CT)*

195. *Order:* Chlorpromazine hydrochloride 35 mg PO

196. *Order:* Demerol (meperidine) 35 mg IM

197. *Order:* Sodium bicarbonate 0.5 mEq per kg IV
Weight: 135 lb

Solve Using Dimensional Analysis (Continued)

198. *Order:* Oxytetracycline 100 mg IM

199. *Order:* Dopamine hydrochloride 125 mg IV

200. *Order:* H.P. Acthar Gel (corticotropin) 70 units IM

201. The client is to receive Demerol 75 mg and Phenergan 12.5 mg IM in the same syringe.

   Label: Demerol (meperidine hydrochloride) 50 mg per mL

   Phenergan (promethazine hydrochloride) 25 mg per mL

   How many mL would contain the total amount of medication ordered?

202. An adult weighing 225 lb is to receive Alfentanil hydrochloride Injection 8 mcg per kg IV.

   Label: Alfentanil hydrochloride Injection 500 mcg per mL

   How many mL of Alfentanil should be administered?

203. The client is to receive Tagamet 800 mg per day IM to be divided in equal doses and given q 6 hr.

   Label: Tagamet (cimetidine hydrochloride) 300 mg per 2 mL

   How many mL should be administered per dose?

PRACTICE

Solve Using Dimensional Analysis (Continued)

204. The client is to receive 125 mL per hr of 0.9% NS IV. How many mL per min will be administered?

205. The client is to receive Heparin sodium 8000 units subcut

Label: Heparin sodium 10,000 units per mL

How many mL should be given?

206. An infant weighing 20 lb is to receive Gantrisin Pediatric 75 mg/kg/day in 4 divided doses PO.

Label: Gantrisin Pediatric (sulfisoxazole) 0.5 g per tsp

How many mL should be given per dose?

207. The client is to receive 1000 mL 5% D/W IV. How many g of glucose does the solution contain?

208. The client has an IV of 1000 mL D5W to which Potassium chloride 10 mEq is to be added.

Label: Potassium chloride 30 mEq per mL

How many mL of KCl should be added to the IV solution?

Solve Using Dimensional Analysis (Continued)

209. The client is to receive Pitocin (oxytocin) 5 units in 500 mL Ringer's lactate solution IV. How many milliunits of Pitocin does 1 mL of the solution contain?

210. The client is to receive NegGram Suspension 2 g per day PO in equal doses q 6 hr.

Label: NegGram (naladaxic acid) 250 mg per tsp

How many mL should each dose contain?

211. The client is to receive 500 mL of 25% D/W. How many kcal of dextrose would the client be receiving?

212. A client weighing 160 lb is to receive Dobutrex (dobutamine hydrochloride) 7.5 mcg/kg/min IV. How many mcg per hr will the client receive?

213. The client is to receive 750 mL of 5% D/NS in 5 hours. How many mL per hr should the client receive?

214. The client receives a total daily dosage of 300 mg Macrobid PO in four equal doses.

Label: Macrobid (nitrofurantoin macrocrystals) 25 mg per cap

How many capsules should the client receive per dose?

Solve Using Dimensional Analysis (Continued)

215. The client is to receive Revimine (dopamine hydrochloride) 400 mg in 1000 mL D5W IV to be administered at a rate of 5 mcg/kg/min.

How many mcg of Revimine does 1 mL of solution contain?

216. A client weighing 150 lb is to receive Dopamine hydrochloride 400 mg in 500 mL of IV solution to be administered at a rate of 5 mcg/kg/min. How many mL per hr should the client receive?

217. A client weighing 154 lb is to receive Dobutrex (dobutamine hydrochloride) 250 mg in 250 mL D5W to infuse at a rate of 5 mcg/kg/min.

a. How many mcg per mL will the mixed solution contain?

b. How many mcg per min should the client receive?

c. How many mL per hr will provide the required dose?

218. A client weighing 160 lb is to receive Dopamine hydrochloride 400 mg in 250 mL D5W to infuse at a rate of 5 mcg/kg/min.

a. How many mcg per mL will the mixed solution contain?

PRACTICE

Solve Using Dimensional Analysis (Continued)

b. How many mcg per min should the client receive?

c. How many mL per hr will provide the required dose?

219. *Order:* Infuse Epinephrine 1 mg in 100 mL at 5 mcg per min.
   a. How many mcg per mL will the mixed solution contain?

   b. How many mL per hr will provide the required dose?

220. *Order:* Infuse Pronestyl 1 g in 250 mL D5W at 3 mg per min.
   a. What is the concentration (mg per mL) of the mixed solution?

   b. How many mL per hr will provide the required dose?

(*Note:* See Appendix G for answer key.)

Arithmetic Review

ROMAN NUMERALS

RULE

1. Letters are used to designate numbers.

I = 1

V = 5

X = 10

L = 50

C = 100

2. Reading from left to right:

(a) if the first Roman numeral is greater than the following numeral(s), then add (all together).

EXAMPLES   VI = 5 + 1 = 6

XII = 10 + 2 = 12

(b) if the first Roman numeral is less than the following numeral(s), then subtract (smaller from the larger).

EXAMPLES   IV = 5 − 1 = 4

XL = 50 − 10 = 40

(c) if a smaller Roman numeral comes between 2 larger ones, subtract, then add.

EXAMPLES   XIV = 10 + (5–1) = 10 + 4 = 14

LIX = 50 + (10–1) = 50 + 9 = 59

A. Express the following Arabic numerals as Roman numerals.

1. 6		**6.** 46
2. 50		**7.** 17
3. 3		**8.** 38
4. 12		**9.** 25
5. 24		**10.** 9

B. Express the following Roman numerals as Arabic numerals.

1. XLVII		**6.** VII
2. XXIX		**7.** II
3. V		**8.** LXVI
4. CXII		**9.** CCCIX
5. MCMXXXIII		**10.** XIII

ADDITION

Add the following whole numbers.

1.
```
   12
 + 16
```

2.
```
   22
 +  3
```

3.
```
   43
 + 15
```

4.
```
   28
   48
 + 69
```

5.
```
   39
   88
 + 16
```

6.
```
   642
    91
 + 357
```

7.
```
   611
   292
 + 386
```

8.
```
    81
   648
 +  43
```

9.
```
   8397
    184
 + 5240
```

10.
```
 31,017
     13
 + 2,377
```

11. 6 + 23 =

12. 13 + 52 =

13. 19 + 32 + 15 =

14. 17 + 231 + 92 =

15. 700 + 26 + 845 =

16. 9 + 47 + 299 =

17. 393 + 209 + 567 =

18. 2,091 + 581 + 6,727 =

19. 8 + 5,496 + 745 =

20. 40 + 50,008 + 9,833 =

SUBTRACTION

Subtract the following whole numbers.

1.
```
   29
 -  6
```

2.
```
   215
 -  38
```

3.
```
 5309
 - 342
```

4.
```
   7333
 - 4281
```

5.
```
   73
 - 41
```

6.
```
   303
 -  55
```

7.
```
 12,965
 -   492
```

8.
```
   138
 -  25
```

9.
```
   8846
 - 8721
```

10.   965
        − 82

11. 42 − 31 =

12. 54 − 36 =

13. 235 − 66 =

14. 465 − 203 =

15. 209 − 65 =

16. 6699 − 301 =

17. 1124 − 908 =

18. 1865 − 1392 =

19. 32,945 − 2,030 =

20. 56,841 − 32,931 =

MULTIPLICATION

Multiply the following numbers.

1.   8
       × 4

2.   24
       × 13

3.   311
       × 252

4.   15
       × 9

5.   143
       × 91

6.   609
       × 23

7.   497
       × 704

8. 2536
       × 219

9. 1551
       × 69

10. 733
       × 300

11. 19 × 4 =

12. 21 × 6 =

13. 34 × 12 =

14. 62 × 18 =

15. 256 × 79 =

16. 689 × 203 =

17. 181 × 117 =

18. 1598 × 200 =

19. 18,452 × 1,501 =

20. 986 × 1000 =

DIVISION

Solve the following division problems. Carry answers to two decimal places and round to nearest tenth.

1. $4\overline{)20}$

2. $25\overline{)295}$

3. $8\overline{)164}$

4. $3\overline{)925}$

5. $13\overline{)2363}$

6. $16\overline{)5493}$

7. $232\overline{)2696}$

8. $473\overline{)9652}$

9. $281\overline{)6795}$

10. $596\overline{)9235}$

11. 105 ÷ 5 =

12. 648 ÷ 8 =

13. 2222 ÷ 11 =

14. 6950 ÷ 30 =

15. 6393 ÷ 16 =

16. 15,321 ÷ 35 =

17. 16,209 ÷ 10 =

18. 18,492 ÷ 933 =

19. 802,495 ÷ 436 =

20. 111,666 ÷ 606 =

FRACTIONS

A. Reduce the following fractions to lowest terms.

RULE

Divide both numerator and denominator by the largest whole number that will go evenly into each.

EXAMPLE $\dfrac{5}{10} = \dfrac{5 \div 5}{10 \div 5} = \dfrac{1}{2}$

PRACTICE

1. $\dfrac{2}{6}$

2. $\dfrac{3}{9}$

3. $\dfrac{4}{8}$

4. $\dfrac{3}{15}$

5. $\dfrac{5}{55}$

6. $\dfrac{12}{48}$

7. $\dfrac{9}{10}$

8. $\dfrac{14}{56}$

9. $\dfrac{18}{80}$

10. $\dfrac{255}{1530}$

B. Convert the following mixed numbers to improper fractions.

RULE

Multiply the whole number by the denominator, add to numerator, and place this sum over the original denominator.

EXAMPLE $5\dfrac{3}{8} = 5 \times 8 = 40 + 3 = \dfrac{43}{8}$

PRACTICE

1. $2\,{}^{3}\!/_{4}$

2. $7\,{}^{8}\!/_{9}$

3. $5\,{}^{3}\!/_{10}$

4. $12\,{}^{1}\!/_{4}$

5. $6\,{}^{2}\!/_{3}$

6. $9\,{}^{2}\!/_{5}$

7. $1\,{}^{2}\!/_{3}$

8. $1\,{}^{1}\!/_{2}$

9. $10\,{}^{2}\!/_{5}$

10. $8\,{}^{3}\!/_{6}$

C. Convert the following improper fractions to mixed numbers. Reduce the fraction to lowest terms.

RULE

Divide the denominator into the numerator and reduce to lowest terms.

EXAMPLE $\quad \dfrac{72}{9} = 72 \div 9 = 8$

$$\dfrac{45}{6} = 45 \div 6 = 7\dfrac{3}{6} = 7\dfrac{1}{2}$$

PRACTICE

1. $\dfrac{25}{6}$

2. $\dfrac{19}{3}$

3. $\dfrac{94}{5}$

4. $\dfrac{62}{8}$

5. $\dfrac{16}{11}$

6. $\dfrac{40}{13}$

PRACTICE (Continued)

7. $\dfrac{122}{9}$

9. $\dfrac{82}{4}$

8. $\dfrac{125}{23}$

10. $\dfrac{99}{2}$

D. Add the following fractions. Convert the answer to mixed numbers when possible and reduce the fraction to lowest terms.

RULE

When the denominators are the same, add the numerators and place this sum over the original denominator.

EXAMPLE

$$\begin{array}{r} \dfrac{1}{8} \\[6pt] + \dfrac{3}{8} \\[6pt] \hline \dfrac{4}{8} = \dfrac{1}{2} \end{array}$$

RULE

1. When the denominators are not the same, determine the least common denominator (LCD) by finding the smallest number divisible by both denominators.

2. Divide each denominator by this LCD and multiply each numerator by its respective quotient.

3. Add the numerators, place over the LCD and reduce to lowest terms.

EXAMPLE

$$\begin{array}{rcl} \dfrac{2}{16} & = & \dfrac{2}{16} \\[8pt] + \dfrac{1}{8} & = & + \dfrac{2}{16} \qquad \text{LCD} = 16 \\[8pt] \hline & & \dfrac{4}{16} = \dfrac{1}{4} \end{array}$$

$$\frac{7}{10} = \frac{49}{70}$$

$$+ \frac{9}{35} = + \frac{18}{70} \qquad \text{LCD} = 70$$

$$\frac{67}{70}$$

PRACTICE

1. $\frac{7}{9}$
$+ \frac{4}{9}$

2. $\frac{3}{4}$
$+ \frac{1}{4}$

3. $\frac{2}{6}$
$+ \frac{5}{6}$

4. $\frac{1}{12}$
$+ \frac{4}{12}$

5. $\frac{1}{15}$
$\frac{2}{15}$
$+ \frac{6}{15}$

6. $\frac{32}{90}$
$+ \frac{16}{90}$

7. $\frac{1}{3}$
$+ \frac{3}{4}$

8. $\frac{2}{5}$
$\frac{6}{10}$
$+ \frac{3}{5}$

9. $\frac{2}{3}$
$\frac{5}{6}$
$+ \frac{4}{6}$

10. $\frac{60}{48}$
$+ \frac{34}{48}$

11. $\frac{1}{2} + \frac{2}{2} =$

12. $\frac{2}{3} + \frac{1}{3} =$

PRACTICE

13. $\dfrac{5}{8} + \dfrac{2}{8} =$

14. $\dfrac{2}{3} + \dfrac{1}{4} + \dfrac{5}{6} =$

15. $\dfrac{2}{12} + \dfrac{3}{18} + \dfrac{2}{2} =$

16. $\dfrac{2}{3} + \dfrac{5}{12} + \dfrac{2}{4} =$

17. $\dfrac{3}{15} + \dfrac{10}{60} + \dfrac{1}{12} =$

18. $\dfrac{1}{4} + \dfrac{16}{64} + \dfrac{8}{32} =$

19. $\dfrac{9}{10} + \dfrac{20}{100} + \dfrac{6}{10} =$

20. $\dfrac{32}{18} + \dfrac{1}{18} + \dfrac{9}{72} =$

E. Subtract the following fractions. Convert the answer to mixed numbers when possible and reduce the fraction to lowest terms.

RULE

When the denominators are the same, subtract the numerators and place this difference over the original denominator.

EXAMPLE

$$\begin{array}{r} \dfrac{7}{10} \\ -\ \dfrac{3}{10} \\ \hline \dfrac{4}{10} = \dfrac{2}{5} \end{array}$$

RULE

1. When the denominators are not the same, determine the least common denominator (LCD) by finding the smallest number divisible by both denominators.

2. Divide each denominator by this LCD and multiply each numerator by its respective quotient.

3. Subtract the numerators, place over the LCD, and reduce to lowest terms.

EXAMPLE

$$\frac{13}{21}$$
$$-\frac{4}{21}$$
$$\frac{9}{21} = \frac{3}{7}$$

PRACTICE

1. $\frac{5}{6}$
$-\frac{1}{6}$

2. $\frac{3}{7}$
$-\frac{2}{7}$

3. $\frac{7}{14}$
$-\frac{3}{14}$

4. $\frac{3}{4}$
$-\frac{2}{4}$

5. $\frac{19}{36}$
$-\frac{6}{36}$

6. $\frac{9}{11}$
$-\frac{2}{33}$

7. $\frac{10}{2}$
$-\frac{4}{5}$

8. $\frac{90}{10}$
$-\frac{12}{6}$

9. $\frac{36}{7}$
$-\frac{2}{3}$

10. $\frac{50}{10}$
$-\frac{30}{40}$

11. $\frac{2}{4} - \frac{1}{4} =$

12. $\frac{8}{12} - \frac{3}{12} =$

13. $\frac{4}{8} - \frac{3}{8} =$

14. $\frac{5}{8} - \frac{1}{2} =$

15. $\frac{14}{18} - \frac{6}{24} =$

16. $\frac{32}{8} - \frac{2}{4} =$

17. $\frac{100}{50} - \frac{3}{5} =$

18. $\frac{20}{15} - \frac{4}{5} =$

19. $\frac{28}{7} - \frac{2}{3} =$

20. $\frac{14}{2} - \frac{4}{6} =$

F. Multiply the following fractions. Convert answer to mixed numbers when possible and reduce the fraction to lowest terms.

> ### RULE
>
> **1.** Convert mixed numbers to improper fractions.
>
> **2.** Use cancellation and division to reduce the size of numbers in numerators or denominators.
>
> **3.** Multiply numerators and denominators and reduce the resulting fraction to lowest terms or convert to a mixed number.

EXAMPLES

$$\frac{1}{\cancel{6}_2} \times \frac{\cancel{3}^1}{5} = \frac{1}{10} \qquad 2\frac{3}{4} \times 4\frac{1}{2} \times \frac{11}{4} \times \frac{9}{2} = \frac{99}{8} = 12\frac{3}{8}$$

Hints on cancellation:

1. Look for powers of 10 (cross out zero[s]).

EXAMPLES

a. $175,\cancel{000} \times \dfrac{1}{200,\cancel{000}} = \dfrac{7}{8}$ (Divide by 5) (then by another 5)

$\overset{7}{\cancel{35}}$ ... $\overset{\cancel{40}}{8}$

OR

$175,\cancel{000}^{\,7} \times \dfrac{1}{200,\cancel{000}_{\,8}}$ (Divide by 25) $= \dfrac{7}{8}$

OR

b. $29\cancel{0} \times \dfrac{1}{1\cancel{000}} \times \dfrac{\cancel{500}}{5\cancel{0}} \times \dfrac{6\cancel{0}}{1} = 29 \times 6 = 174$

Cross out zeros.

OR

$\cancel{290}^{58} \times \dfrac{1}{1\cancel{000}_2} \times \dfrac{\cancel{500}}{5\cancel{0}_1} \times \dfrac{6\cancel{0}}{1} = 58 \times 6 = \dfrac{348}{2} = 174$

2. Any even numbers—such as 58, 2, or 6—can always be divided by 2.

EXAMPLE

$$\overset{58}{\cancel{290}} \times \frac{1}{\cancel{1000}} \times \frac{\overset{1}{\cancel{500}}}{\cancel{50}} \times \frac{\overset{3}{\cancel{60}}}{1} = 58 \times 3 = 174 \quad \text{OR} \quad 29 \times 6 = 174$$

either divide the 2 into 6 or 2 into 58

3. If the sum of the digits in a number can be divided by a certain number, then that number divides into the original number.

EXAMPLE

$$84 \times \frac{1}{2.2} \times \frac{8}{1} \times \frac{\overset{1}{\cancel{5}}}{\cancel{75}} \times \frac{5}{1}$$

If the sum of the digits in a number can be divided by 3, then 3 divides into the original number.

84 is 8 + 4 = 12

since 12 ÷ 3 is 4 (not a fraction)

then

$$\begin{array}{r} 28 \\ 3\overline{)84} \\ \underline{6} \\ 24 \\ \underline{24} \end{array}$$

$$\overset{28}{\cancel{84}} \times \frac{1}{2.2} \times \frac{8}{1} \times \frac{\overset{1}{\cancel{5}}}{\cancel{75}} \times \frac{\overset{1}{\cancel{5}}}{1}$$

now divide 28 or 8 and 2.2 by 2 (Example shows 8 and 2.2 divided by 2)

$$\overset{28}{\cancel{84}} \times \frac{1}{\underset{1.1}{\cancel{2.2}}} \times \frac{\overset{4}{\cancel{8}}}{1} \times \frac{\overset{1}{\cancel{5}}}{\cancel{75}} \times \frac{\overset{1}{\cancel{5}}}{1} = \frac{112}{1.1} = 1.1\overline{)112.0.000}$$

$$\begin{array}{r} 101.818 \\ 1.1\overline{)112.0.000} \\ \underline{11} \\ 20 \\ \underline{11} \\ 90 \\ \underline{88} \\ 20 \\ \underline{11} \\ 90 \end{array}$$

$$\frac{112}{1.1} = 102$$

or 101.8

or 101.82

PRACTICE

1. $\dfrac{6}{7} \times \dfrac{3}{5} =$

2. $\dfrac{1}{4} \times \dfrac{3}{5} =$

3. $\dfrac{8}{10} \times \dfrac{1}{4} =$

4. $6\dfrac{2}{3} \times 5\dfrac{1}{2} =$

5. $5 \times 3\dfrac{2}{10} =$

6. $9 \times 3\dfrac{2}{3} =$

7. $6\dfrac{3}{7} \times 8 =$

8. $3\dfrac{2}{5} \times 20 =$

9. $4\dfrac{1}{6} \times 5\dfrac{1}{4} =$

10. $2\dfrac{6}{10} \times 1\dfrac{9}{10} =$

G. Divide the following fractions. Convert the answer to mixed numbers when possible and reduce the fraction to lowest terms.

RULE

1. Convert mixed numbers to improper fractions.

2. Invert the second fraction.

3. Cancel the numerator and denominator wherever possible.

4. Multiply the numerator and denominator and reduce the resulting fraction to lowest terms or convert to a mixed number.

EXAMPLES

$$\dfrac{1}{10} \div \dfrac{35}{5} = \dfrac{1}{10} \times \dfrac{\overset{1}{\cancel{5}}}{3} = \dfrac{1}{6}$$

$$5\dfrac{3}{4} \div 3\dfrac{1}{6} = \dfrac{23}{\underset{2}{\cancel{4}}} \times \dfrac{\overset{3}{\cancel{6}}}{19} = \dfrac{69}{38} = 1\dfrac{31}{38}$$

PRACTICE

1. $\dfrac{1}{4} \div \dfrac{2}{16} =$

2. $\dfrac{1}{2} \div \dfrac{3}{2} =$

3. $\dfrac{3}{6} \div \dfrac{22}{23} =$

4. $\dfrac{32}{4} \div 2 =$

5. $6\dfrac{2}{4} \div 4 =$

6. $2\dfrac{2}{5} \div 1\dfrac{3}{15} =$

7. $4\dfrac{2}{4} \div 3\dfrac{1}{2} =$

8. $2\dfrac{2}{8} \div 3\dfrac{4}{8} =$

9. $4\dfrac{6}{18} \div \dfrac{4}{8} =$

10. $20\dfrac{1}{2} \div 6\dfrac{1}{6} =$

Note: When multiplying complex fractions, it is necessary to use both the multiplication and division rules for fractions.

EXAMPLES

a. $\dfrac{1}{6} \times \dfrac{20}{1/4} \times \dfrac{1}{15}$

Take $\dfrac{20}{1/4}$ to the side and get a simpler fraction.

$\dfrac{20}{1/4}$ means 20 divided by $\dfrac{1}{4}$ or

$20 \div \dfrac{1}{4} = 20 \times \dfrac{4}{1} = 80$

So, $\dfrac{1}{6} \times \dfrac{20}{1/4} \times \dfrac{1}{15}$ becomes $\dfrac{1}{\cancel{6}_3} \times \cancel{80}^{\overset{\displaystyle 8}{\cancel{16}}} \times \dfrac{1}{\cancel{15}_3} = \dfrac{8}{9}$

or 0.889 or 0.89 or 0.9

OR change $\dfrac{1}{4}$ to 0.25

$$\dfrac{1}{6} \times \dfrac{20}{1/4} \times \dfrac{1}{15} = \dfrac{1}{\cancel{6}_{3}} \times \dfrac{\overset{2}{\cancel{20}}}{.25} \times \dfrac{1}{\cancel{15}_{3}} = \dfrac{2}{2.25}$$

$$
\begin{array}{r}
.88 \\
2.25\overline{)2.00.00} \\
\underline{180} \\
2000 \\
\underline{1800} \\
\end{array}
$$

b. $\dfrac{1}{100} \times \dfrac{1}{1/150} \times \dfrac{15}{1}$

$$1 \div \dfrac{1}{150} = 1 \times \dfrac{150}{1} = 150$$

$$= \dfrac{1}{\cancel{100}_{2}} \times \dfrac{\overset{3}{\cancel{150}}}{1} \times \dfrac{15}{1} = \dfrac{45}{2} = 22.5$$

OR change $\dfrac{1}{150}$ to a decimal as shown in the previous example

$$\dfrac{1}{100} \times \dfrac{1}{1/150} \times \dfrac{15}{1}$$

$$
\dfrac{1}{150} = 150\overline{)1.0000}
\begin{array}{l}
.0066 \\
\end{array}
$$
$$
\begin{array}{r}
.0066 \\
150\overline{)1.0000} \\
\underline{900} \\
1000 \\
\underline{900} \\
\end{array}
$$

Because $\dfrac{1}{150}$ equals a repeating decimal, it is not a good idea to use this method here.

Note: To multiply fractions containing decimals in the numerator or denominator, see the following examples.

a. $0.2 \times \dfrac{1000}{1} \times \dfrac{1}{400}$

Divide 200 into 1000 and 400

$$0.2 \times \dfrac{\overset{5}{\cancel{1000}}}{1} \times \dfrac{1}{\underset{2}{\cancel{400}}}$$

either divide 2 into 0.2 (see section on dividing decimals)

$$2\overline{)\overset{.1}{.2}}$$

$$\overset{0.1}{0.2} \times \dfrac{\overset{5}{\cancel{1000}}}{1} \times \dfrac{1}{\underset{\underset{1}{2}}{\cancel{400}}} = 0.5$$

OR

multiply 0.2×5 to 1.0 (see section on multiplying decimals)

$$0.2 \times \dfrac{\overset{5}{\cancel{1000}}}{1} \times \dfrac{1}{\underset{2}{\cancel{400}}}$$

$$1.0 \times \dfrac{1}{2} = \dfrac{1}{2}$$

b.

$$.006 \times \dfrac{\overset{15}{\cancel{60}}}{1} \times \dfrac{1}{\underset{.1}{\cancel{0.4}}} \text{ divide 4 into 60 and 0.4}$$

$$= \dfrac{.090}{0.1} = 0.9 \qquad \overset{15}{\underset{.090}{\times\ .006}} \qquad .1\overline{)\overset{.90}{0.90}} \text{ or } 0.9$$
$$\qquad\qquad\qquad\qquad\qquad \underline{\ 9\ }$$

c. $\overset{3}{\cancel{150}} \times \dfrac{1}{\underset{2}{\cancel{1000}}} \times \dfrac{1}{\underset{0.25}{\cancel{0.75}}} \times \dfrac{\overset{1}{\cancel{30}}}{1} = \dfrac{3}{.50} = 6 \quad .50\overline{)\overset{6}{3.00}}$
$$\qquad\qquad\qquad\qquad\qquad\qquad\qquad\qquad \underline{300}$$

DECIMALS

A. Write the following decimals in numbers.

> ## RULE
>
> Whole numbers are placed to the left of the decimal point; decimal fractions*
> are placed to the right of the decimal point.
>
> *A decimal fraction is defined by its location to the right of the decimal point
> (e.g., one place = tenths, two places = hundredths, three places =
> thousandths, four places = ten-thousandths).

EXAMPLES   one and two tenths = 1.2

three and five hundredths = 3.05

Note: The decimal point is read as "and."

PRACTICE

1. twenty-four and two tenths

2. ten and four tenths

3. sixteen and twenty-nine hundredths

4. thirty and fifteen hundredths

5. two hundred sixty-one thousandths

6. three and three thousandths

7. nine ten-thousandths

8. thirty-two and twenty-seven ten-thousandths

PRACTICE

9. six hundred-thousandths

10. twenty-five and eighty-five hundred-thousandths

B. Change the following decimals to fractions.

RULE

1. The numerator consists of the number(s) to the right of the decimal point.

2. The denominator consists of the decimal fraction (i.e., number of places to the right of the decimal point).

EXAMPLE   1 = tenths (10), 2 = hundredths (100), etc.

Note: The number of zeros in the denominator is always the same as the number of digits in the numerator.

EXAMPLES $0.1 = \dfrac{1}{10}$ $0.01 = \dfrac{1}{100}$

PRACTICE

1. 0.5

2. 0.4

3. 0.53

4. 0.25

5. 0.16

6. 0.35

7. 0.548

8. 0.973

9. 0.4535

10. 0.7246

C. Change the following fractions to decimals. Carry each answer to two decimal places and round to the nearest tenth.

> **RULE**
>
> Divide the numerator by the denominator.

EXAMPLE

$$\frac{5}{8} = 5 \div 8 = 8\overline{)5.000}$$

$$\begin{array}{r} .625 \\ 8\overline{)5.000} \\ \underline{48} \\ 20 \\ \underline{16} \\ 40 \\ \underline{40} \end{array}$$

$\frac{5}{8} = 0.625$ or 0.6 to nearest tenth

PRACTICE

1. $\frac{1}{3}$

2. $\frac{1}{6}$

3. $\frac{2}{5}$

4. $\frac{5}{6}$

5. $\frac{3}{4}$

6. $\frac{12}{14}$

7. $\frac{8}{16}$

8. $\frac{5}{12}$

9. $\frac{1}{4}$

10. $\frac{14}{35}$

D. Add the following decimals.

RULE

1. Place decimals to be added in a column with decimal points one under the other.

2. Add the columns and place the decimal point directly under the line of decimal points.

EXAMPLE

$$\begin{array}{r} 0.4 \\ + 8.95 \\ \hline 9.35 \end{array}$$

PRACTICE

1.
$$\begin{array}{r} 0.2 \\ + 1.76 \\ \hline \end{array}$$

2.
$$\begin{array}{r} .50 \\ 22.80 \\ + 7.00 \\ \hline \end{array}$$

3.
$$\begin{array}{r} .30 \\ 3.615 \\ 11.2 \\ \hline \end{array}$$

4.
$$\begin{array}{r} 16. \\ 2.345 \\ 0.750 \\ + 12.000 \\ \hline \end{array}$$

5.
$$\begin{array}{r} 13.2 \\ 6.215 \\ 7.20 \\ + 185.6 \\ \hline \end{array}$$

6.
$$\begin{array}{r} 9.276 \\ 10.31 \\ 146.200 \\ + 8.3 \\ \hline \end{array}$$

7.
$$\begin{array}{r} 6.03 \\ 28.1 \\ 7.2106 \\ + 48.1 \\ \hline \end{array}$$

8.
$$\begin{array}{r} 2470.50316 \\ 4.3922 \\ 61.74 \\ + .111 \\ \hline \end{array}$$

9.
$$\begin{array}{r} 0.000396 \\ 21.25976 \\ 8.71 \\ + 6.31256 \\ \hline \end{array}$$

10.
$$\begin{array}{r} 62.132 \\ 7.9204 \\ 9.1 \\ 168.0074 \\ + .2183 \\ \hline \end{array}$$

E. Subtract the following decimals.

RULE

1. Place the decimals to be subtracted in a column with decimal points one under the other.

2. Subtract the columns and place the decimal point directly under the line of decimal points.

EXAMPLES

```
 0.300*
-0.106
 0.194
```

*Zeros may be added after decimal numbers without changing the value.

PRACTICE

1.   28.25
  − 6.10

2. 386.152
  − 4.06

3.   5.6
  − 3.92

4. 92.0064
  − 2.84

5.   201.6002
  − 29.364

6.   0.921
  − 0.070352

7.   24.92
  − 8.0286

8.   17
  − 6.2813

9.   793
  − 24.008

10. 693.4228
  − 16.111

F. Round off the following decimals to the place indicated.

RULE

1. Carry computation to one decimal place beyond the desired place.
2. If the final digit is 4 or less, leave the prior digit the same.
3. If the final digit is 5 or more, increase the prior digit by 1.

EXAMPLES   Round to the nearest tenth:

$$7.01 = 7$$

Round to the nearest hundredth.

$$10.106 = 10.11$$

PRACTICE

1. 2.32 to nearest tenth

2. 3.44 to nearest tenth

3. 32.66 to nearest tenth

4. 16.791 to nearest hundredth

5. 41.105 to nearest hundredth

6. 15.4038 to nearest hundredth

7. 3.2896 to nearest thousandth

8. 291.6345 to nearest thousandth

9. 782.5211 to nearest tenth

10. 2.6859 to nearest tenth

G. Multiply the following decimals.

RULE

1. Multiply as whole numbers.
2. Count the total number of decimal places in the problem.
3. Starting from the right, count off the same number of places in the answer.
4. If necessary, add zeros to provide enough places in the answer.

EXAMPLE

$$
\begin{array}{rl}
3.9 & \text{(1 decimal place)} \\
\times\ 0.005 & \text{(3 decimal places)} \\
\hline
0.0195 & \text{(4 decimal places)}
\end{array}
$$

PRACTICE

1.   16.3
$\times\ 0.8$

2.   32.6
$\times\ 0.25$

3.   93.6
$\times\ 3.2$

4.   17.81
$\times\ 6.02$

5.   71.3
$\times\ 84.2$

6.   0.025
$\times\ 0.2$

7.   0.087
$\times\ 0.6$

8.   0.09302
$\times\ 2.4$

9.   0.234
$\times\ 7$

10.   2.361
$\times\ 9$

H. Divide the following decimals. Carry to two decimal places and round to the nearest tenth.

RULE

1. If the divisor is a whole number, proceed as in division of whole numbers. In the answer, place the decimal point directly above its position in the dividend.

2. If the divisor is a decimal, move the decimal point to the right end, making the divisor a whole number. Move the decimal point in the dividend the same number of places to the right (adding zeros if necessary). Then proceed as in division of whole numbers.

EXAMPLE

$$
\begin{array}{r}
3\ 33.33 \\
0.24\overline{)80.00.00} \\
\underline{72} \\
80 \\
\underline{72} \\
80 \\
\underline{72} \\
80 \\
\underline{72} \\
80 \\
\underline{72} \\
8
\end{array}
$$

PRACTICE

1. $2.5\overline{)100.0}$

2. $3.24\overline{)9.1006}$

3. $0.6\overline{)1.75}$

4. $2.0\overline{)9.0}$

5. $7.3\overline{)62.59}$

6. $0.423 \div 3 =$

7. $1.5 \div 0.5 =$

8. $326.5 \div 22 =$

9. $222 \div 0.11 =$

10. $1.843 \div 20 =$

(**Note:** See Appendix G for answer key.)

APPENDIX B

Conversion between Celsius and Fahrenheit Temperatures

Although electronic digital thermometers are replacing the use of glass thermometers in health care settings, the latter are still commonly enough used that health care workers should be able to convert between Celsius and Fahrenheit temperatures. Figure B-1 compares these two scales.

Note that the Fahrenheit degree is smaller than the Celsius, that is, 180 Fahrenheit degrees between the boiling and freezing points of water, as compared to 100 degrees on the Celsius. The factor 1.8 is used to convert from one degree size to the other.

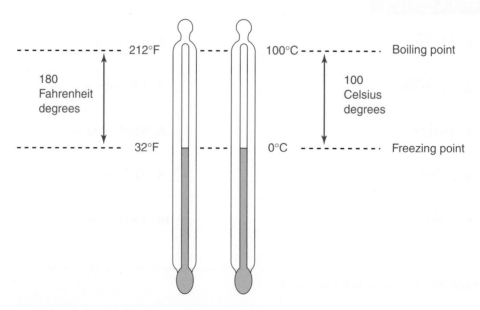

Figure B-1 *Fahrenheit and Celsius scales*

It can be seen that 0°C is not the same as 0°F. In fact, 32°F = 0°C. The factor 32 is used to account for the different zero points.

From this information, the following formulas have been derived for converting between the two scales.

$$C° = \frac{F° - 32}{1.8}$$

$$F° = 1.8\ C° + 32$$

Obviously, either formula can be used to determine either C or F, so only one need be memorized.

EXAMPLE   Convert 101°F to C.

$$C = \frac{F - 32}{1.8}$$

$$C = \frac{101 - 32}{1.8}$$

$$C = 38.3°$$

EXAMPLE   Convert 42°C to F.
$$F = 1.8\ C + 32$$
$$F = 1.8 \times 42 + 32$$
$$F = 107.6°$$

PRACTICE

Convert the following temperatures, rounding answers to tenths.

1. 104°F = _____ C

2. 28°C = _____ F

3. 99°F = _____ C

4. 9°C = _____ F

5. 110°F = _____ C

6. 37°C = _____ F

7. 95°F = _____ C

8. 52°C = _____ F

9. 98.6°F = _____ C

10. 34°C = _____ F

(*Note:* See Appendix G for answer key.)

Measuring and Recording Fluid Balance

Accurate measurement and recording of fluid intake and output is an important aspect of health care. Intake consists of all fluids ingested by mouth or by tube feeding plus fluids given parenterally, that is, IV. Output consists of urine excreted plus fluids lost during emesis and diarrhea, if measurable. In addition, diaphoresis and rapid breathing should be noted in the medical record as these are forms of fluid loss that are not typically measured but should be documented.

Measurements are recorded in mL or oz, depending on hospital policy, on some type of fluid balance sheet.

A. Calculate the total fluid intake in mL for 24 hours and record below.

Breakfast	6 ounces milk
	4 ounces apple juice
	4 ounces water
	450 mL 5% D/W IV
Lunch	6 ounces soup
	6 ounces coffee
	4 ounces ice cream
Snack	6 ounces ginger ale
	5 ounces water
Dinner	6 ounces vegetable juice
	6 ounces milk
	5 ounces coffee
	4 ounces gelatin
Snack	4 ounces sherbet
	8 ounces water
	500 mL 5% D/W IV

Night   6 ounces water

                             550 mL lactated Ringer's IV

                                                    Total = _____ mL

B. Calculate the total fluid output in mL for 24 hours and record below.

7–3   400 mL

                             300 mL

                             250 mL

3–11   200 mL

                             300 mL

                             250 mL

11–7   250 mL

                             350 mL

                             300 mL

                                                    Total = _____ mL

(**Note:** See Appendix G for answer key.)

APPENDIX D

Dimensional Analysis Variation

Some learners who have previously learned the technique of dimensional analysis have been taught to identify as starting factor the desired unit to which the known quantity will be converted, preceded by a question mark.

EXAMPLE Express 1.32 yards in inches.

First, write down the desired unit preceded by a question mark. Then, set it equal to the known quantity.

$$? \text{ inches} = 1.32 \text{ yards}$$

Then, choose appropriate units for conversion factors that will lead from the given units (yards) to the desired units (inches).

yards → feet → inches (or yards → inches)

$$? \text{ inches} = 1.32 \text{ yards} \times \frac{3 \text{ feet}}{1 \text{ yard}} \times \frac{12 \text{ inches}}{1 \text{ foot}} = 47.52 \text{ inches}$$

OR

$$(\text{inches} = 1.32 \text{ yards} \times \frac{36 \text{ inches}}{1 \text{ yard}} = 47.52 \text{ inches})$$

It can be seen that since ? inches and 1.32 yards are equivalent values, interchanging them as starting factor and answer unit does not change the result; therefore the practice is acceptable.

Furthermore, some learners may have been taught that it is not necessary to arrange corresponding units sequentially (diagonally) in the conversion equation so that cancellable labels are in sequential conversion factors. The rationale for this is that as long as conversion factors remain 1:1 relationships, the placement of factors does not affect the result. The writers feel that this practice increases the chance for error and should be discouraged. It is strongly recommended that conversion factors be arranged as taught in Step II of dimensional analysis methodology in Chapter 1, so that units are cancelled sequentially in a consistent manner until the desired unit for the answer, which is in the final conversion factor, is reached.

Twenty-Four Hour Clock

Most health care institutions are using the 24-hour clock for documenting medication administration, especially with the use of computerized MARs. The chance for error is greatly reduced because the same numbers are never repeated.

EXAMPLE

	AM	PM
Traditional time	10	10
24-hour time	1000	2200

Refer to Figure E-1.

The inside numbers represent the hours from 1:00 A.M. to 12 noon (A.M. time). The outside numbers represent the hours between 1:00 P.M. and midnight (P.M. time).

From 12 midnight to 1:00 A.M., the time is stated in minutes, for example, 0001, 0002, 0015, 0030, and so on, to 0059. After 0059, hours are stated in 100s, for example, 0100 (1 A.M.), 0200 (2 A.M.), and so on, to 2400 (midnight). See Table E-1.

RULE

To convert from traditional to 24-hour clock:

between 1:00 A.M. and 12 noon—delete the colon and precede single digit numbers with a zero.

Between 12 noon and 12 midnight—add 12 hours to the traditional time.

To convert from 24-hour clock to traditional:

between 0100 and 1200—replace colon and drop zero preceding single digit numbers.

between 1300 and 2400—subtract 1200 (12 hours) and replace the colon.

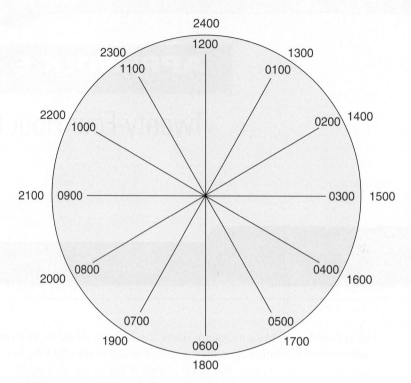

Figure E-1 *24-hour clock*

Table E-1 *Comparison of Traditional and 24-Hour Clocks*			
	A.M.		P.M.
Traditional	**24-Hour**	**Traditional**	**24-Hour**
12 midnight	2400	12 noon	1200
1	0100	1	1300
2	0200	2	1400
3	0300	3	1500
4	0400	4	1600
5	0500	5	1700
6	0600	6	1800
7	0700	7	1900
8	0800	8	2000
9	0900	9	2100
10	1000	10	2200
11	1100	11	2300

EXAMPLE   Convert 9:00 A.M. to 24-hour time.

9:00 = 0900 hours

EXAMPLE   Convert 1:15 P.M. to 24-hour time.

1:15 + 1200 = 1315 hours

EXAMPLE   Convert 0100 hours to traditional time.

0100 = 1:00 A.M.

EXAMPLE   Convert 2030 hours to traditional time.

2030 − 1200 = 8:30 P.M.

PRACTICE

Convert traditional to 24-hour time

1. 3:00 P.M. = _____

2. 10:00 A.M. = _____

3. 5:00 P.M. = _____

4. 12 midnight = _____

5. 9:30 P.M. = _____

6. 7:00 A.M. = _____

7. 9:00 P.M. = _____

8. 10:00 P.M. = _____

9. 8:00 A.M. = _____

10. 6:15 P.M. = _____

Convert 24-hour time to traditional time

1. 1600 hours = _____

2. 0815 hours = _____

3. 1700 hours = _____

4. 2015 hours = _____

5. 2245 hours = _____

6. 1030 hours = _____

7. 0800 hours = _____

8. 1115 hours = _____

9. 1200 hours = _____

10. 0930 hours = _____

(**Note:** See Appendix G for answer key.)

APPENDIX F

Percentage Solutions

A solution is a liquid preparation containing one or more dissolved or diluted substances. The diluting fluid is called the *solvent* and the drug or other substance being dissolved is called the *solute*.

To prepare a specified percentage strength of a solution, it is necessary to calculate the exact amount of drug that must be added to a certain volume of liquid to produce a solution of the desired strength.

As a rule, percentage solutions are prepared by the pharmacist if they are not commercially available. Occasionally, it may be necessary for the nurse to prepare a percentage solution to be used for client care or for disinfection (e.g., mouth rinse, throat irrigation, wet dressing, enema, douche) or for terminal disinfection of hospital equipment and contaminated areas. Dimensional analysis can be used to calculate the amounts of solvent and solute necessary to prepare these solutions.

EQUIVALENT UNITS FOR SOLIDS AND LIQUIDS

In solutions, the word "percent" or the symbol % means the *parts of substance per 100 parts of solution*. For example, 2% indicates two parts of 100 parts total. The measured parts either must be units of the *same kind* or else must be *equivalents*. Certainly 2 grams of salt in 100 pounds of mixture could not be called a 2% mixture, as grams and pounds are not equivalent units. The parts can be minims, drams, fluid ounces, cups, milliliters, or liters, for instance. For example, a 10% solution of alcohol means 10 parts of alcohol to 100 parts of solution. Because they are both liquids, the parts that measure both the alcohol and the total solution would be of the same kind. For instance, the solution could have 10 minims of alcohol for 100 minims of solution, 10 fluid ounces of alcohol for 100 fluid ounces of solution, or 10 pints of alcohol for 100 pints of solution. However, if a dry substance were to be placed into solution, equivalent units relating dry measure to liquid measure must be used. For example, a 5% salt solution would require 5 grains of salt for 100 minims of solution, 5 grams of salt for 100 milliliters of solution, or 5 ounces of salt for 100 fluid ounces of solution.

Table F-1 *Equivalents*

Dry Units	Fluid Units
grain	minim
gram	milliliter
dram	fluid dram
ounce	fluid ounce
kilogram	liter

It is important in this case to know the equivalents for dry and liquid measure, which are listed in Table F-1.

CALCULATION OF PERCENTAGE SOLUTIONS USING DIMENSIONAL ANALYSIS

The percentage strength of a desired solution is expressed as a conversion factor that contains the relationship between solute and solvent.

EXAMPLE   Find the quantity of alcohol needed to prepare 200 mL of a 15% alcohol solution. The parts (solute and solvent) will be measured in mL. The conversion factor can be written as:

$$\frac{15 \text{ mL alcohol}}{100 \text{ mL solution}} \quad \text{or} \quad \frac{100 \text{ mL solution}}{15 \text{ mL alcohol}}$$

Problem: Find the quantity of alcohol needed to prepare 200 mL of solution.

Definite quantity: 200 mL of solution. This is the starting factor and the problem proceeds as follows:

Starting Factor	Answer Unit
200 mL solution	mL alcohol

Equivalent: 15 mL alcohol = 100 mL solution

Conversion Equation:

$$200 \text{ mL solution} \times \frac{15 \text{ mL alcohol}}{100 \text{ mL solution}} = 30 \text{ mL alcohol}$$

(**Note:** In this problem, not only are the units labeled as mL, but also the substances are clearly identified.)

REMEMBER

It is extremely important that the quantity of total solution is not confused with the quantity of substance dissolved; therefore, the descriptive label should be used.

EXAMPLE Find the quantity of 25% solution needed to supply 15 grains of drug.

Starting Factor   Answer Unit
15 gr drug   minims solution

Equivalent: 25 gr drug = 100 minims solution
Conversion Equation:

$$15 \text{ gr drug} \times \frac{100 \text{ minims solution}}{25 \text{ gr drug}} = 60 \text{ minims solution}$$

(**Note:** In the second factor, grains of drug has to appear in the denominator to *cancel the label* of the first factor. However, the relationship 100 minims of solution to 25 grains of drug is an equivalent expression and gives a true relationship even when inverted.)

EXAMPLE Find the number of grams of dry drug needed to prepare 60 mL of 5% solution.

Starting Factor   Answer Unit
60 mL solution   g drug

Equivalent: 5 g drug = 100 mL solution
Conversion Equation:

$$60 \text{ mL solution} \times \frac{5 \text{ g drug}}{100 \text{ mL solution}} = 3 \text{ g}$$

EXAMPLE Find the volume of 10% solution that can be made using four 5-grain tablets of drug.

Starting Factor   Answer Unit
4 tablets   minims solution

Equivalents: 5 gr drug = 1 tab, 10 gr drug = 100 minims solution
Conversion Equation:

$$4 \text{ tabs} \times \frac{5 \text{ gr drug}}{1 \text{ tab}} \times \frac{100 \text{ minims solution}}{10 \text{ gr drug}} = 200 \text{ minims solution}$$

EXAMPLE Find the number of 10 grain tablets needed to make a pint of 2% solution of drug.

Starting Factor   Answer Unit
1 pt solution   tablets

Equivalents: 1 pt = 1 oz, 2 oz drug = 100 oz solution, 1 oz = 8 dr, 1 dr = 60 gr, 10 gr = 1 tab
Conversion Equation:

$$1 \text{ pt solution} \times \frac{16 \text{ oz}}{1 \text{ pt}} \times \frac{2 \text{ oz drug}}{100 \text{ oz solution}} \times \frac{8 \text{ dr}}{1 \text{ oz}} \times \frac{60 \text{ gr}}{1 \text{ dr}} \times \frac{1 \text{ tab}}{10 \text{ gr}} = 15.3$$

or 15 tablets

EXAMPLE Prepare 2500 mL of a 1:1000 solution using 1 g tablets.

Starting Factor	Answer Unit
2500 mL solution	tablets

Equivalents: 1 g = 1000 mL, 1 g = 1 tab
Conversion Equation:

$$2500 \text{ mL solution} \times \frac{1 \text{ g drug}}{1000 \text{ mL solution}} \times \frac{1 \text{ tab}}{1 \text{ g drug}} = 2.5 \text{ tablets}$$

(**Note:** Solution strength may be expressed either as percentage or as a ratio. The ratio 1:1000 means there is one part solute in 1000 parts of solvent, and the conversion factor in the above problem is written as $\frac{1 \text{ g drug}}{1000 \text{ mL solution}}$.)

SELF-QUIZ—EQUIVALENTS

Match dry units with equivalent fluid units.

_____ **1.** grain	**A.** fluid dram
_____ **2.** gram	**B.** fluid ounce
_____ **3.** dram	**C.** liter
_____ **4.** ounce	**D.** milliliter
_____ **5.** kilogram	**E.** minim

PRACTICE

Calculation of Percentage Solutions

1. How many mL of solute are needed to prepare 4000 mL of a 2% Lysol solution?

2. How many grams of solute are needed to prepare 2 oz of 8% iodine solution?

3. Prepare 1000 mL of 70% alcohol solution.

4. Prepare 1000 mL of 1% Neomycin solution from 5 g Neomycin tablets.

5. Prepare 4000 mL 1:1000 bichloride of mercury solution using 500 mg tablets.

6. Prepare 500 mL 1:2000 potassium permanganate solution using potassium permanganate crystals (measure in g).

PRACTICE

Calculation of Percentage Solutions (Continued)

7. Prepare 1000 mL 1:100 potassium permanganate solution using potassium permanganate crystals (measure in g).

8. Prepare 250 mL 1% acetic acid solution from a 10% solution.

9. Prepare 2000 mL of 1:1000 bichloride of mercury solution using 0.5 g tablets.

10. How many mL of alcohol are needed to prepare 1 qt of 40% alcohol solution?

Answer Keys

CHAPTER 1 DIMENSIONAL ANALYSIS

Practice: Identifying the Starting Factor and Answer Unit (pages 4–5)

	Starting Factor	Answer Unit
1.	gr 3	mg
2.	5 kg	lb
3.	250 mg	tab
4.	0.5 g	cap
5.	250 mg	mL
6.	650 pennies	quarters
7.	9 dimes	nickels
8.	5.08 cm	inches
9.	26.2 mi	kilometers
10.	350 mi	dollars

Practice: Identifying Equivalents (page 8)

1. 3 ft = 1 yd
2. 12 in = 1 ft
3. 4 quarters = 1 dollar
4. 2 nickels = 1 dime
5. 2.5 cm = 1 in
6. 60 mg = 1 gr
7. 2.2 lb = 1 kg
8. 1000 mg = 1 g
9. 1000 mg = 1 g
10. 5 mL = 1 tsp

Practice: Setting Up Conversion Equations (pages 12–13)

1. Equivalents: 500 mg = 1 tsp, 1 tsp = 5 mL

   Conversion Equation: $250 \ \cancel{mg} \times \dfrac{1 \ \cancel{tsp}}{500 \ \cancel{mg}} \times \dfrac{5 \ mL}{1 \ \cancel{tsp}} = $ _____ mL

2. Equivalents: 250 mg = 5 mL

   Conversion Equation: $125 \text{ mg} \times \dfrac{5 \text{ mL}}{250 \text{ mg}} =$ _____ mL

3. Equivalents: 0.5 g = 1 dr, 1 dr = 4 mL

   Conversion Equation: $0.75 \text{ g} \times \dfrac{1 \text{ dr}}{0.5 \text{ g}} \times \dfrac{4 \text{ mL}}{1 \text{ dr}} =$ _____ mL

4. Equivalents: gr 1 = 60 mg, 1 tab = 15 mg

   Conversion Equation: $\text{gr } \frac{1}{8} \times \dfrac{60 \text{ mg}}{\text{gr } 1} \times \dfrac{1 \text{ tab}}{15 \text{ mg}} =$ _____ tab

5. Equivalents: 5 mL = 1 tsp, 1 tsp = 300 mg

   Conversion Equation: $15 \text{ mL} \times \dfrac{1 \text{ tsp}}{5 \text{ mL}} \times \dfrac{300 \text{ mg}}{1 \text{ tsp}} =$ _____ mg

6. Equivalents: 12 in = 1 ft

   Conversion Equation: $84 \text{ in} \times \dfrac{1 \text{ ft}}{12 \text{ in}} =$ _____ ft

7. Equivalents: 2.2 lb = 1 kg

   Conversion Equation: $6.5 \text{ lb} \times \dfrac{1 \text{ kg}}{2.2 \text{ lb}} =$ _____ kg

8. Equivalents: 1 oz = 30 mL

   Conversion Equation: $675 \text{ mL} \times \dfrac{1 \text{ oz}}{30 \text{ mL}} =$ _____ oz

9. Equivalents: 1 L = 1000 mL

   Conversion Equation: $2.5 \text{ L} \times \dfrac{1000 \text{ mL}}{1 \text{ L}} =$ _____ mL

10. Equivalents: 5 mL = 1 tsp

    Conversion Equation: $10 \text{ mL} \times \dfrac{1 \text{ tsp}}{5 \text{ mL}} =$ _____ tsp

Practice: Solving Conversion Equations (pages 15–17)

1. Equivalents: 0.125 mg = 1 tab

   Conversion Equation: $0.250 \text{ mg} \times \dfrac{1 \text{ tab}}{0.125 \text{ mg}} = 2 \text{ tab}$

2. Equivalents: 30 mg = 1 cap, 60 mg = gr 1

   Conversion Equation: $\text{gr } \frac{1}{2} \times \dfrac{60 \text{ mg}}{\text{gr } 1} \times \dfrac{1 \text{ cap}}{30 \text{ mg}} = 1 \text{ cap}$

3. Equivalents: 0.5 g = 1 tab, 1000 mg = 1 g

   Conversion Equation: $250 \text{ mg} \times \dfrac{1 \text{ g}}{1000 \text{ mg}} \times \dfrac{1 \text{ tab}}{0.5 \text{ g}} = 0.5 \text{ tab}$

4. Equivalents: gr $\frac{1}{4}$ = 1.4 mL

   Conversion Equation: $\text{gr } \frac{1}{6} \times \dfrac{1.4 \text{ mL}}{\text{gr } \frac{1}{4}} = 0.9 \text{ mL}$

5. Equivalents: gr $^1/_{150}$ = 1 mL

   Conversion Equation: $\text{gr } ^1/_{100} \times \dfrac{1 \text{ mL}}{\text{gr } ^1/_{150}} = 1.5 \text{ mL}$

   OR

   $\text{gr } 0.01 \times \dfrac{1 \text{ mL}}{\text{gr } 0.007} = 1.4 \text{ mL}$

6. Equivalents: gr $7^1/_2$ = 5 mL, 15 gr = 1 g

   Conversion Equation: $1 \text{ g} \times \dfrac{\text{gr } 15}{1 \text{ g}} \times \dfrac{5 \text{ mL}}{\text{gr } 7.5} = 10 \text{ mL}$

7. Equivalents: 20 mg = 1 tsp, 5 mL = 1 tsp

   Conversion Equation: $10 \text{ mL} \times \dfrac{1 \text{ tsp}}{5 \text{ mL}} \times \dfrac{20 \text{ mg}}{1 \text{ tsp}} = 40 \text{ mg}$

8. Equivalents: 125 mg = 5 mL

   Conversion Equation: $250 \text{ mg} \times \dfrac{5 \text{ mL}}{125 \text{ mg}} = 10 \text{ mL}$

9. Equivalents: 30 mg = 5 mL

   Conversion Equation: $75 \text{ mg} \times \dfrac{5 \text{ mL}}{30 \text{ mg}} = 12.5 \text{ mL}$

10. Equivalents: gr $1^1/_2$ = 1 tab, gr 1 = 60 mg

    Conversion Equation: $90 \text{ mg} \times \dfrac{\text{gr } 1}{60 \text{ mg}} \times \dfrac{1 \text{ tab}}{\text{gr } 1.5} = 1 \text{ tab}$

CHAPTER 2 THE METRIC SYSTEM OF MEASUREMENT

Practice: Convert within the Metric System (page 24)

1. 3.2 L
2. 0.4 g
3. 2 kg
4. 5 mg
5. 0.3 m
6. 750 mL
7. 220 mg
8. 2500 g
9. 2.5 cm
10. 12,000 mcg

CHAPTER 3 THE APOTHECARIES SYSTEM OF MEASUREMENT

Practice: Abbreviations (page 27)

1. dr
2. gr
3. pt
4. lb
5. oz

Practice: Convert within the Apothecaries System (page 29)

1. 1.7 qt
2. $^1/_2$ oz
3. 24 oz
4. $^1/_2$ dr
5. 90 minims
6. 10 dr
7. 0.3 oz
8. 256 dr
9. 56 oz
10. 3.9 lb

CHAPTER 4 THE HOUSEHOLD SYSTEM OF MEASUREMENT

Practice: Abbreviations (page 32)

1. gtt
2. gal
3. pt
4. tbs
5. tsp

Practice: Convert within the Household System (page 33)

1. 48 tsp
2. 256 oz
3. 16 cups
4. 5.7 ft
5. 2 oz
6. 18 tsp
7. 2.8 gal
8. 8 tbs
9. 8.3 oz
10. 12 tbs

CHAPTER 5 CONVERSION OF METRIC, APOTHECARIES, AND HOUSEHOLD UNITS

Practice: Equivalents (page 36)

A. Fill in the Blanks (page 36)
   1. gr 1
   2. 1 g
   3. 1000 mg
   4. 1000 g
   5. 2.2 lb
   6. 1 gtt
   7. 1000 mL
   8. 2.5 cm
   9. 39.4 in
   10. $\frac{1}{2}$ oz

B. Match Equivalent Amounts (page 36)
   1. d
   2. c
   3. e
   4. b
   5. a

Practice: Carry Each Answer to Two Decimal Places (pages 38–39)

1. 1250 mL
2. 88 lb
3. 2.5 cups
4. 10 mL
5. 30 mg
6. 1.4 kg
7. 1.3 mL
8. 8 tbs
9. 19.2 oz
10. gr 30
11. 90 gtt
12. 75 minims
13. gr 2
14. 0.7 mL
15. 2.5 tsp
16. 22.5 mL
17. 480 mL
18. 7.5 dr
19. 8 g
20. 71.4 kg
21. 180 mg
22. 45 minims
23. 11.4 lb
24. 12 cm
25. 24 in
26. 64 dr
27. gr 1.5
28. gr 82.5
29. 4 tbs
30. 300 mg

CHAPTER 6 CALCULATION OF ORAL MEDICATIONS

Practice: Reading Medicine Cups (pages 42–43)

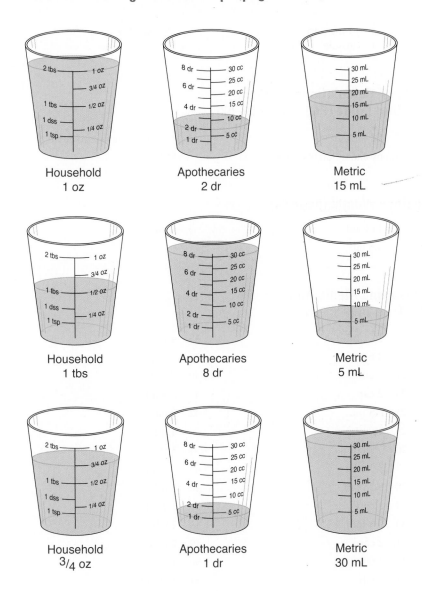

Household
1 oz

Apothecaries
2 dr

Metric
15 mL

Household
1 tbs

Apothecaries
8 dr

Metric
5 mL

Household
3/4 oz

Apothecaries
1 dr

Metric
30 mL

Practice: Reading Labels (pages 47–49)

A. Figure 6-6
   1. Inderal LA 80
   2. propranolol hydrochloride

3. 80 mg per cap
4. capsule
5. Ayerst

6. 1
7. 2

B. Figure 6-7
   1. None
   2. potassium chloride

3. 15 mEq per 11.25 mL
4. liquid
5. Roxane

6. 11.25 mL
7. 7.5 mL

C. Figure 6-8
1. Percocet
2. oxycodone and
   acetaminophen

3. 5 mg per 325 mg
4. tablet

5. Endo Laboratories

D. Figure 6-9
1. Restoril
2. temazepam

3. 15 mg/cap
4. capsule

5. Sandoz

Practice: Reading Labels and Clinical Calculations Involving Medications Administered by the Oral Route (PO) (pages 50–52)

1. 2 tab
2. 2 tab

3. 12 mL
4. nystatin, 500,000 units

5. prochlorperazine maleate, 2 tab

Practice: Oral Dosage Based on Body Weight (page 54)

1. 2 tab
2. 3 cap

3. 14.6 mL
4. 4.5 tab

5. 2 tab

Practice: Clinical Calculations Involving Medications Administered by the Oral Route (PO) (pages 55–65)

1. 2 cap
2. 2 tab
3. 2 tab
4. 3 tab
5. 4 cap
6. 3 tab
7. 2 cap
8. 1 cap
9. 8 mL
10. ½ tab
11. 3 tab
12. 6 mL
13. 2 tab
14. 2.4 mL
15. 2 tab
16. 0.5 tab
17. 0.5 tab
18. 2 dr
19. 15 mL

20. 14.1 mL
21. 3 tab
22. 3 tab
23. 2 cap
24. 6.8 mL
25. 10 mL
26. 3 tab
27. 0.5 tab
28. 0.25 tab
29. 2 cap
30. 7.5 mL
31. 2 cap
32. 1 tab
33. 1 tab
34. 1 cap
35. 2.5 mL
36. 1 cap
37. 8 mL

38. 4 tab
39. 0.5 tab
40. 7.5 mL
41. 2.5 mL
42. 2 tab
43. 4 mL
44. 3 tsp
45. 2.5 mL
46. 8 mL
47. 1.2 mL
48. 2 tab
49. 2 cap
50. 1 tab
51. 12.5 mL
52. 4 tab
53. 1 tab
54. 2 tab
55. 2 tab

CHAPTER 7 ADMINISTRATION OF ORAL MEDICATIONS

Self-Quiz—Abbreviations (pages 70–71)

A. Match the abbreviations with the correct meaning.
1. c
2. b
3. i
4. e
5. a
6. l
7. f
8. n
9. h
10. d

B. Write the term.
1. before meals
2. capsule
3. gram
4. after meals
5. every three hours
6. without
7. elixir
8. whenever necessary
9. four times a day
10. milliliter

C. Identify the route.
1. intramuscular
2. intravenous
3. subcutaneous
4. left eye
5. right eye
6. both eyes
7. by mouth
8. sublingual
9. intradermal

Practice: Simulated Medication Administration Using MAR (pages 78–82)

1.

Medication	Amount to Be Given
Dexamethasone	2 mg
K-Lor	20 mEq
Alupent Syrup	1.5 tsp
Erythromycin D-R	500 mg
Haldol	1.5 mg or 0.75 mL

2. 2 tab at 7:30 A.M.

3. • water or juice
   • 120 mL

4. • 20 mg per tab
   • 1 tab

5. • 7.5 mL
   • 15 mg
   • yes

6. • 15 mL
   • 20 doses

7. • 100 mg per cap
   • 1 cap

8. • 4 mg
   • 2 mg

9. • Darvocet-N 100
   • every 4 hours as needed
   • 1 tab

CHAPTER 8 CALCULATION OF PARENTERAL MEDICATIONS

Shade in the Dosage (page 88)

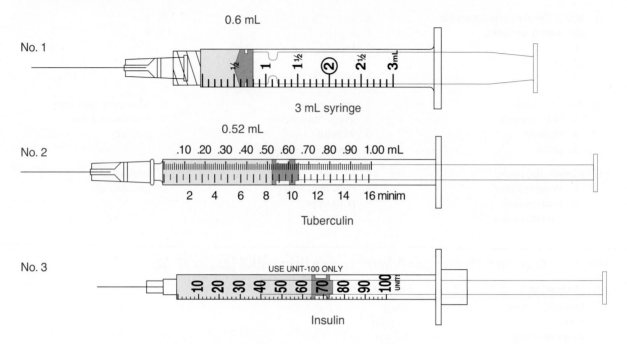

0.6 mL

No. 1

3 mL syringe

0.52 mL

No. 2

.10 .20 .30 .40 .50 .60 .70 .80 .90 1.00 mL

2   4   6   8   10 12 14 16 minim

Tuberculin

No. 3

USE UNIT-100 ONLY

Insulin

Practice: Reading Labels (pages 95–98)

1. (cyclophosphamide)
   a. 1 g
   b. 50 mL
   c. 50 mL = 1 g

2. (10)
   a. IV or IM
   b. Keep covered in carton until time of use.
   c. Baxter, Elkins-Sinn Inc, Lederle, A.H. Robins Co.

3. (20 mg)
   a. 10 mg per mL
   b. gentamycin sulfate injection
   c. Schering

4. (Cefazolin Sodium)
   a. 2 mL
   b. 225 mg per mL
   c. refrigerator

5. (IM)
   a. 100 mg
   b. hydroxyzine hydrochloride
   c. Vistaril

6. (400 mcg per mL or 0.4 mg per mL)
   a. 1 mL
   b. IM, subcut, IV
   c. Package Insert

7. (Sodium chloride)
   a. single
   b. 15–30° C (59–86° F)
   c. 4m Eq/mL

8. (10 mL)
   a. 50 mg per mL
   b. oxytetracycline
   c. Roerig Pfizer

9. (thiothixene hydrochloride)
   a. IM
   b. no
   c. 2 mL

Practice: Calculating Dosages from Premixed Solutions (pages 102–108)

1. 0.6 mL

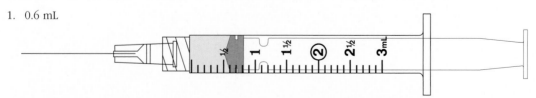

2. hydroxyzine hydrochloride, 1.5 mL

3. 1.5 mL or 1.7 mL

OR

4. glycopyrrolate, 0.5 mL

5. 1.5 mL

6. cefazolin sodium, 0.6 mL

7. IV, 0.4 mL

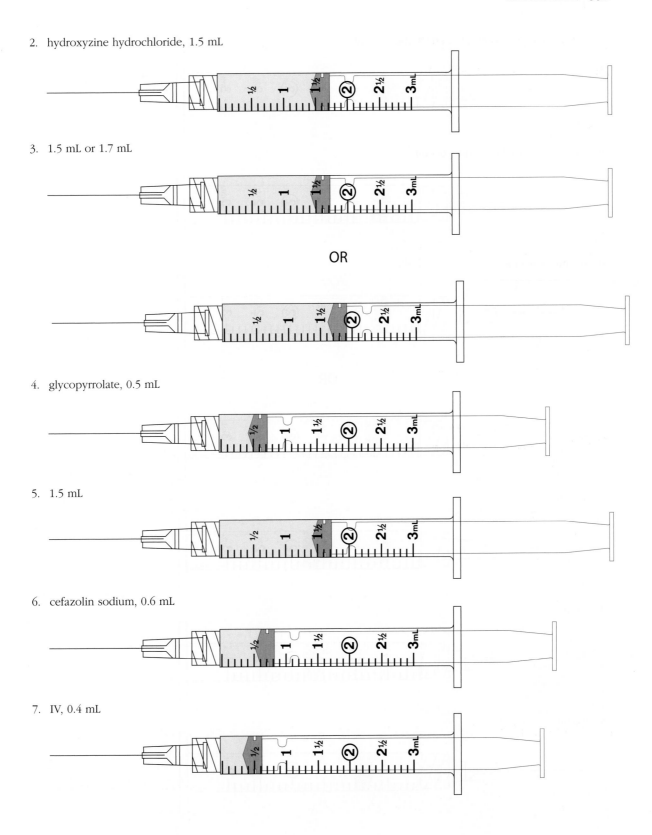

8. American Pharmaceutical Partners, Inc., 0.5 mL

9. hydroxyzine hydrochloride, 0.5 mL

10. 0.5 mL or 0.6 mL

OR

11. 1.6 mL

12. 1.6 mL

13. 0.8 mL

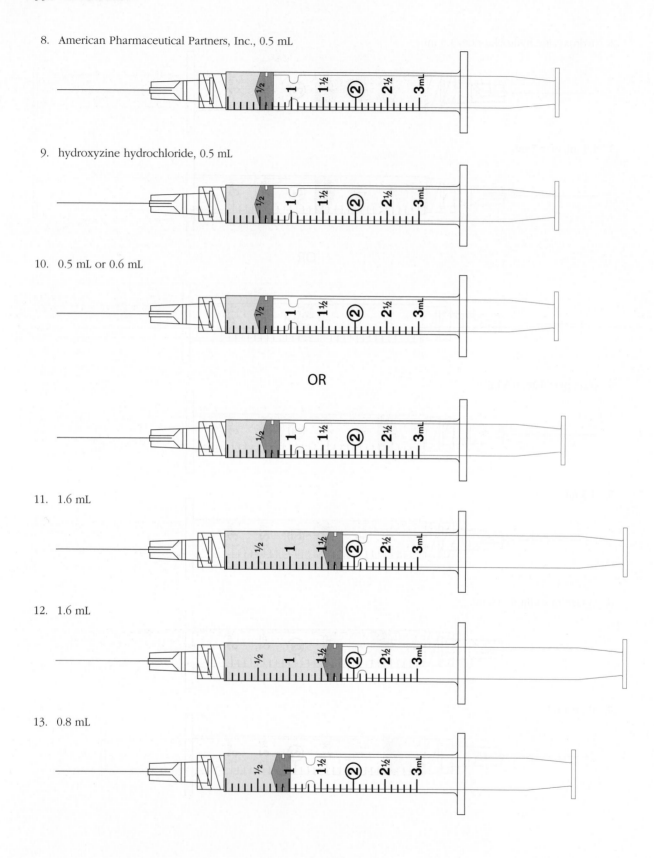

14. 2 mL

15. 1 mL

16. 1.8 mL

17. 0.8 mL

18. 0.8 mL

19. 1.5 mL

20. 1 mL

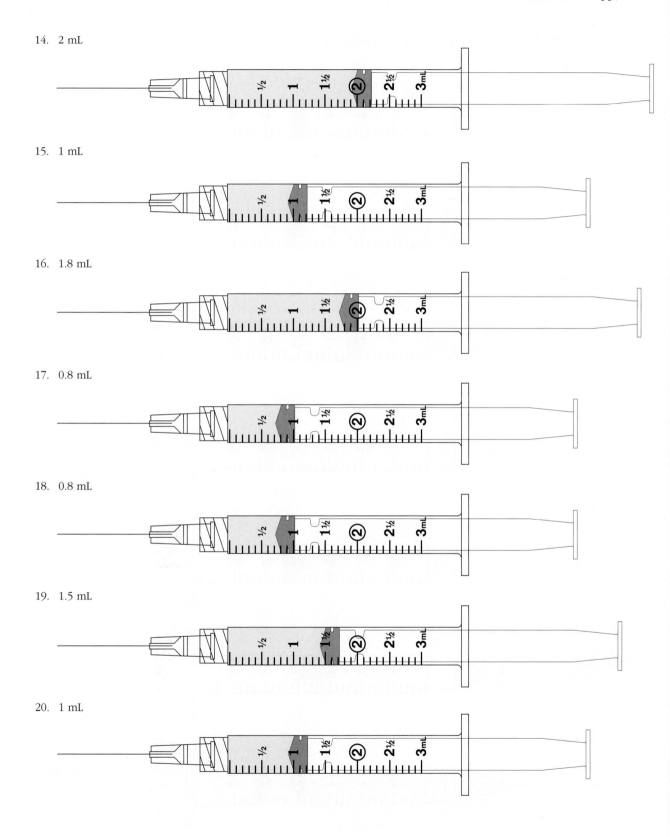

Practice: IM Calculations Based on Body Weight (pages 109–112)

1. 1.9 mL

2. 2 mL

3. 1 mL

4. 2.4 mL

5. 2 mL

6. 1.7 mL

7. 2.5 mL

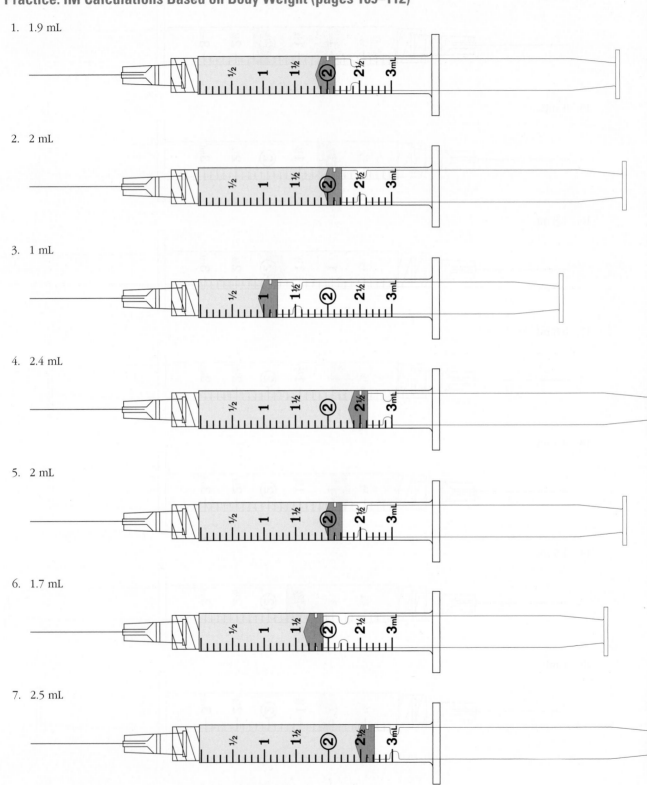

8. 0.8 mL

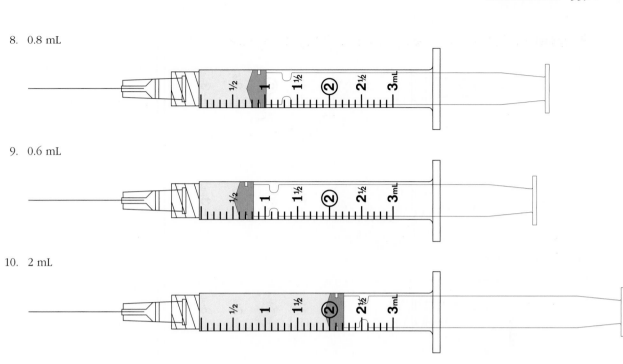

9. 0.6 mL

10. 2 mL

Practice: Medications Dispensed in Units (pages 113–116)

1. 0.8 mL

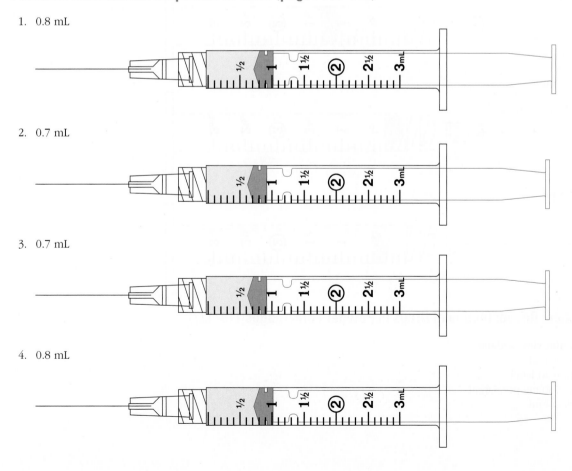

2. 0.7 mL

3. 0.7 mL

4. 0.8 mL

5. 0.8 mL

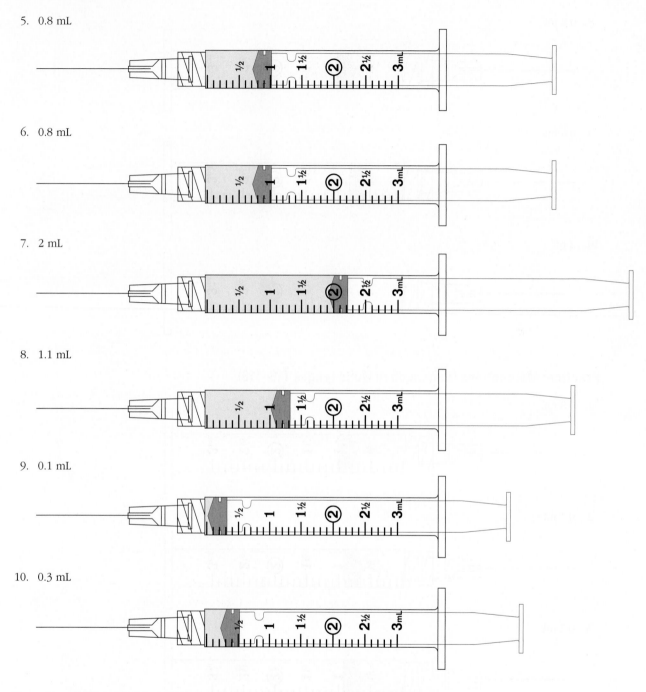

6. 0.8 mL

7. 2 mL

8. 1.1 mL

9. 0.1 mL

10. 0.3 mL

Practice: Reconstitution of Drugs in Powder Form (pages 119–127)

1. cefuroxime sodium
   a. 3.6 mL
   b. read label
   c. 750 mg per 3.6 mL
   d. 2.4 mL

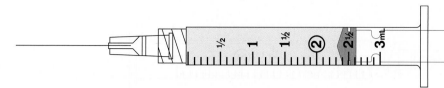

2. methylprednisolone sodium succinate for injection
   a. Bacteriostatic Water for Injection with Benzyl Alcohol
   b. 8 mL
   c. 62.5 mg per mL
   d. 1.3 mL

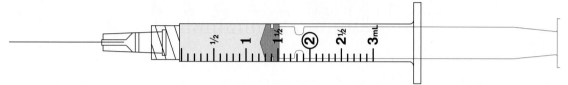

   e. 10 A.M. on 9/18
   f. 20°–25°C or 68°–77°F

3. ticarcillin disodium
   a. Sterile Water for Injection or 1% Lidocaine Hydrochloride sol (without epinephrine)
   b. 1 g per 2.6 mL
   c. 1.8 mL

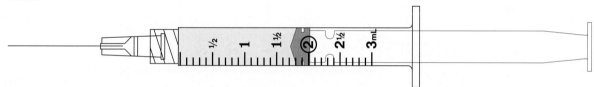

   d. IV

4. ceftazidime
   a. Sterile Water for Injection, Sodium Chloride for Injection or Bacteriostatic Water for Injection
   b. 2.6 mL
   c. 1.3 mL

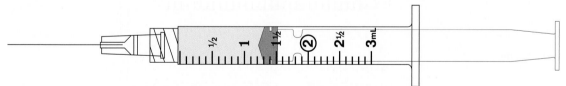

   d. 0.75 g
   e. 2 g q 8 hr
   f. 9 A.M. on 11/16
   g. within 24 hr

5. a. 1.6 mL

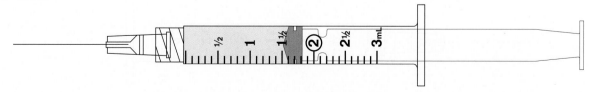

b. 0.8 mL

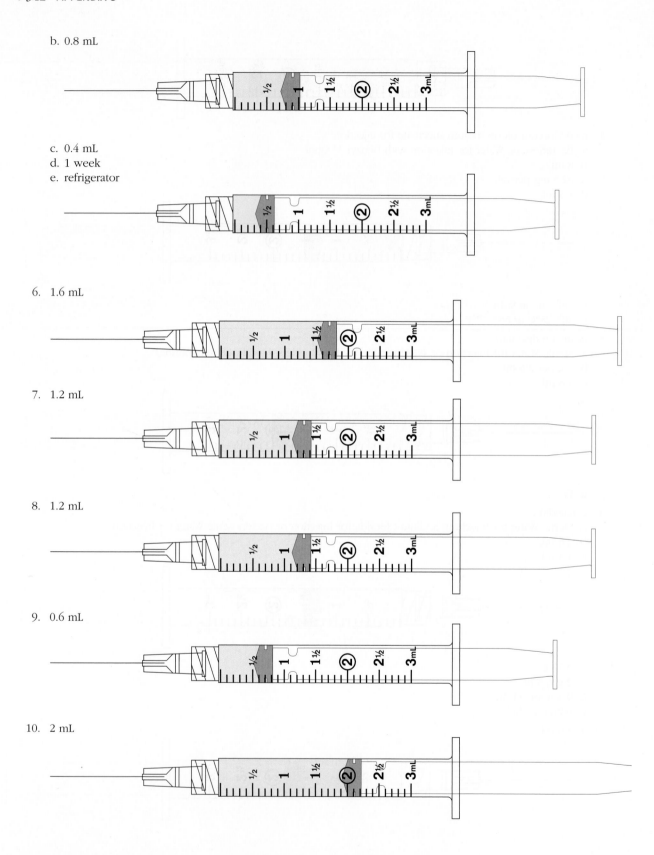

c. 0.4 mL
d. 1 week
e. refrigerator

6. 1.6 mL

7. 1.2 mL

8. 1.2 mL

9. 0.6 mL

10. 2 mL

11. 1.5 mL

12. 1.5 mL

13. 1.3 mL

14. 1.6 mL

15. 2 mL

16. 1.9 mL

17. 2.3 mL

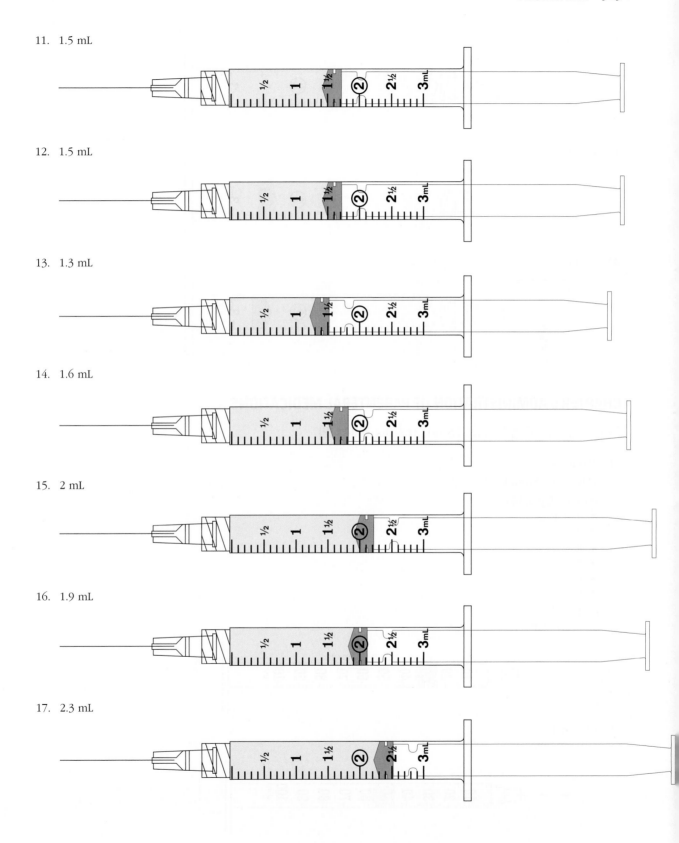

18. 1.1 mL

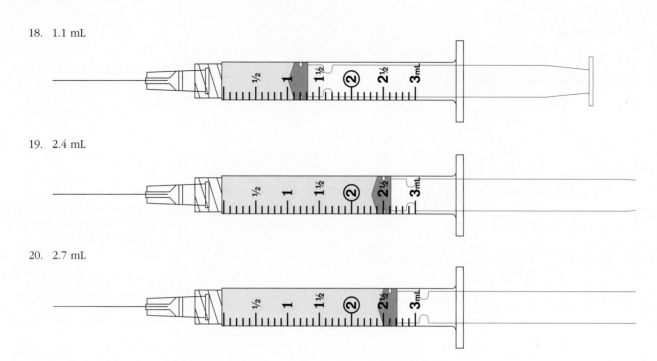

19. 2.4 mL

20. 2.7 mL

CHAPTER 9 ADMINISTRATION OF PARENTERAL MEDICATIONS

Practice: Reading Insulin Labels (pages 140–142)

1. 100 units
2. Lilly, Novo Nordisk
3. • a, b, d, e, f, h, i, j
   • d, e, g
   • e, g
4. • R
   • N
   • L
   • U
5. a. 1. a
      2. 24 units

b. 1. h, f
   2. 46 units

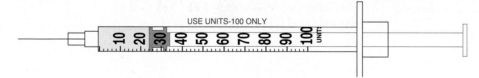

c. 1. a or b and i
   2. Regular
   3. 52 units

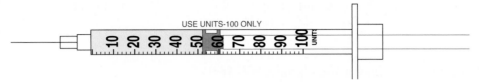

d. 1. c or f and h
   2. Lente
   3. 66 units

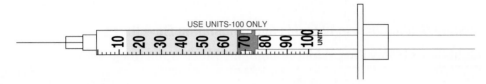

CHAPTER 10 CALCULATION OF INTRAVENOUS MEDICATIONS AND SOLUTIONS

Reading Labels: Drop Factor (page 150)

Section I: Intravenous Equipment

A. Figure 10-4
    1. a. 10
       b. 15
       c. 60

2. a, b
3. c

Reading IV Labels (pages 151–152)

Figure 10-5

1. 1,000 mL
2. 5%
3. Abbott

Figure 10-6

1. 250 mL
2. 0.9%

Figure 10-7

1. 1000 mL
2. 5%
3. NaCl, NaLactate, KCl, CaCl

Section II: Calculation of IV Flow Rates and Infusion Times

Practice: Calculation of IV Flow Rate in gtt per min (pages 161–163)

1. 31 gtt
2. 25 gtt
3. 50 gtt
4. 23 gtt
5. 35 gtt
6. 52 gtt

7. 28 gtt
8. 6 gtt
9. 100 gtt
10. 13 gtt
11. 31 gtt
12. 17 gtt

13. 38 gtt
14. 21 gtt
15. 125 gtt
16. 20 gtt
17. 13 gtt

Practice: Calculation of the Number of mL per hr That Will Infuse (pages 164–165)

1. 125 mL
2. 83 mL
3. 125 mL
4. 125 mL
5. 104 mL
6. 83 mL
7. 125 mL

Practice: Calculation of Infusion Time (pages 166–167)

1. 12 hr 30 min
2. 8 hr 54 min
3. 4 hr
4. 14 hr 42 min
5. 7 hr 12 min

Section III: Adding Medications to IV Fluids and Calculating Flow Rates
Practice: Calculation of Flow Rate When IV Contains Medication (page 168)

1. 63 gtt
2. 125 gtt
3. 25 gtt
4. 50 gtt
5. 33 gtt

Practice: Adding Drugs to IVs and Calculating Flow Rate in gtt per min (pages 170–175)

1. cefazolin sodium
   a. 2 mL
   b. 1.6 mL
   c. 25 gtt
2. a. 2.4 mL
   b. 125 gtt
3. Omnipen-N
   a. 3 mL
   b. 38 gtt
4. a. 15 mL
   b. 28 gtt
5. a. 3 mL
   b. 150 gtt
6. 100 gtt
7. a. 1 mL
   b. 17 gtt
8. a. 1.3 mL
   b. 25 gtt
9. a. 3.1 mL
   b. 167 gtt
10. a. 10 mL
    b. 25 gtt

Section IV: Special Applications of IV Therapy
Practice: Calculation of the Volume of Solution or Concentration of Drug (pages 177–182)

1. a. 2.5 mL
   b. 100 mL
2. 25 mL
3. 8 mL
4. 50 mL
5. 100 mL
6. 100 mL
7. 100 mL
8. 200 mL
9. a. 300 mL
   b. 10 min
10. 50 mL
11. 4 mg
12. 3 mcg
13. 61.2 mg
14. 96 mg
15. a. 10 mL
    b. 267 mL
    c. 2 hr 54 min
16. a. 40 mL
    b. 0.13 g
    c. 400 mL
    d. 8 hr
17. a. 15 mL
    b. 0.3 mg
    c. 20 mL
    d. 30 mL
    e. 40 mL

Practice: IV Flow Rate and Dosages Based on Body Weight (pages 184–187)

1. a. 459.1 mcg per min
    b. 55 mL per hr
    c. 55 gtt per min
    d. 8.3 mcg per gtt
2. a. 515.2 mcg per min
    b. 31 mL per hr
    c. 31 gtt per min
    d. 16.6 mcg per gtt
3. a. 135 mcg per min
    b. 41 mL per hr
    c. 41 gtt per min
    d. 3.3 mcg per gtt
4. a. 582.4 mcg per min
    b. 11 mL per hr
    c. 11 gtt per min
    d. 52.9 mcg per gtt
5. a. 416 mcg per min
    b. 15 mL per hr
    c. 15 gtt per min
    d. 27.7 mcg per gtt

Practice: Titration Infusions (pages 189–192)

1. a. Lower: 3181.8 mcg per min
       Upper: 6363.6 mcg per min
    b. Lower: 19 mL per hr or 19 gtt per min
       Upper: 38 mL per hr or 38 gtt per min
    c. 4000 mcg per min
2. a. Lower: 397.7 mcg per min
       Upper: 795.5 mcg per min
    b. Lower: 30 mL per hr or 30 gtt per min
       Upper: 60 mL per hr or 60 gtt per min
    c. 530.7 mcg per min
3. a. Lower: 350 mcg per min
       Upper: 700 mcg per min
    b. Lower: 4 mL per hr or 4 gtt per min
       Upper: 8 mL per hr or 8 gtt per min
    c. 583.3 mcg per min
4. a. Lower: 136.4 mcg per min
       Upper: 272.7 mcg per min
    b. Lower: 82 mL per hr or 82 gtt per min
       Upper: 164 mL per hr or 164 gtt per min
    c. 128.3 mcg per min
5. a. Lower: 150 mcg per min
       Upper: 375 mcg per min
    b. Lower: 23 mL per hr or 23 gtt per min
       Upper: 56 mL per hr or 56 gtt per min
    c. 186 mcg per min

Practice: IV Bolus (pages 193–196)

1. a. 5 mL
    b. 100 sec or 1 min 40 sec
2. a. 1.5 mL
    b. 72 sec or 1 min 12 sec
3. a. 0.6 mL
    b. 1 min 12 sec
4. a. 3.5 mL
    b. 1 min 48 sec
5. a. 9.6 mL
    b. 9 min 36 sec
6. a. 306.8 mg
    b. 0.6 mL
    c. 12 min 18 sec or 12 min
7. a. 77.3 mg
    b. 7.7 mL
    c. 2 min 12 sec
    d. 5 mL
    e. 30 mL

Practice: Nutrition Calculations (pages 198–200)

1. 255 kcal
2. 140 kcal
3. 110 kcal
4. 42.5 kcal
5. 420 kcal
6. 850 kcal
7. 600 kcal
8. 2040 kcal
9. a. 200 kcal
    b. 425 kcal
10. a. 170 kcal
    b. 340 kcal

Section V: Assessment and Adjustment of IVs

Practice: Adjusting IVs (pages 202–205)

1. a. 35 gtt
   b. 33 gtt

2. a. 42 gtt
   b. 44 gtt

3. a. 42 gtt
   b. 33 gtt

4. a. 21 gtt
   b. 27 gtt

5. a. 63 gtt
   b. 50 gtt

6. a. 31 gtt
   b. 33 gtt

7. a. 28 gtt
   b. 32 gtt

8. a. 50 gtt
   b. 40 gtt

9. a. 35 gtt
   b. 31 gtt

10. a. 63 gtt
    b. 60 gtt

CHAPTER 12 PEDIATRIC DOSAGE

Practice: Calculating Pediatric Dosage Based on Body Weight—Oral Medications (pages 215–219)

1. Vantin 4.5 mL
2. 6 mL
3. 9.7 mL
4. 6.8 mL
5. 5 mL, 4.7 mL

6. 7.5 mL
7. 5 mL
8. 9.3 mL
9. 9.5 mL
10. 4.5 mL

11. 5.1 mL
12. 13.2 mL
13. 1.7 mL
14. 5.2 mL
15. 2.4 mL

Practice: Calculating Pediatric Dosage—Injections (pages 220–222)

1. Clindamycin, 0.5 mL
2. furosemide, 3.4 mL
3. 0.38 mL
4. 0.34 mL

5. 1.6 mL
6. 0.12 mL
7. 0.59 mL

8. 1.1 mL
9. 2.3 mL
10. 0.045 mL or 0.05 mL

Practice: Calculating Pediatric Dosage—IVs (pages 224–228)

1. a. 7.5 mL
   b. 978 mcg
   c. 58.7 mg
   d. 49 mL
   e. 5 hr 6 min

2. a. 1.2 mL
   b. 37 mcg
   c. 2.2 mg
   d. 18 mL per hr or 19 mL per hr

3. a. 6.1 mg
   b. 0.24 mL

4. 0.4 mL

5. 3.3 mL

6. a. 10 mL
   b. 50 mg per mL
   c. 7.3 mL
   d. 100 mL per hr
   e. 14 days

7. a. 0.76 mL
   b. 300 gtt

8. a. 0.87 mL
   b. 200 gtt

Practice: Use the Nomogram to Determine the Child's Body Surface Area (page 230)

1. 1.22 M^2
2. 0.8 M^2

3. 1.1 M^2
4. 0.47 M^2

5. 0.53 M^2

Practice: Use Nomogram and Dimensional Analysis to Calculate Pediatric Dosages (pages 231–232)

1. 10.3 mg
2. 4.4 mg
3. 101.2 mg
4. 161.8 mg
5. 185.3 mg

CHAPTER 13 CLINICAL CALCULATIONS

Practice: Solve Using Dimensional Analysis (pages 234–290)

1. 2 cap
2. 0.5 tab
3. 0.5 tab
4. 10 mL
5. 1 tab
6. 2 tab
7. 2 cap
8. 3 tab
9. 12.5 mL
10. 2 tab
11. 2.5 mL
12. 10 mL
13. 2 tab
14. 2.5 mL
15. 2 tsp
16. 2 tab
17. 3 tab
18. 22.5 mL
19. 2 tab
20. 1 tab
21. 20 mL
22. 2 tab
23. 18 mL
24. 2 tab
25. 2 tab
26. 0.5 tab
27. 2 tab
28. 2 cap
29. 1 tab
30. 3 tab
31. 2 tab
32. 2 tab
33. 1 tab

34. 10 mL
35. 15 mL
36. 10 mL
37. 1 tab
38. 2 tab
39. 2 cap
40. 4 tab
41. 2 tab
42. 3 cap
43. 12 mL
44. 2 tab
45. 4 tab
46. 1 tab
47. 3 cap
48. 5 mL
49. 1.3 mL
50. 1 mL
51. 2 mL
52. 0.5 mL
53. 0.8 mL
54. 1.4 mL
55. 1.2 mL
56. 0.75 mL
57. 0.6 mL
58. 0.4 mL
59. 0.9 mL
60. 1.5 mL
61. 0.5 mL
62. 1 mL
63. 0.4 mL
64. 1.5 mL
65. 4 mL
66. 0.6 mL

67. 1 mL
68. 0.8 mL
69. 0.8 mL
70. 0.6 mL
71. 1.5 mL
72. 0.5 mL
73. 1.3 mL
74. 0.7 mL
75. 1.1 mL
76. 2.7 mL
77. 0.6 mL
78. 0.5 mL
79. 1 mL
80. 0.67 mL
81. Give 1.3 mL, Discard 0.7 mL.
82. 3 mL
83. 1.5 mL
84. 1.2 mL
85. 2.3 mL
86. 0.7 mL
87. 1.6 mL
88. 0.75 mL
89. 0.75 mL
90. 0.9 mL
91. 0.3 mL
92. 1.3 mL
93. 1.6 mL
94. 1.4 mL
95. 0.4 mL
96. 1.3 mL
97. 1.7 mL
98. 0.8 mL
99. 1.2 mL

100. 1.4 mL

101. 1.1 mL

102. a. 1.3 mL
   b. 2.5 mL

103. 2.4 mL

104. 3 mL

105. 0.6 mL

106. 1.5 mL

107. 1.4 mL

108. 0.05 mL

109. 0.4 mL

110. 0.7 mL

111. 31 gtt

112. 31 gtt

113. 26 gtt

114. 42 gtt

115. 63 gtt

116. 31 gtt

117. 10 gtt

118. 36 gtt

119. 21 gtt

120. 6 gtt

121. 8 gtt

122. 28 gtt

123. 21 gtt

124. 38 gtt

125. 25 gtt

126. 36 gtt

127. 14 gtt

128. 42 gtt

129. 31 gtt

130. 83 gtt

131. 25 gtt

132. 42 gtt

133. 7 gtt

134. 16 gtt

135. 30 gtt

136. a. 30 mL
   b. 10 gtt

137. 10 hr 24 min

138. a. 7 mL
   b. 100 gtt

139. 35 gtt

140. a. Add 21 mL
   b. 25 gtt

141. 100 gtt

142. a. 1.5 mL
   b. 10 gtt

143. a. Flow rate: 12 gtt
   b. 8 hr 18 min

144. 60 units

145. 30 gtt

146. a. 375 mcg per min
   b. 28 mL
   c. 28 gtt
   d. 13.4 mcg per gtt

147. a. 23.5 units per min
   b. 50 mL
   c. 50 gtt

148. a. 310.4 mcg per min
   b. 93 mL
   c. 93 gtt
   d. 3.3 mcg per gtt

149. a. 822.7 mcg per min
   b. 99 mL
   c. 99 gtt
   d. 8.3 mcg per gtt

150. a. 886 mcg per min
   b. 66 mL
   c. 66 gtt
   d. 13.4 mcg per gtt

151. a. 198.2 mcg per min
   b. 59 mL
   c. 59 gtt
   d. 3.4 mcg per gtt

152. a. 200 mcg per mL
   b. Lower: 45 mcg per min
      Upper: 135 mcg per min
   c. Lower: 14 mL per hr or 14
      gtt per min
      Upper: 41 mL per hr or 41
      gtt per min
   d. 3.2 mcg per gtt
   e. 60.8 mcg per min

153. 21 mL

154. a. 8 mL
   b. 25 gtt

155. 7 hr 6 min

156. a. 6 mL
   b. 100 gtt

157. a. 5.9 mL
   b. 100 gtt

158. a. 21 mL
   b. 25 gtt

159. 60 min

160. a. 150 gtt
   b. 75 gtt

161. 24,000 units

162. a. 1.5 mL
   b. 3 min

163. 70 mg

164. a. 7.5 mL
   b. 5 min

165. a. 1.1 mL
   b. 1 min 6 sec

166. 1.2 mL

167. 400 kcal

168. 170 kcal

169. 70 kcal

170. 165 kcal

171. 1 tab

172. 7.5 mL

173. 3 tab

174. 0.4 mL

175. 7 mL

176. 7 mL

177. 0.6 mL

178. 1 mL

179. 0.07 mL

180. 6 mL

181. 0.7 mL

182. a. 325 mcg per min
   b. 39 mL per hr

183. 2.8 mL

184. 0.7 mL

185. 7.7 mL

186. 32.9 mg

187. 1.9 mL

188. 0.16 mg

189. 0.07 mg

190. 0.38 mg

191. 0.7 mL

192. 7 mL

193. 2.5 mL

194. 0.6 mL

195. 1.4 mL

196. 0.7 mL

197. 31 mL

198. 2 mL

199. 3.1 mL

200. 0.88 mL

201. 2 mL

202. 1.6 mL

203. 1.3 mL per dose

204. 2 mL

205. 0.8 mL

206. 1.7 mL

207. 50 g

208. 0.3 mL

209. 10 milliunits

210. 10 mL

211. 500 kcal

212. 32,730 mcg

213. 150 mL

214. 3 cap

215. 400 mcg

216. 26 mL

217. a. 1000 mcg per mL
    b. 350 mcg per min
    c. 21 mL per hr

218. a. 1600 mcg per mL
    b. 363.6 mcg per min
    c. 14 mL per hr

219. a. 10 mcg per mL
    b. 30 mL per hr

220. a. 4 mg per mL
    b. 45 mL per hr

APPENDIX A ARITHMETIC REVIEW

Roman Numerals (page 292)

A. Express as Roman numerals.
1. VI
2. L
3. III
4. XII
5. XXIV
6. XLVI
7. XVII
8. XXXVIII
9. XXV
10. IX

B. Express as Arabic numerals
1. 47
2. 29
3. 5
4. 112
5. 1933
6. 7
7. 2
8. 66
9. 309
10. 13

Addition (page 292)

Add Whole Numbers

1. 28
2. 25
3. 58
4. 145
5. 143
6. 1090
7. 1289
8. 772
9. 13,821
10. 33,407
11. 29
12. 65
13. 66
14. 340
15. 1571
16. 355
17. 1169
18. 9399
19. 6249
20. 59,881

Subtraction (pages 292–293)

Subtract Whole Numbers

1. 23
2. 177
3. 4967
4. 3052
5. 32
6. 248
7. 12,473
8. 113
9. 125
10. 883
11. 11
12. 18
13. 169
14. 262
15. 144
16. 6398
17. 216
18. 473
19. 30,915
20. 23,910

Multiplication (page 293)

Multiply Numbers

1. 32
2. 312
3. 78,372
4. 135
5. 13,013
6. 14,007
7. 349,888

8. 555,384
9. 107,019
10. 219,900
11. 76
12. 126
13. 408
14. 1116
15. 20,224

16. 139,867
17. 21,177
18. 319,600
19. 27,696,452
20. 986,000

Division (page 293)

Division Problems

1. 5
2. 11.8
3. 20.5
4. 308.3
5. 181.8
6. 343.3

7. 11.6
8. 20.4
9. 24.2
10. 15.5
11. 21
12. 81
13. 202

14. 231.7
15. 399.6
16. 437.7
17. 1620.9
18. 19.8
19. 1840.6
20. 184.3

Fractions (pages 294–305)

A. Reduce to lowest terms.

1. $\frac{1}{3}$
2. $\frac{1}{3}$
3. $\frac{1}{2}$
4. $\frac{1}{5}$
5. $\frac{1}{11}$
6. $\frac{1}{4}$
7. $\frac{9}{10}$
8. $\frac{1}{4}$
9. $\frac{9}{40}$
10. $\frac{1}{6}$

B. Convert to improper fractions.

1. $\frac{11}{4}$
2. $\frac{71}{9}$
3. $\frac{53}{10}$
4. $\frac{49}{4}$
5. $\frac{20}{3}$
6. $\frac{47}{5}$
7. $\frac{5}{3}$
8. $\frac{3}{2}$
9. $\frac{52}{5}$
10. $\frac{51}{6}$

C. Convert to mixed numbers (reduce to lowest terms).

1. $4\frac{1}{6}$
2. $6\frac{1}{3}$
3. $18\frac{4}{5}$
4. $7\frac{3}{4}$
5. $1\frac{5}{11}$
6. $3\frac{1}{13}$
7. $13\frac{5}{9}$
8. $5\frac{10}{23}$
9. $20\frac{1}{2}$
10. $49\frac{1}{2}$

D. Add fractions (change to mixed numbers and reduce to lowest terms).

1. $\dfrac{11}{9} = 1\dfrac{2}{9}$

2. $\dfrac{4}{4} = 1$

3. $\dfrac{7}{6} = 1\dfrac{1}{6}$

4. $\dfrac{5}{12}$

5. $\dfrac{9}{15} = \dfrac{3}{5}$

6. $\dfrac{48}{90} = \dfrac{8}{15}$

7. $\dfrac{13}{12} = 1\dfrac{1}{12}$

8. $\dfrac{16}{10} = 1\dfrac{3}{5}$

9. $\dfrac{13}{6} = 2\dfrac{1}{6}$

10. $\dfrac{94}{48} = 1\dfrac{23}{24}$

11. $\dfrac{3}{2} = 1\dfrac{1}{2}$

12. $\dfrac{3}{3} = 1$

13. $\dfrac{7}{8}$

14. $\dfrac{21}{12} = 1\dfrac{3}{4}$

15. $\dfrac{48}{36} = 1\dfrac{1}{3}$

16. $\dfrac{19}{12} = 1\dfrac{7}{12}$

17. $\dfrac{27}{60} = \dfrac{9}{20}$

18. $\dfrac{48}{64} = \dfrac{3}{4}$

19. $\dfrac{170}{100} = 1\dfrac{7}{10}$

20. $\dfrac{141}{72} = 1\dfrac{23}{24}$

E. Subtract fractions (change to mixed numbers and reduce to lowest terms).

1. $\dfrac{4}{6} = \dfrac{2}{3}$

2. $\dfrac{1}{7}$

3. $\dfrac{4}{14} = \dfrac{2}{7}$

4. $\dfrac{1}{4}$

5. $\dfrac{13}{36}$

6. $\dfrac{25}{33}$

7. $\dfrac{42}{10} = 4\dfrac{1}{5}$

8. $\dfrac{210}{30} = 7$

9. $\dfrac{94}{21} = 4\dfrac{10}{21}$

10. $\dfrac{170}{40} = 4\dfrac{1}{4}$

11. $\dfrac{1}{4}$

12. $\dfrac{5}{12}$

13. $\dfrac{1}{8}$

14. $\dfrac{1}{8}$

15. $\dfrac{114}{216} = \dfrac{19}{36}$

16. $\dfrac{28}{8} = 3\dfrac{1}{2}$

17. $\dfrac{70}{50} = 1\dfrac{2}{5}$

18. $\dfrac{8}{15}$

19. $\dfrac{70}{21} = 3\dfrac{1}{3}$

20. $\dfrac{38}{6} = 6\dfrac{1}{3}$

F. Multiply fractions.

1. $\dfrac{18}{35}$

2. $\dfrac{3}{20}$

3. $\dfrac{1}{5}$

4. $36\dfrac{2}{3}$

5. 16

6. 33

7. $51\dfrac{3}{7}$

8. 68

9. $21\dfrac{7}{8}$

10. $4\dfrac{47}{50}$

G. Divide fractions.

1. 2

2. $\dfrac{1}{3}$

3. $\dfrac{23}{44}$

4. 4

5. $1\dfrac{5}{8}$

6. 2

7. $1\dfrac{2}{7}$

8. $\dfrac{9}{14}$

9. $8\dfrac{2}{3}$

10. $3\dfrac{12}{37}$

Decimals (page 306)

A. Write in numbers.
1. 24.2
2. 10.4
3. 16.29
4. 30.15
5. 0.261
6. 3.003
7. 0.0009
8. 32.0027
9. 0.00006
10. 25.00085

B. Change to fractions (reduce to lowest terms).

1. $\dfrac{5}{10} = \dfrac{1}{2}$

2. $\dfrac{4}{10} = \dfrac{2}{5}$

3. $\dfrac{53}{100}$

4. $\dfrac{25}{100} = \dfrac{1}{4}$

5. $\dfrac{16}{100} = \dfrac{4}{25}$

6. $\dfrac{35}{100} = \dfrac{7}{20}$

7. $\dfrac{548}{1000} = \dfrac{137}{250}$

8. $\dfrac{973}{1000}$

9. $\dfrac{4535}{10,000} = \dfrac{907}{2000}$

10. $\dfrac{7246}{10,000} = \dfrac{3623}{5000}$

C. Change to decimals.
1. 0.3
2. 0.2
3. 0.4
4. 0.8
5. 0.8
6. 0.9
7. 0.5
8. 0.4
9. 0.3
10. 0.4

D. Add decimals.
1. 1.96
2. 30.30
3. 15.115
4. 31.095
5. 212.215
6. 174.086
7. 89.4406
8. 2536.74636
9. 36.282716
10. 247.3781

E. Subtract decimals.
1. 22.15
2. 382.092
3. 1.68
4. 89.1664
5. 172.2362
6. 0.850648
7. 16.8914
8. 10.7187

9. 768.992
10. 677.3118

F. Round off decimals.
1. 2.3
2. 3.4
3. 32.7
4. 16.79
5. 41.11
6. 15.40
7. 3.290
8. 291.635
9. 782.5
10. 2.7

G. Multiply decimals.
1. 13.04
2. 8.15
3. 229.52
4. 107.2162
5. 6003.46
6. 0.005
7. 0.0522
8. 0.223248
9. 1.638
10. 21.249

H. Divide decimals.
1. 40
2. 2.8
3. 2.9
4. 4.5
5. 8.6
6. 0.1
7. 3
8. 14.8
9. 2018.2
10. 0.1

APPENDIX B CONVERSION BETWEEN CELSIUS AND FAHRENHEIT TEMPERATURES

Practice: Convert Temperatures (page 315)

1. 40°C
2. 82.4°F
3. 37.2°C
4. 48.2°F

5. 43.3°C
6. 98.6°F
7. 33.3°C

8. 125.6°F
9. 37°C
10. 93.2°F

APPENDIX C MEASURING AND RECORDING FLUID BALANCE

Calculate Fluid Balance (pages 316–317)

A. Intake: 3950 mL

B. Output: 2600 mL

APPENDIX E TWENTY-FOUR HOUR CLOCK

Practice: Convert traditional to 24-hour time (page 321)

1. 1500 hours
2. 1000 hours
3. 1700 hours
4. 2400 hours
5. 2130 hours
6. 0700 hours
7. 2100 hours
8. 2200 hours
9. 0800 hours
10. 1815 hours

Practice: Convert 24-hour time to traditional time (page 321)

1. 4:00 P.M.
2. 8:15 A.M.
3. 5:00 P.M.
4. 8:15 P.M.
5. 10:45 P.M.
6. 10:30 A.M.
7. 8:00 A.M.
8. 11:15 A.M.
9. 12 noon
10. 9:30 A.M.

APPENDIX F

Self-Quiz—Equivalents (page 325)

1. E
2. D
3. A
4. B
5. C

Practice: Calculation of Percentage Solutions (pages 325–326)

1. 80 mL Lysol/3920 mL water
2. 4.8 g iodine
3. 700 mL alcohol/300 mL water
4. 2 Neomycin tab/1000 mL water
5. 8 bichloride of mercury tab/4000 mL water
6. 0.25 g potassium permanganate crystals/500 mL water
7. 10 g potassium permanganate crystals/1000 mL water
8. 25 mL acetic acid/225 mL water
9. 4 bichloride of mercury tab/2000 mL water
10. 400 mL alcohol/600 mL water

APPENDIX H

Performance Criteria

Student Name _____ Date _____

Performance Criteria: Administration of Oral Medications
Chapter 7: Administration of Oral Medications

	S	U	Comments
A. Prior to administration			
1. Obtains MAR to confirm medication order regarding dose, route, and time of administration			
2. Checks for any known allergies			
3. Washes hands			
B. Administration of tablets or capsules			
1. Obtains correct medication			
2. Checks the label against the MAR			
3. a. Pours the correct dose into bottle cap and then into cup; recaps medicine bottle and rechecks label against the MAR **OR** b. Selects prepackaged unit dose, checks label against MAR, then places wrapped medication in cup			
4. If controlled drugs are dispensed, maintains security of storage area and documents (records) in appropriate manner			
5. Uses two methods of ID to confirm client's identity: asks or states client's name, examines the wristband, compares information on wristband to the			

(continues)

356

Student Name _____   Date _____

	S	U	Comments
MAR, sensor-checks client and medication bar codes for matching			
6. If necessary, assesses pulse, blood pressure, and so on, as appropriate, for medication being administered			
7. Elevates head, as necessary			
8. Hands the medicine cup to the client or taps the medicine into the client's hand or directly into the client's mouth			
9. Gives water or juice to assist in swallowing medication			
10. For sublingual medication, instructs client to place tablet under tongue and hold in place until it is absorbed			
11. For buccal medication, instructs client to place tablet between cheek and teeth, close mouth, and hold tablet against cheek until absorbed			
C. Administration of liquid medications			
1. Obtains correct medication and checks the label against the MAR			
2. Shakes well, if in suspension			
3. Uncaps the bottle and places the cap open side up on a clean surface			
4. Holds the medicine cup at eye level			
5. Places thumbnail on the correct marking on medicine cup			
6. Pours correct amount of medication, measuring at lowest point of meniscus			
7. Rechecks the poured dosage by setting cup on level surface and reading meniscus at eye level			
8. Rechecks the label against the MAR			
9. Wipes the bottle top with a damp paper towel and replaces cap			
10. Uses two methods of ID to confirm client's identity: asks or states client's name, examines the wristband, compares information on wristband to the MAR, sensor-checks client and medication bar codes for matching			
11. Elevates head, as necessary			
12. Hands medicine cup to client or assists as needed			
a. Uses a straw for medications that stain the teeth (iron, hydrochloric acid, etc.)			

(continues)

Student Name _____ **Date** _____

	S	U	Comments
b. Follows medication with water, if indicated			
c. Omits water if contraindicated			
D. Administration of liquid medications via syringe			
1. Obtains correct medication and checks the label against the MAR			
2. Selects correct size syringe according to desired dosage			
3. a. Pours medication into a medicine cup and withdraws the dosage into the syringe **OR**			
b. Withdraws the medication into the syringe via a sterile needle, then discards the needle			
4. Obtains correct dose			
5. Checks dosage in syringe, making sure there are no air bubbles displacing medication			
6. Rechecks the label against the MAR			
7. Uses two methods of ID to confirm client's identity: asks or states client's name, examines the wristband, compares information on wristband to the MAR, sensor-checks client and medication bar codes for matching			
8. Places syringe tip in client's mouth and instills the medication slowly			
E. Following administration of medication			
1. Remains with client until medication is taken			
2. Records accurately on MAR or nurse notes, or both. Identifies initials by entering full name and title			
3. Records fluids given, if indicated			
4. Provides proper after care of equipment			
F. Maintains principles of asepsis throughout the procedure			
G. Maintains principles of safety and comfort throughout the procedure			

S = Satisfactory   U = Unsatisfactory   **Evaluator** _____

Student Name _____   Date _____

Performance Criteria: Administration of Injections
Chapter 9: Administration of Parental Medications

	S	U	Comments
A. Preparing the medication			
1. Obtains medication MAR to confirm medication order regarding dose, route, and time of administration			
2. Checks for any known allergies			
3. Washes hands			
4. Selects appropriate size syringe and needle			
a. Intradermal injection: 1 mL tuberculin syringe with 25–27 gauge, $\frac{1}{4}''$ to $\frac{5}{8}''$ needle			
b. Subcutaneous injection: 1–3 mL syringe with 25–28 gauge, $\frac{1}{4}''$ to $\frac{5}{8}''$ needle			
c. Intramuscular injection: 1–3 mL syringe with 20–22 gauge, $1''$ to $1\frac{1}{2}''$ needle			
d. Filter needle if obtaining medication from ampule			
5. Obtains correct medication (vial, ampule, or cartridge)			
6. Checks medication label against MAR			
7. Checks for expiration date of medication			
8. Withdraws medication into syringe			
a. *Vial:*			
1. cleanses stopper with antiseptic wipe			
2. injects air into vial equal to amount of medication to be withdrawn			
3. withdraws accurate dosage of medication, changes needle where appropriate			
b. *Glass Ampule:*			
1. wraps ampule in gauze or antiseptic wipe			
2. snaps off top of ampule			
3. places filter needle into open ampule and withdraws required dosage			
4. replaces filter needle with sterile needle for administration			
c. *Double Vial Technique:* (Mixing two medications in one syringe)			
1. cleanses stoppers on both vials with antiseptic wipe			

(continues)

Student Name _____   Date _____

	S	U	Comments
2. placing first vial on a flat surface, injects air into air space equal to the desired dose			
3. injects air into second vial equal to the desired dose and then withdraws this amount of medication			
4. recleanses top of first vial, reinserts needle, and withdraws desired dose, being careful not to inject any medication from second vial			
5. returns or disposes of drug container properly			
6. rechecks label(s) against the MAR			
d. *Prefilled Cartridge:*			
1. inserts into cartridge holder			
2. ejects excess air			
B. Administering the injection			
1. *Intradermal*			
a. Uses two methods of ID to confirm client's identity: asks or states client's name, examines the wristband, compares information on wristband to the MAR, sensor-checks client and medication bar codes for matching			
b. Selects correct site			
—ventral forearm			
—upper chest area			
—subscapular area			
c. Places glove on nondominant hand			
d. Cleanses site with antiseptic wipe and allows to dry			
e. Spreads the site to hold tissue taut			
f. Positions syringe so needle is at 10° to 15° angle to the client's skin; bevel up			
g. Inserts needle ⅛″ below skin's surface with point visible through skin			
h. Injects medication slowly until wheal forms			
i. Withdraws needle, blots gently with antiseptic wipe, avoiding massage			
j. Places used syringe and needle (without recapping) into puncture-resistant container			

(continues)

Student Name _____   **Date** _____

	S	U	Comments
2. *Subcutaneous*			
a. Uses two methods of ID to confirm clients's identity; asks or states client's name, examines the wristband, compares information on wristband to the MAR, sensor-checks client and medication bar codes for matching			
b. Provides privacy			
c. Selects correct site			
—outer aspects of upper arms			
—anterior and outer aspects of thighs			
—abdomen, above iliac crests ($1\frac{1}{2}$–2″ away from umbilicus)			
—subscapular region of back			
d. Places glove on nondominant hand			
e. Cleanses site with antiseptic wipe			
f. Grasps skin between thumb and forefinger to elevate subcutaneous tissue			
g. Inserts $\frac{1}{2}$″ needle at 90° angle to skin and $\frac{5}{8}$″ or longer needle at 45° angle with bevel up			
h. Releases skin and grasps hub of syringe to stabilize needle			
i. Injects medication slowly			
j. Places antiseptic wipe adjacent to the needle without applying pressure			
k. Removes needle quickly and immediately applies pressure with antiseptic wipe			
l. Discards used syringe and needle (without recapping) into puncture-resistant container			
3. *Intramuscular*			
a. Uses two methods of ID to confirm clients's identity: asks or states client's name, examines the wristband, compares information on wristband to the MAR, sensor-checks client and medication bar codes for matching			
b. Provides privacy			
c. Selects correct site			
—ventrogluteal			
—dorsogluteal			

(continues)

Student Name _____   Date _____

	S	U	Comments
—deltoid			
—vastus lateralis			
—rectus femoris			
d. Positions client and exposes site			
e. Places glove on nondominant hand			
f. Cleanses site with antiseptic wipe			
g. Stretches skin taut at injection site			
h. Quickly injects needle at 90° angle, using a dartlike thrust			
i. Releases skin and grasps hub of syringe to stabilize needle			
j. Aspirates for blood, keeping needle and syringe steady. If blood appears, withdraws needle, discards medication, obtains new syringe, needle, and dose, and selects a new site			
k. Injects medication slowly			
l. Places antiseptic wipe adjacent to site			
m. Withdraws needle quickly and immediately applies antiseptic wipe			
n. Massages site gently, unless contraindicated			
o. Discards used syringe and needle (without recapping) into puncture-resistant container			
C. Following injection			
1. Leaves client comfortable, call light within reach, siderails up, if necessary			
2. Disposes of equipment according to hospital policy			
3. Records accurately			
D. Maintains principles of asepsis throughout the procedure			
E. Maintains principles of client safety and comfort throughout the procedure			

S = Satisfactory   U = Unsatisfactory   Evaluator _____

Student Name _____   Date _____

Performance Criteria: Z-Track Method—Deep Intramuscular Injection

(*Note:* Follows usual procedure for intramuscular injection with the following modifications.)

Chapter 9: Administration of Parental Medications

	S	U	Comments
1. Selects appropriate size syringe with suitable needle for withdrawing medication (This needle will be discarded.)			
2. After obtaining medication, pulls back plunger to add 0.5 mL air lock			
3. Replaces needle with sterile needle, 20 or 21 gauge, $1\frac{1}{2}''-1\frac{1}{2}''$ long (for iron—19 or 20 gauge, 2″–3″ long)			
4. Uses ventrogluteal site, unless another site is specified			
5. Places glove on nondominant hand			
6. Displaces skin firmly to one side, then cleanses selected site with antiseptic wipe			
7. Inserts needle at 90° angle			
8. While maintaining retracted skin, aspirates for blood for at least 5–10 seconds, then injects medication at a rate of 1 mL every 10 seconds			
9. Waits 10 seconds (still maintaining skin retraction)			
10. Withdraws needle quickly, simultaneously releasing retracted skin			
11. Does *NOT* massage site			
12. Discards used syringe and needle (without recapping) into puncture-resistant container			
13. Records location of injection site (rotates site)			

S = Satisfactory   U = Unsatisfactory   **Evaluator** _____

Student Name _____   Date _____

Performance Criteria: Administration of Heparin

(*Note:* Follows usual procedure for subcutaneous injection with the following modifications.)

Chapter 9: Administration of Parental Medications

	S	U	Comments
1. Selects appropriate size syringe with 25–27 gauge needle, $\frac{1}{2}$"–$\frac{5}{8}$" long plus second sterile needle for injection			
2. Obtains correct dose and changes needle			
3. Selects correct site: abdomen, above the anterior iliac spines and 2″ away from umbilicus, scars, or ecchymoses			
4. Places glove on nondominant hand			
5. Gently bunches a well-defined roll of tissue without pinching			
6. Wipes site with antiseptic wipe (avoids rubbing)			
7. While maintaining roll, inserts needle at a 90° angle into subcutaneous fatty tissue. Does *NOT* aspirate for blood. While still maintaining roll of tissue and keeping needle steady, slowly injects medication			
8. Withdraws needle in same direction of insertion while simultaneously releasing tissue roll			
9. Holds antiseptic wipe at injection site for $\frac{1}{2}$–1 minute. Does *NOT* massage site			
10. Discards used syringe and needle (without recapping) into puncture-resistant container			
11. Records location of injection site (rotates injection sites)			

S = Satisfactory   U = Unsatisfactory   Evaluator _____

Student Name _____ Date _____

Performance Criteria: Administration of Insulin

(**Note:** Follows usual procedure for subcutaneous injection with the following modifications.)

Chapter 9: Administration of Parental Medications

	S	U	Comments
1. Selects appropriate size (0.5 or 1 mL) insulin syringe with $\frac{1}{2}$″ needle			
2. Rolls vial of modified insulin between hands to mix (avoids shaking)			
*3. When mixing two insulins in one syringe, withdraws regular insulin into syringe first, then modified insulin (clear to cloudy)			
4. Withdraws correct dose			
5. Selects correct site according to previously established plan for rotation of sites			
6. Places glove on nondominant hand			
7. Pinches cleansed site between thumb and forefinger and inserts needle at 90° angle or at angle appropriate to administer insulin in subcutaneous tissue			
8. Does not aspirate for blood unless hospital policy indicates			
9. Upon withdrawal of needle, places antiseptic wipe over site and presses lightly. Does *NOT* massage			
10. Discards used syringe and needle (without recapping) into puncture-resistant container			
11. Records administration on diabetic record, if appropriate, as well as on medication record or site selection plan			

S = Satisfactory   U = Unsatisfactory   **Evaluator** _____

*See procedure for mixing insulins in accompanying box.

PROCEDURE FOR MIXING INSULINS (clear to cloudy)

1. Obtain correct insulin vials and correct insulin syringe/needle. Roll modified insulin to mix.

2. Cleanse top of modified (cloudy) insulin and inject air into air space equal to desired dose

3. Cleanse top of regular (clear) insulin and inject air into air space equal to desired dose, then withdraw desired dose of regular insulin

4. Insert needle into vial of modified insulin and withdraw desired dose, being careful not to introduce any regular insulin into vial

5. Gently rotate syringe to mix insulins

Student Name _____ Date _____

Performance Criteria: Setting Up an IV
Chapter 11: Administration of Intravenous Medications and Solutions

	S	U	Comments
1. Washes hands			
2. Gathers equipment			
a. Bottle or bag of prescribed IV solution			
b. Proper tubing (micro or macrodrip)			
c. IV pole			
3. Examines the container			
a. Correct solution			
b. Correct amount			
c. Expiration date			
d. Glass bottle, intact			
e. Plastic bag (absence of dimples or puncture marks)			
f. Solution, clear			
4. Examines the tubing			
a. Spike cover, intact and secure			
5. Slides flow clamp along tubing until it is directly under drip chamber and closes the clamp			
6. Spikes the container			
a. Bottle with rubber stopper (uses vented tubing). Removes metal cap, swabs stopper with alcohol; places bottle on stable surface, steadies by holding stopper between finger and thumb; removes plastic cover from spike and pushes spike firmly into rubber stopper, avoiding contamination; hangs on IV pole			
b. Bottle with indwelling vent and a latex diaphragm. Removes protective metal cap and diaphragm; notes release of vacuum; removes spike cover and inserts spike in proper opening; hangs on IV pole			
c. Plastic bag: hangs on IV pole before spiking; steadies port with one hand and removes protective cap by pulling smoothly to the right; removes spike cover and inserts spike into port with one quick motion			
7. Gently squeezes drip chamber until half full (or full, depending on equipment instructions)			
8. Primes the tubing			
a. Holds end over sink, wastebasket, etc.			
b. Removes protective cap, without contaminating inside (does not discard cap)			

(continues)

Student Name _____ **Date** _____

	S	U	Comments
c. Unclamps tubing and lets fluid run through until it fills the tubing and all air bubbles have been expelled. Maintains sterility of end of tubing			
d. If small bubbles appear at top of tubing or in drip chamber, lightly taps area until bubbles rise into chamber			
e. Clamps off tubing and replaces protective cap			
9. Loops tubing over IV pole until ready to perform venipuncture			
10. Labels container and tubing with date, time of insertion, and any medication added			

S = Satisfactory   U = Unsatisfactory   **Evaluator** _____

Student Name _____ Date _____

Performance Criteria: Preparation and Administration of IV Piggyback (IVPB) through Infusing IV

Chapter 11: Administration of Intravenous Medications and Solutions

	S	U	Comments
A. Preparation for procedure			
1. Checks medication order on medex and checks for drug allergies			
2. Obtains IV medication			
3. Washes hands			
B. Assessment of client			
1. Assesses IV site for redness, swelling, and temperature			
2. Checks for compatibility between primary solution and medication to be added			
C. Preparation of medication			
1. Fills in medication label and tubing sticker with appropriate information			
2. Prepares medication			
3. Checks order again with the prepared medication			
4. Cleanses port of IVPB container and adds medication; squeezes container and inverts several times to fully mix the medication			
5. Affixes medication label to container			
6. Calculates flow rate			
7. Connects medication bag to IVPB tubing			
8. Primes tubing			
D. Administration of medication			
1. Identifies client and rechecks site			
2. Prepares tape for securing IVPB			
3. Identifies primary line tubing			
For compatible IVPB			
4. Selects appropriate port			
5. Cleanses port well with alcohol			
6. Attaches secondary tubing to primary IV port			
7. Lowers primary container to stop infusion of primary solution			
8. Initiates flow rate			

(continues)

Student Name _____   Date _____

	S	U	Comments
For incompatible IVPB			
9. Clamps primary line off			
10. Flushes primary line with normal saline			
11. Initiates IVPB infusion			
12. On completion of infusion, flushes primary line with normal saline			
13. Restarts primary infusion at appropriate rate			
E. Follow-up			
1. Charts medication on record and charts I & O			
2. Within 15 minutes, assesses infusion rate and site			
3. When IVPB is completed, adjusts primary IV, if necessary			

S = Satisfactory   U = Unsatisfactory   **Evaluator** _____

Student Name _____ Date _____

Performance Criteria: Administration of IV Push Medication via Port in an Infusing IV

Chapter 11: Administration of Intravenous Medications and Solutions

	S	U	Comments
A. Preparation for procedure			
1. Checks medication order on medex			
2. Checks for drug allergies			
3. Obtains IV medication			
4. Washes hands			
B. Assessment of client			
1. Assesses IV site for redness, swelling, and temperature			
2. Checks for compatibility between primary solution and medication to be added			
C. Preparation of medication			
1. *Prepares medication			
2. Rechecks order and prepared medication			
D. Administration of medication			
1. Identifies client and rechecks site			
For compatible IV on a controller			
2. Cleanses port closest to the site with alcohol			
3. Connects needleless syringe to port and proceeds to give medication at designated rate			
For compatible IV infusing by gravity			
4. Cleanses the port closest to the site and inserts the needleless syringe			
5. While injecting the medication at the designated rate, alternately pinches and releases the tubing to prevent retrograde flow of the drug			
For incompatible IV infusing by gravity			
6. Prepares two flushes			
7. Uses port closest to the IV site			
8. Clamps off primary line tubing			
9. Flushes port with 5 mL of flushing solution			

*If medication needs to be diluted, draw up diluent in a 5 or 10 mL syringe. Draw air into syringe to accommodate the anticipated amount of medication that will be added and 0.5 mL of air to allow space for mixing medication. Draw up correct dosage of medication in another syringe; remove the needle from the diluent syringe and add medication through hub of diluent syringe. *Invert several times to mix.*

(continues)

Student Name _____ **Date** _____

	S	U	Comments
10. Injects medication at recommended rate			
11. Follows medication with flush of 5 mL at same rate			
12. Observes client for any reaction and for desired effect			
E. Follow-up			
1. Disposes of all equipment properly			
2. Charts medication			
3. Visits client at appropriate time to determine if desired outcome has been achieved.			

S = Satisfactory   U = Unsatisfactory   **Evaluator** _____

Student Name _____   Date _____

Performance Criteria: Starting IV (with an Over-the-Stylet Type Catheter)

Chapter 11: Administration of Intravenous Medications and Solutions

	S	U	Comments
1. Washes hands			
2. Obtains equipment and sets up IV			
3. Identifies and prepares client for procedure			
4. Selects vein; clips hair at site, if necessary			
5. Applies tourniquet			
6. Puts on gloves			
7. Preps insertion site with antiseptic			
8. Removes protective shield from catheter			
9. Grasps client's arm so that the thumb below the insertion site increases skin tension and stabilizes the vein			
10. Places catheter at 30° angle with stylet about 1 cm distal to venipuncture site			
11. Punctures the skin so that the stylet approaches the vein from the side			
12. Advances the stylet into the vein at a slight angle to the vein, with slow, steady pressure			
13. Aligns the stylet with the vein and follows the vein until about $\frac{1}{8}$" of the plastic catheter is within the lumen			
14. After blood flows into the body of the catheter, releases thumb pressure on client's arm, holds the stylet firmly in place with one hand, and advances the catheter smoothly into the vein			
15. Continues to advance the catheter until the catheter hub is approximately $\frac{1}{4}$" from the puncture site			
16. Loosens the tourniquet, holds the catheter steady and retracts stylet			
17. Removes cap from the IV tubing and joins the catheter and tubing adapters firmly together			
18. Opens the clamp on the IV tubing to a fast rate to check for free-flow, then partially closes clamp			
19. Tapes the catheter hub to the client's arm			
20. Applies dressing in such a manner that dressing can be changed without disturbing the catheter			
21. Forms a loose loop in the tubing and tapes to client's arm			

(continues)

Student Name _____ **Date** _____

	S	U	Comments
22. Adjust the IV flow to the prescribed rate			
23. Indicates the size of the catheter and date on the tape			
24. If necessary, immobilize the site in such a manner that circulation and comfort are not impaired			

S = Satisfactory   U = Unsatisfactory   **Evaluator** _____

Student Name _____ Date _____

Performance Criteria: Assessment, Adjustment, and Termination of IV

	S	U	Comments
1. Assesses by observing			
a. Patency of tubing			
b. Rate of flow			
c. Amount remaining			
d. Injection site			
e. Client's reaction			
2. Adjust flow rate to correct number of drops per minute or mL per hour			
3. Terminates when indicated, applying principles of asepsis, safety, and comfort			
a. Puts on gloves			
b. Clamps off			
c. Removes tape and dressing			
d. Places sterile gauze pad over site			
e. Withdraws catheter, immediately applies pressure to site for 2–3 minutes			
f. Tapes gauze securely over site			
g. Discards catheter into designated container			

S = Satisfactory   U = Unsatisfactory   Evaluator _____

INDEX

GETTING STARTED WITH CLINICAL CALCULATIONS PRACTICE SOFTWARE, 5TH EDITION

System Requirements

Operating system: Microsoft Windows 98, Windows Me, Windows NT 4.0, Windows 2000, Windows XP, or newer

Processor: Pentium II processor or faster

Memory: 32–64 MB

Hard disk space: 16 MB

Monitor: SVGA-compatible color

Graphics adapter: SVGA or higher; 800 x 600, True Color (24-bit or 32-bit) or High Color (16-bit) modes

CD-ROM drive: 8x or faster

An Internet connection and Netscape Navigator 6.2 or Microsoft Internet Explorer 5.5, or newer, are required.

Microsoft is a registered trademark, and Windows and Windows NT are trademarks of Microsoft Corporation.

Set-Up Instructions

1. Insert disc into CD-ROM drive. The program should start. If it does not, go to step 2.
2. From My Computer, double-click the icon for the CD drive.
3. Double click the *index.htm* file to start the program.

Technical Support

Telephone: 1-800-648-7450, 8:30 AM–5:30 PM Eastern Time

Fax: 1-518-881-1247

E-mail: delmar.help@cengage.com

Delmar Cengage Learning End User License Agreement

IMPORTANT! READ CAREFULLY: This End User License Agreement ("Agreement") sets forth the conditions by which Delmar Cengage Learning will make electronic access to the Delmar Cengage Learning-owned licensed content and associated media, software, documentation, printed materials, and electronic documentation contained in this package and/or made available to you via this product (the "Licensed Content"), available to you (the "End User"). BY CLICKING THE "I ACCEPT" BUTTON AND/OR OPENING THIS PACKAGE, YOU ACKNOWLEDGE THAT YOU HAVE READ ALL OF THE TERMS AND CONDITIONS, AND THAT YOU AGREE TO BE BOUND BY ITS TERMS, CONDITIONS, AND ALL APPLICABLE LAWS AND REGULATIONS GOVERNING THE USE OF THE LICENSED CONTENT.

1.0 SCOPE OF LICENSE

1.1 <u>Licensed Content</u>. The Licensed Content may contain portions of modifiable content ("Modifiable Content") and content which may not be modified or otherwise altered by the End User ("Non-Modifiable Content"). For purposes of this Agreement, Modifiable Content and Non-Modifiable Content may be collectively referred to herein as the "Licensed Content." All Licensed Content shall be considered Non-Modifiable Content, unless such Licensed Content is presented to the End User in a modifiable format and it is clearly indicated that modification of the Licensed Content is permitted.

1.2 Subject to the End User's compliance with the terms and conditions of this Agreement, Delmar Cengage Learning hereby grants the End User, a nontransferable, nonexclusive, limited right to access and view a single copy of the Licensed Content on a single personal computer system for noncommercial, internal, personal use only. The End User shall not (i) reproduce, copy, modify (except in the case of Modifiable Content), distribute, display, transfer, sublicense, prepare derivative work(s) based on, sell, exchange, barter or transfer, rent, lease, loan, resell, or in any other manner exploit the Licensed Content; (ii) remove, obscure, or alter any notice of Delmar Cengage Learning's intellectual property rights present on or in the Licensed Content, including, but not limited to, copyright, trademark, and/or patent notices; or (iii) disassemble, decompile, translate, reverse engineer, or otherwise reduce the Licensed Content.

2.0 TERMINATION

2.1 Delmar Cengage Learning may at any time (without prejudice to its other rights or remedies) immediately terminate this Agreement and/or suspend access to some or all of the Licensed Content, in the event that the End User does not comply with any of the terms and conditions of this Agreement. In the event of such termination by Delmar Cengage Learning, the End User shall immediately return any and all copies of the Licensed Content to Delmar Cengage Learning.

3.0 PROPRIETARY RIGHTS

3.1 The End User acknowledges that Delmar Cengage Learning owns all rights, title and interest, including, but not limited to all copyright rights therein, in and to the Licensed Content, and that the End User shall not take any action inconsistent with such ownership. The Licensed Content is protected by U.S., Canadian and other applicable copyright laws and by international treaties, including the Berne Convention and the Universal Copyright Convention. Nothing contained in this Agreement shall be construed as granting the End User any ownership rights in or to the Licensed Content.

3.2 Delmar Cengage Learning reserves the right at any time to withdraw from the Licensed Content any item or part of an item for which it no longer retains the right to publish, or which it has reasonable grounds to believe infringes copyright or is defamatory, unlawful, or otherwise objectionable.

4.0 PROTECTION AND SECURITY

4.1 TThe End User shall use its best efforts and take all reasonable steps to safeguard its copy of the Licensed Content to ensure that no unauthorized reproduction, publication, disclosure, modification, or distribution of the Licensed Content, in whole or in part, is made. To the extent that the End User becomes aware of any such unauthorized use of the Licensed Content, the End User shall immediately notify Delmar Cengage Learning. Notification of such violations may be made by sending an e-mail to delmarhelp@cengage.com.

5.0 MISUSE OF THE LICENSED PRODUCT

5.1 In the event that the End User uses the Licensed Content in violation of this Agreement, Delmar Cengage Learning shall have the option of electing liquidated damages, which shall include all profits generated by the End User's use of the Licensed Content plus interest computed at the maximum rate permitted by law and all legal fees and other expenses incurred by Delmar Cengage Learning in enforcing its rights, plus penalties.

6.0 FEDERAL GOVERNMENT CLIENTS

6.1 Except as expressly authorized by Delmar Cengage Learning, Federal Government clients obtain only the rights specified in this Agreement and no other rights. The Government acknowledges that (i) all software and related documentation incorporated in the Licensed Content is existing commercial computer software within the meaning of FAR 27.405(b)(2); and (2) all other data delivered in whatever form, is limited rights data within the meaning of FAR 27.401. The restrictions in this section are acceptable as consistent with the Government's need for software and other data under this Agreement.

7.0 DISCLAIMER OF WARRANTIES AND LIABILITIES

7.1 Although Delmar Cengage Learning believes the Licensed Content to be reliable, Delmar Cengage Learning does not guarantee or warrant (i) any information or materials contained in or produced by the Licensed Content, (ii) the accuracy, completeness or reliability of the Licensed Content, or (iii) that the Licensed Content is free from errors or other material defects. THE LICENSED PRODUCT IS PROVIDED "AS IS," WITHOUT ANY WARRANTY OF ANY KIND AND DELMAR CENGAGE LEARNING DISCLAIMS ANY AND ALL WARRANTIES, EXPRESSED OR IMPLIED, INCLUDING, WITHOUT LIMITATION, WARRANTIES OF MERCHANTABILITY OR FITNESS FOR A PARTICULAR PURPOSE. IN NO EVENT SHALL DELMAR CENGAGE LEARNING BE LIABLE FOR: INDIRECT, SPECIAL, PUNITIVE OR CONSEQUENTIAL DAMAGES INCLUDING FOR LOST PROFITS, LOST DATA, OR OTHERWISE. IN NO EVENT SHALL DELMAR CENGAGE LEARNING'S AGGREGATE LIABILITY HEREUNDER, WHETHER ARISING IN CONTRACT, TORT, STRICT LIABILITY OR OTHERWISE, EXCEED THE AMOUNT OF FEES PAID BY THE END USER HEREUNDER FOR THE LICENSE OF THE LICENSED CONTENT..

8.0 GENERAL

8.1 Entire Agreement. This Agreement shall constitute the entire Agreement between the Parties and supercedes all prior Agreements and understandings oral or written relating to the subject matter hereof.

8.2 Enhancements/Modifications of Licensed Content. From time to time, and in Delmar Cengage Learning's sole discretion, Delmar Cengage Learning may advise the End User of updates, upgrades, enhancements and/or improvements to the Licensed Content, and may permit the End User to access and use, subject to the terms and conditions of this Agreement, such modifications, upon payment of prices as may be established by Delmar Cengage Learning.

8.3 No Export. The End User shall use the Licensed Content solely in the United States and shall not transfer or export, directly or indirectly, the Licensed Content outside the United States.

8.4 Severability. If any provision of this Agreement is invalid, illegal, or unenforceable under any applicable statute or rule of law, the provision shall be deemed omitted to the extent that it is invalid, illegal, or unenforceable. In such a case, the remainder of the Agreement shall be construed in a manner as to give greatest effect to the original intention of the parties hereto.

8.5 Waiver. The waiver of any right or failure of either party to exercise in any respect any right provided in this Agreement in any instance shall not be deemed to be a waiver of such right in the future or a waiver of any other right under this Agreement.

8.6 Choice of Law/Venue. This Agreement shall be interpreted, construed, and governed by and in accordance with the laws of the State of New York, applicable to contracts executed and to be wholly preformed therein, without regard to its principles governing conflicts of law. Each party agrees that any proceeding arising out of or relating to this Agreement or the breach or threatened breach of this Agreement may be commenced and prosecuted in a court in the State and County of New York. Each party consents and submits to the nonexclusive personal jurisdiction of any court in the State and County of New York in respect of any such proceeding.

8.7 Acknowledgment. By opening this package and/or by accessing the Licensed Content on this Web site, THE END USER ACKNOWLEDGES THAT IT HAS READ THIS AGREEMENT, UNDERSTANDS IT, AND AGREES TO BE BOUND BY ITS TERMS AND CONDITIONS. IF YOU DO NOT ACCEPT THESE TERMS AND CONDITIONS, YOU MUST NOT ACCESS THE LICENSED CONTENT AND RETURN THE LICENSED PRODUCT TO DELMAR CENGAGE LEARNING (WITHIN 30 CALENDAR DAYS OF THE END USER'S PURCHASE) WITH PROOF OF PAYMENT ACCEPTABLE TO DELMAR CENGAGE LEARNING, FOR A CREDIT OR A REFUND. Should the End User have any questions/comments regarding this Agreement, please contact Delmar Cengage Learning at delmarhelp@cemgage.com.